Release Your Body
RESOLVING
PLANTAR FASCIITIS

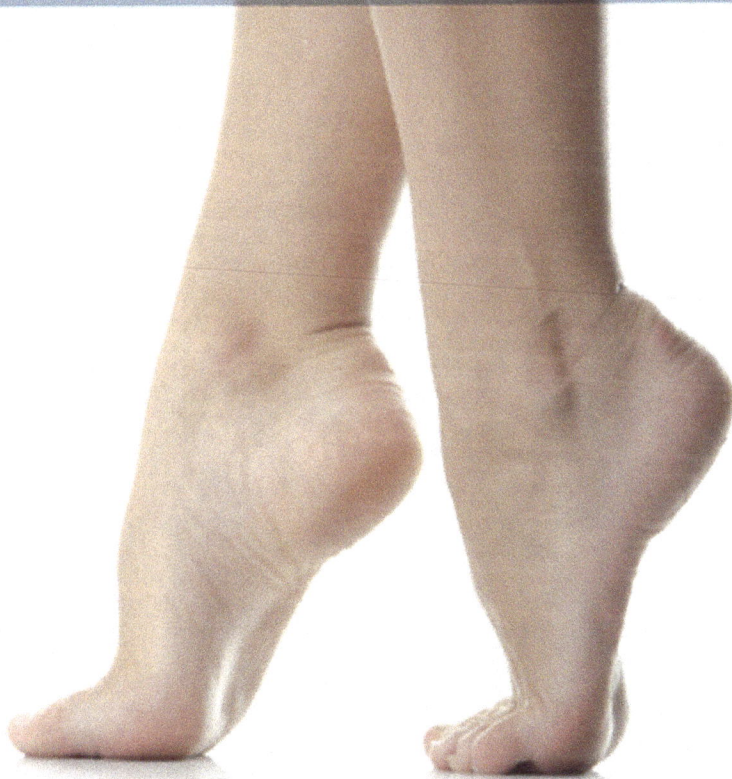

A Roadmap to Success

Dr. Brian Abelson, DC   Kamali T. Abelson, BSc

With Contributions by
Dr. Evangelos Mylonas, DC

Canadian Cataloguing in Publication Data

Abelson, Brian and Abelson, Kamali

Resolving Plantar Fasciitis - Volume 1 of the Release Your Body Series of Books©

Includes index and table of contents.

Copyright Registration 2015	1118729
ISBN-13 - Hardcopy	978-0-9733848-8-8
ISBN-13 - E-Copy	978-0-9733848-9-5

First Printing: 2015, Published by Rowan Tree Books Ltd.
Printed in Canada 10 9 8 7 6 5 4 3 2 1

Kinetic Health®

Web Sites: *www.releaseyourbody.com* – *www.kinetichealth.ca* – *www.activerelease.ca*
Kinetic Health books are available at a special discount for bulk purchase by practitioners, corporations, institutions, and other organizations. For details, see our website or contact the Special Sales Manager at Kinetic Health.

Address: Kinetic Health®
Bay #10, 34 Edgedale Drive NW, Calgary, AB, Canada, T3A-2R4
403-241-3772 (bus)   403-241-3846 (fax)

Credits

Production, Book Design, Editor: Kamali T. Abelson
Proofreading and Technical Editor: Kamali T. Abelson, Dr. Evangelos Mylonas DC
Junior Copy Writer: Kathryn McCallum
Photographs and Videos: Dr. Brian Abelson DC
Cover Artwork: Lavanya Balasubramaniyam
Illustrations: Kamali Abelson, Lavanya Balasubramaniyam, Thara Abelson, Rowan Tree Books Ltd
123RF Limited, Shutterstock

Health Disclaimer

This book provides information about wellness management in an informational and educational manner only, with information that is general in nature and that is not specific to you, the reader. The contents of this book are intended to assist you and other readers in your personal wellness efforts.

Nothing in this book should be construed as personal advice or diagnosis, and must *not* be used in this manner. The information provided about conditions is general in nature. This information does not cover all possible uses, actions, precautions, side-effects, or interactions of medicines, or medical procedures. The information in this book should not be considered as complete and does *not* cover all diseases, ailments, physical conditions, or their treatment.

You should consult with your physician before beginning any exercise, weight loss, or health care program. This book should *not* be used in place of a call or visit to a competent health-care professional. You should consult a health care professional before adopting any of the suggestions in this book or before drawing inferences from it. Any decision regarding treatment and medication for your condition should be made with the advice and consultation of a qualified health care professional. If you have, or suspect you have, a health-care problem, then you should immediately contact a qualified health care professional for treatment.

No Warranties

The authors, publishers, and/or their respective directors, shareholders, officers, employees, agents, trainers, contractors, representatives, or successors do not guarantee or warrant the quality, accuracy, completeness, timeliness, appropriateness or suitability of the information in this book, or of any product or services referenced by this book. The information in this book is provided on an "as is" basis and the authors and publishers make no representations or warranties of any kind with respect to this information. This book may contain inaccuracies, typographical errors, or other errors.

Liability Disclaimer

The publishers, authors, and any other parties involved in the creation, production, provision of information, or delivery of this book specifically disclaim any responsibility, and shall not be liable for any damages, claims, injuries, losses, liabilities, costs, or obligations, including any direct, indirect, special, incidental, or consequential damages (collectively known as "Damages") whatsoever and howsoever caused, arising out of, or in connection with, the use or misuse of the book and the information contained within it, whether such Damages arise in contract, tort, negligence, equity, statute law, or by way of any other legal theory.

Exercise Disclaimer...Please read!

Exercise is not without its risks, and this or any other exercise program may result in injury. Risks include but are not limited to: aggravation of a pre-existing condition, risk of Injury, or adverse effect of over-exertion such as muscle strain, abnormal blood pressure, fainting, disorders of heartbeat, and in very rare instances, of heart attack.

To reduce the risk of injury in your case, consult your doctor before beginning this exercise program. The instruction and advice presented here are in no way intended as a substitute for medical consultation. The authors and publisher disclaim any liability from, and in connection with this program.

The exercises in this document are provided for educational purposes only, and are not to be interpreted as a recommendation for a specific treatment plan, product, or course
of action.

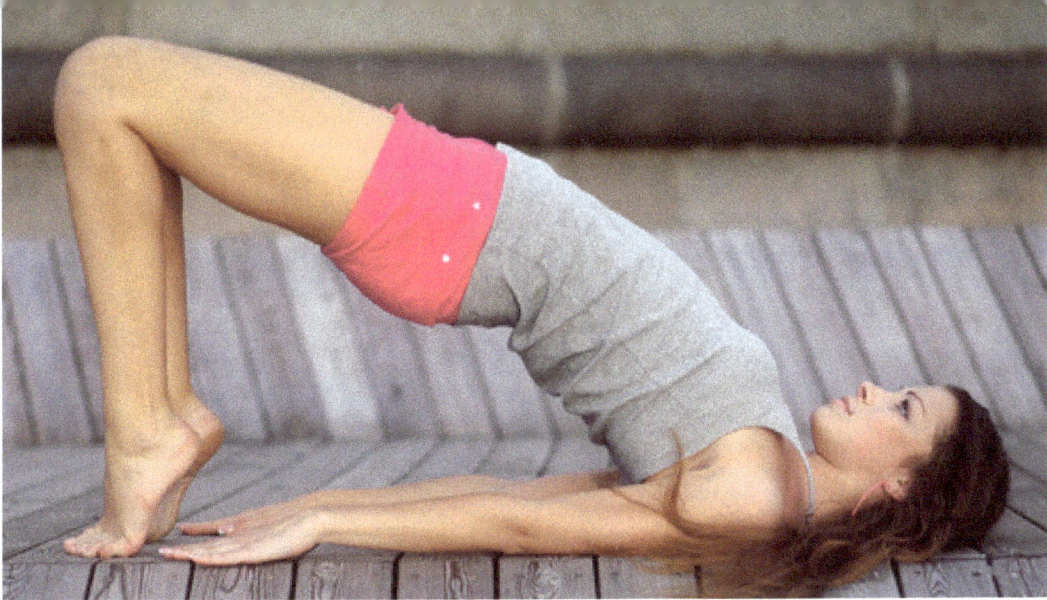

Exercise Disclaimer... Please Read!

Exercise is not without its risks, and this or any other exercise program may result in injury. Risks include, but are not limited to:

- Aggravation of a pre-existing condition.
- Risk of injury during exercise.
- Adverse effects of over-exertion (muscle strain, pain, and stiffness).
- Abnormal blood pressure.
- Fainting.
- Erratic heartbeat.
- Heart attack (in very rare instances).

The instruction and advice presented here are in no way intended as a substitute for medical consultation. The authors and publisher disclaim any liability, from/or/ and in connection, with this program/book.

The exercises in this book are provided for educational purposes only, and are not to be interpreted as a recommendation for a specific treatment plan, product, or course of action, or as a substitute for professional supervision or advice. To reduce the risk of injury in your case, consult your doctor before beginning this or any exercise program.

The authors, publishers, and technical experts use reasonable effort to include accurate and up-to-date information in its information sources; however, all information appearing is general in nature. Kinetic Health, the authors, publishers, and practitioners do not assume liability or give any warranty of any kind for the information and data contained or omitted from this document, or for any action or inaction made in reliance thereon. Information presented in this book and associated web sites may be changed at any time. Specific advice should be obtained in respect of specific situations.

Any programs involving weights, intense workouts, and apparatus may put strong physical demands on any child who is still growing – supervision is obligatory in such cases.

If you have, or have had asthma, growth condition, heart condition, or have experienced chest pains or dizziness in the last month, we strongly advise you NOT to try any of our workouts.

This book is NOT a medical facility and no information contained in our book should be used to prevent, treat or diagnose medical conditions of any kind. As with any exercise program, if at any point during your workout you begin to feel faint, dizzy, or have physical discomfort, you should stop immediately and consult a physician.

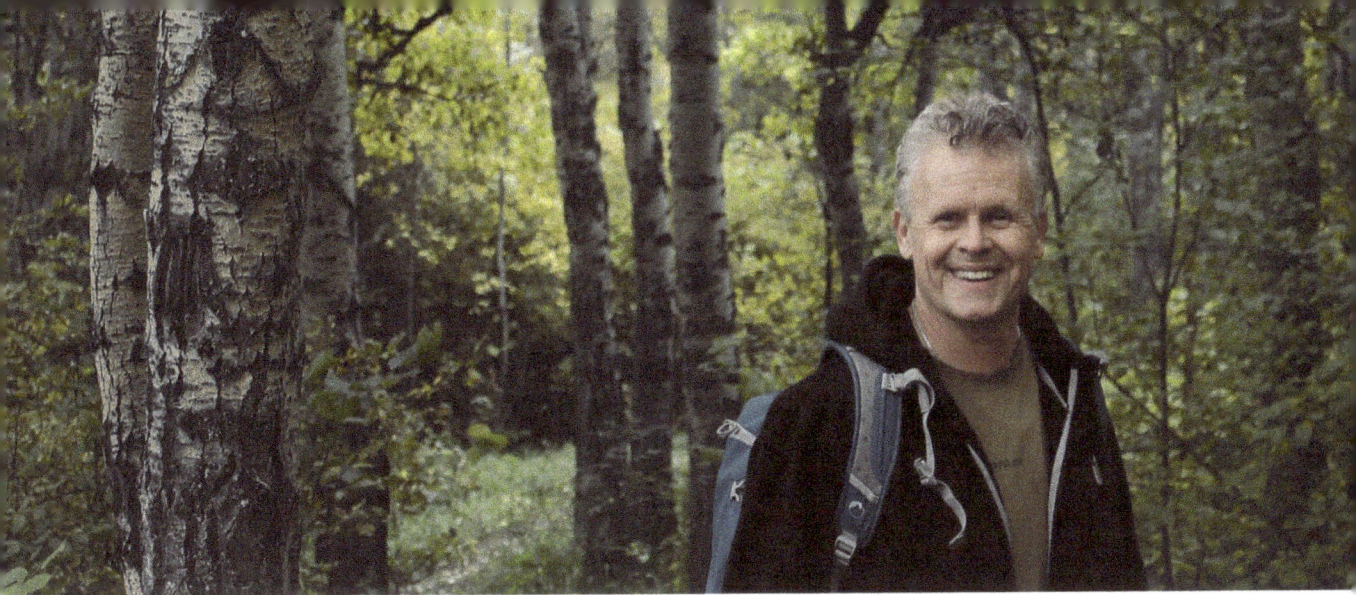

Preface by Dr. Abelson

Plantar Fasciitis (PF) is one of the most common conditions that we successfully treat at our clinic. In fact, between the general public and members of the running community, I find that I am treating several cases of Plantar Fasciitis every day.

Resolving Plantar Fasciitis can be a very frustrating process for many people. Often, when I review my patient case histories, I find that most of my patients have already tried a wide range of other therapies, ranging from orthotics, ultrasound, stretching, ice, heat, manipulation, various soft-tissue techniques, acupuncture, electrical stimulation, steroid injections, and on to a plethora of ointments and creams. Not surprisingly, most of these patients are very skeptical when I tell them that their Plantar Fasciitis really can be resolved (in the majority of cases).

The scepticism of these patients is usually short-lived once they start on our *Plantar Fasciitis Program*. The information provided in this book *really works* and will help to resolve almost 90% of Plantar Fasciitis cases.

Don't get me wrong, this program requires lots of work and dedication on your part, but the results will be well worth it. Just be sure that you complete each aspect of this program, and follow the suggestions I have put forth to you.

In this Book

There is a very important point that I would like to make at this time. Although this entire book is about Plantar Fasciitis and how to resolve this particular condition, it also contains a great deal of information that can help you to prevent a host of other maladies from ever manifesting in your body.

Let me explain. From a practitioner's perspective, musculoskeletal conditions such as Plantar Fasciitis do not occur unless numerous other areas of your body are also involved. These can include biomechanical compensations in areas that you normally would never relate to your primary condition, and of which you may not be aware. (See *Plantar Fasciitis and the Kinetic Web - page 37*.)

For example, one common finding in our patients with Plantar Fasciitis is that a significant percentage of these patients have weak, unstable hips. This is a significant finding when you consider how a decrease in hip function is directly related to conditions such as low back pain, muscular imbalances, poor proprioception and balance, and osteoarthritis of the back, hips, knees, ankles, and of course, the feet.

Bottom line, be diligent with every section as you progress through each component of our program. Every test is important; every exercise is provided to address specific problems. By following our advice, you will significantly increase your odds of fully resolving of Plantar Fasciitis, and also prevent a host of other injuries from occurring.

Our Program

Our program uses specific strengthening, stretching, and self-myofascial release techniques. This is NOT a one-size-fits-all program. Instead, we will show you how to analyze and identify your personal strengths and weakness (throughout your kinetic chain) and help you to build a customized program that addresses *your specific problems.*

Our *Plantar Fasciitis Program* requires you to identify *which* structures (muscles, ligaments, tendons, connective tissues, fascia, or nerves) are affected, and then determine the *extent* to which these structure's *associated kinetic chains and movement patterns* have been impacted.

The Importance of Customizing Your Treatment

The number and type of anatomical structures that need to be addressed varies greatly from case-to-case. Some cases require treatment of just the structures of the foot, while other cases require treatment of structures ranging through the foot, ankle, knee, hip, and core. This is why *generic* treatment protocols often fail to achieve success.

The ability to determine exactly which structures are involved requires a good understanding of the anatomy, neurology, and kinetic chain relationships within your body. In this book, we start you on the path to understanding the impact that your body's **Kinetic Web** – a linked, three-dimensional series of kinetic chains – has upon resolving your Plantar Fasciitis.

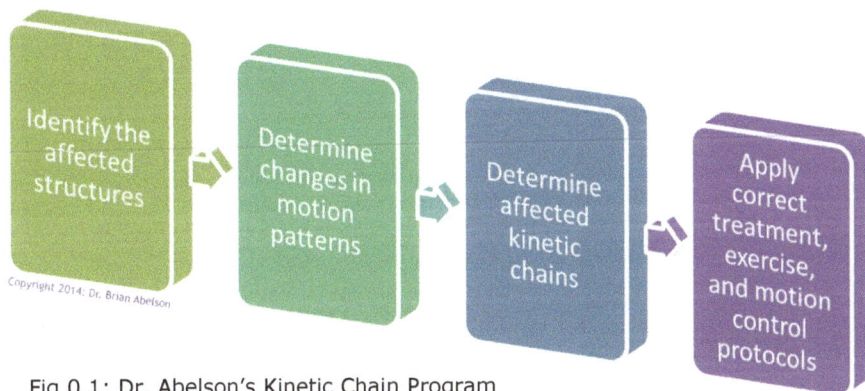

Fig 0.1: Dr. Abelson's Kinetic Chain Program

We will briefly review how each kinetic chain is made up of individual structural links (the joints, bones, muscles, ligaments, tendons, fascia, and various neurological structures) that are connected to each other to form a three-dimensional **Kinetic Web**. Any weak link in these kinetic chains can cause its own set of problems, and can also generate further motion and biomechanical compensations, eventually resulting in the development of new problems throughout the Kinetic Web.

Enjoy the Benefits of Our High Success Rate

My perspectives in this book are based upon a combination of over 21 years of clinical observation, research, and practical experience. I certainly acknowledge that much more hard research needs to be conducted in this area in order to confirm my perspectives about Plantar Fasciitis. On the other hand, after helping to achieve the successful resolution of hundreds of Plantar Fasciitis cases at our clinic, I don't recommend waiting for this research to come in before addressing this condition. So, get started on healing your Plantar Fasciitis.

I hope you enjoy this book. I think you will find it to be an excellent resource for resolving your Plantar Fasciitis. The techniques and recommendations provided in this book have given our clinic an almost 90% success rate. So even if you have unsuccessfully tried just about any imaginable type of therapy – don't be discouraged – as the majority of Plantar Fasciitis cases *can* be resolved.

Wishing you a fast and permanent resolution of your Plantar Fasciitis!

Dr. Brian Abelson

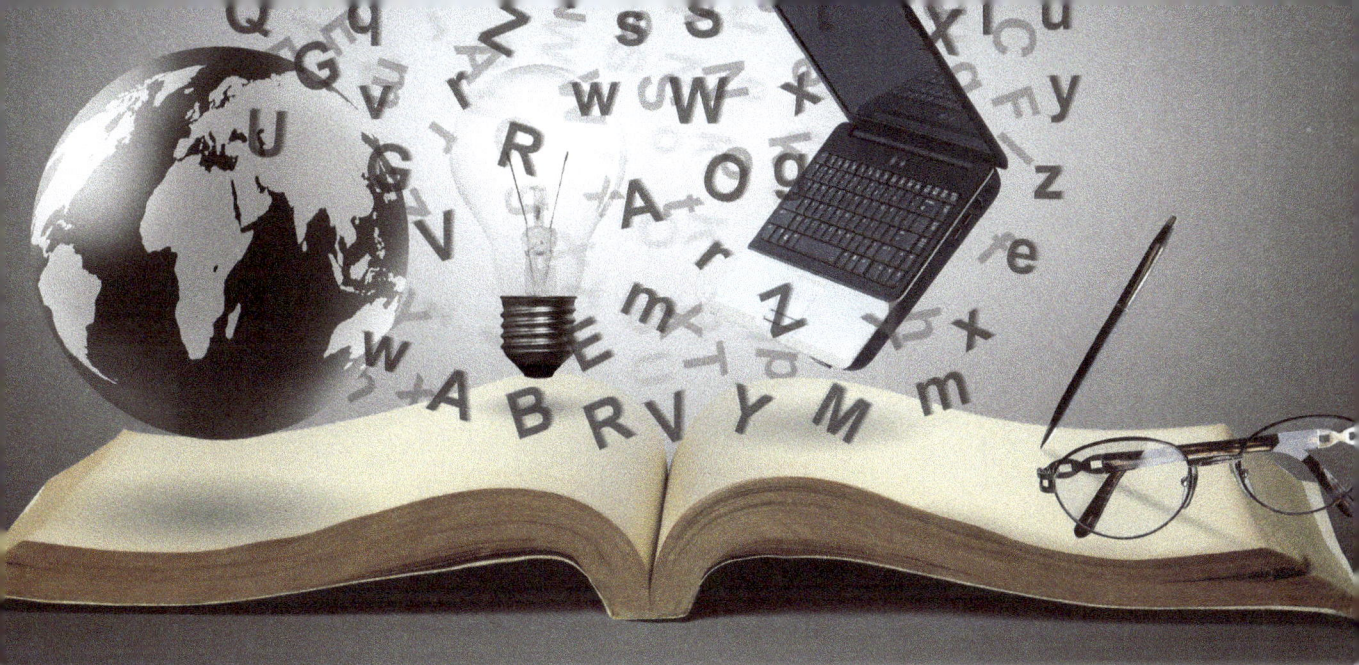

Table of Contents

Table of Contents

Plantar Fasciitis

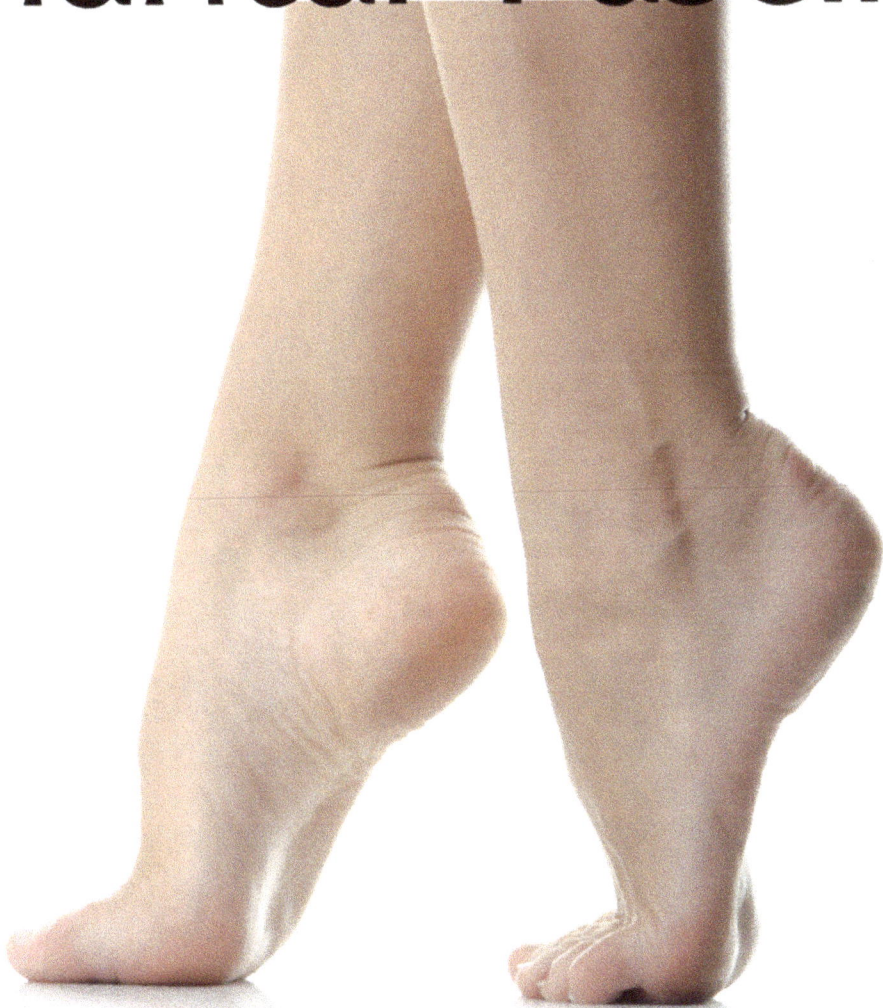

Understanding

Plantar Fasciitis

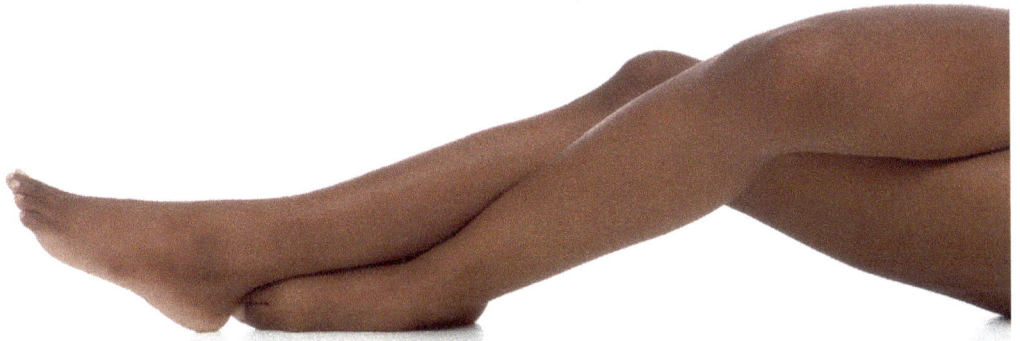

About Plantar Fasciitis

In this chapter

Plantar Fasciitis (PF) affects about 10% of the population over the course of their lives, and commonly occurs in a wide cross-section of athletes (especially runners and dancers). Since there are over seven billion people in the world, this means over 700 million individuals will eventually suffer from this condition at some point in their life. Plantar Fasciitis usually affects:

- One foot, but about a third of those suffering from this condition experience PF in both feet. [1]
- Both females and males equally.

Symptoms of Plantar Fasciitis

Symptomatically, people suffering from Plantar Fasciitis often experience:

- Severe foot and heel pain when their feet first touch the floor in the morning. Many of these patients avoid stepping on their heels, and end up walking on their toes.
- Decreased pain with motion as their day progresses.

---

1.   Irving DM, Cook JL, Young MA, Menz HB. *Obesity and Pronated Foot Type May Increase the Risk of Chronic Heel Pain: a Matched Case-Control Study.* BMC Musculoskelet Disord 2007; 8:41.

- Pain, typically in the front or center of the heel, that increases with extended periods of standing or weight-bearing.
- Dull aching or sharp burning pain in the heel.
- A pulling sensation in the heel.
- Difficulty walking or running on hard surfaces or up stairways.
- Numbness, tingling, or pain along the nerve pathways of the lower leg and foot.

Typically, these people find a point of extreme tenderness when they palpate or touch the inside of their heel (*medial tubercle* of the *calcaneus*). Due to the altered motion patterns caused by their foot pain, persons who suffer from Plantar Fasciitis often complain about accompanying ankle, knee, hip, and back pain.

Plantar Fasciitis...What Does it Mean?

The term 'Plantar Fasciitis' can be very misleading since the suffix "*itis*" implies "*inflammation*". This can be confusing since Plantar Fasciitis can occur both with, and without, inflammatory changes within the tissue. A more accurate term would be **Plantar Fasciosis** ("osis" means *abnormal state*), but since Plantar Fasciitis is the most commonly known term, we will continue to use this term throughout this book.

In medical literature, Plantar Fasciitis is most often described as "*an inflammation of the plantar aponeurosis or plantar fascia*". The *plantar fascia* is a thin band of fibrous tissue that runs from the heel bone (*calcaneus*) to the base of the toes. Interestingly, the actual *plantar fascia* is rarely tender to palpation and touch.[2] Instead, it is the deeper soft-tissue structures that show signs of injury, and which cause the pain felt by patients. It is important to remember that the area of pain does NOT indicate the SOURCE of the problem. It is often just the area where the pain manifests.

In the medical community, the general consensus is that Plantar Fasciitis is a degenerative condition, often caused by repetitive motion.[3] Degenerative histopathological findings of the *plantar fascia* combined with the lack of pro-inflammatory cells have confirmed the degenerative hypothesis. [4]

While I agree that repetitive strain is a common *cause* of Plantar Fasciitis, I do not agree with the general consensus when it comes to *which* soft-tissue structures need to be addressed in order to resolve Plantar Fasciitis. For example, most

---

2. Dr. Michael Leahy DC, "*Active Release Techniques - Soft Tissue Management Systems for the Lower Extremity, 2nd Edition*", 2008
3. Lemont H, Ammirati KM, Usen N. Plantar fasciitis. *A degenerative process (fasciosis) without inflammation.* J Am Podiatr Med Assoc 2003;93(3):234-237.
4. Khan KM, Cook JL, Taunton JE, Bonar F. *Overuse tendinosis, not tendinitis: a new paradigm for a difficult clinical problem (part 1).* Phys Sportsmed. 2000; 28:38–48.

traditional methods of treatment address only the structures of the foot. I believe that this minimal approach is insufficient to truly resolve Plantar Fasciitis.

> **TIP:** In this book, we will show why it is important to treat *all* the associated structures of the foot's kinetic chain in order to obtain long-term resolution of this condition.

For those of you who just can't wait to understand these kinetic chain relationships, you can jump ahead to the following sections:

- See *"The Workings of the Plantar Fascia"* - page 39.
- See *"Fascia and the Kinetic Web"* - page 41.
- See *"Fascial Connections for Plantar Fasciitis"* - page 43.

What Causes Plantar Fasciitis?

Plantar Fasciitis (PF) can be caused by a broad range of factors, varying from direct trauma, repetitive strain, and congenital defects to motion compensations that have occurred as a result of earlier injuries.

It is common for Plantar Fasciitis (like many repetitive strain injuries) to develop over a long period of time. Keep in mind that the fascia and soft tissues of the feet can be stressed by a combination of factors such as:

- Alterations in normal foot biomechanics (caused by motion compensations that have developed due to earlier injuries).
- Development of scar-tissue or adhesions anywhere along the kinetic chain (from the bottom of the feet, right up into the hips).
- Repetitive motions that stress the feet, ankles, knees, and hips.
- Standing on hard surfaces for long periods of time.
- Existing muscle and biomechanical imbalances.
- Increased physical activity.
- Shoes that provide inadequate support such as high heels.
- Acute trauma to the feet.

Common Causes of Plantar Fasciitis

The following sections of the book summarize some of the most common causes for the development of Plantar Fasciitis, some of which are obvious, while others become apparent only when important kinetic chain relationships are acknowledged and addressed. Read the following topics to identify and understand the cause of your Plantar Fasciitis.

- *Congenital Causes of Plantar Fasciitis - page 24.*
- *Soft-Tissue Restrictions Can Cause Plantar Fasciitis - page 25.*
- *Nerve Compression Can Cause Plantar Fasciitis - page 27.*
- *Decreased Joint Function Can Cause Plantar Fasciitis - page 27.*
- *Repetitive Actions Can Cause Plantar Fasciitis - page 28.*
- *Poor Arch Support Can Cause Plantar Fasciitis - page 29.*
- *Acute Trauma to the Feet Can Cause Plantar Fasciitis - page 31.*
- *Poor Hip Stability Can Cause Plantar Fasciitis - page 31.*
- *Poor Core Stability Can Cause Plantar Fasciitis - page 32.*
- *Environmental and Lifestyle Factors Can Cause PF - page 33.*
- *Heel Spurs Do Not Cause Plantar Fasciitis - page 34.*

Congenital Causes of Plantar Fasciitis

Some people are born with conditions that predispose them to Plantar Fasciitis. For example:

- People with very high (or very low) arches in their feet often develop Plantar Fasciitis due to altered biomechanics and lack of appropriate shock absorption.
- People who pronate excessively (*forefoot varus*) often develop PF.[5] [6]

Many of these congenital problems can be minimized through the use of appropriate functional exercise routines in combination with good orthotic foot support.

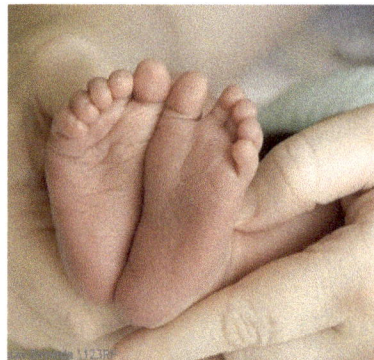

---

5. Irving DM, Cook JL, Young MA, Menz HB. *Obesity and pronated foot type may increase the risk of chronic heel pain: a matched case-control study.* BMC Musculoskelet Disord 2007;8:41.

6. Taunton JE, Ryan MB, Clement DB, et al. *A retrospective case-control analysis of 2002 running injuries.* Br J Sports Med 2002;36(2):95-101.

TIP: Orthotics should only be prescribed **after** functional exercise routines have been properly implemented, and sufficient time has elapsed for muscle strengthening. For example: If the gluteal muscles are strengthened, then almost half the abnormal motion patterns in the feet will go away. But, if you make orthotics without first strengthening these elements of the kinetic chain, you may well *lock-in* the dysfunction. Performed correctly, the appropriate functional exercises may even *eliminate the need* for orthotic supports.

Soft-Tissue Restrictions Can Cause Plantar Fasciitis

Most of us are unaware that we are walking around with a considerable collection of scar-tissue, adhesions, and fascial thickenings embedded within our soft-tissues (muscles, ligaments, tendons, and fascia). This scar-tissue may form due to previous or current injuries, poor posture, deconditioned muscles, or simply as a consequence of activities in your daily life.

Inflammatory processes cause the body to lay down restrictive scar-tissue across the injured structures, which results in:

- Binding together of adjacent tissue layers.
- Tethering of nerves.
- Decreased circulatory function.
- Development of abnormal motion patterns.

Together, these factors can combine and cascade to cause the development of yet more abnormal motion patterns in other parts of the body.

Scar Tissue Can Cause All Kinds of Problems - When ligaments, tendons, or muscle fibers are torn or injured, the body lays down collagen in an attempt to *support, reconnect,* and *reinforce* the damaged tissue. This collagen is commonly referred to as *scar-tissue.*

Scar-tissue is weak and inflexible because the new tissue is often laid down in a random pattern and does not follow the same *fiber orientation* as the surrounding normal tissue.

Although the initial intention of the body was to *stabilize* the injured area with the scar-tissue, the random orientation of these new fibers can instead have the effect of de-stabilizing other surrounding structures. Since the structures and muscles of the body act as a single functional unit, any alteration in tissue consistency can create imbalance in muscle operation, and often results in the development of abnormal motion patterns.

These restrictive fibers also bind the layers of adjacent soft tissues together, and prevent them from *translating* or moving freely across each other. This entrapment causes further friction, inflammation, fascial thickening, and the development of even more abnormal motion patterns.

In fact, ultrasound measurements of tissues of symptomatic and non-symptomatic patients shows the symptomatic tissue to have increased thickening due to the various soft-tissue layers becoming adhesed together.[7]

With Plantar Fasciitis, this includes structures in both the feet[8], as well as structures further up the kinetic chain, such as:

Copyright: Shutterstock /azure

- Calf muscle restrictions in the *gastrocnemius* and *soleus.*
- Hamstring restrictions in the *biceps femoris, semitendinosus,* and *semimembranosus* muscles.
- Restrictions in the hip flexors (*iliacus* and *psoas*).
- Restrictions in the hip extensors (*gluteals*).

Fortunately, these restrictions can often be dealt with through a process of self-myofascial release or some type of soft-tissue therapy (for the more extreme cases). See *"The Anatomy Behind Plantar Fasciitis" - page 49* for more information about how these structures affect or cause your Plantar Fasciitis.

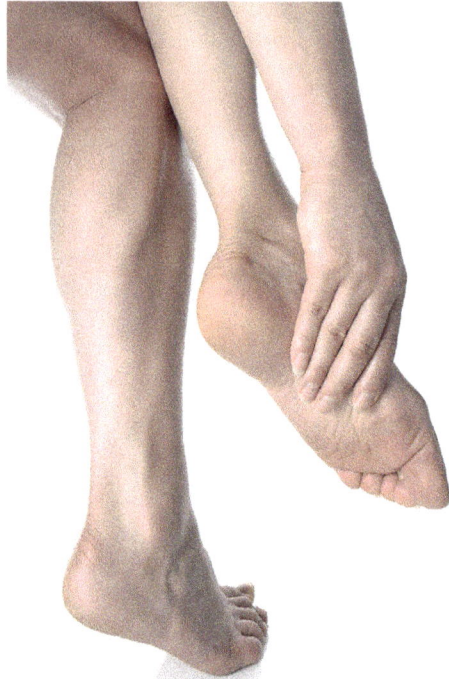

---

7.   Wall, J., Harkness, M., & Cook, B. (1993). Ultrasound diagnosis of plantar fasciitis. Foot Ankle Int, 14(8), 465-470

8.   Kwong, P., Kay, D., & White, M. (1988). Plantar Fasciitis: Mechanics and pathomechanics of treatment. Clinical Sports Medicine, 7(1), 119-126

Nerve Compression Can Cause Plantar Fasciitis

Nerves can become compressed by scar tissue. When practitioners consider the consequences of nerve compression, they usually think about symptoms such as tingling, burning, or pain. However they often fail to consider several other important consequences of nerve compression.

Soft tissue restrictions can also reduce *nerve or neurological function* along the entire kinetic chain. Think of it this way. Nerves pass through all your soft-tissue structures. If a soft-tissue structure develops restrictions, then any nerve that passes through it can become compressed, trapped or tethered to other structures, and therefore experience reduced function. This neurological deficit can exhibit in a number of ways:

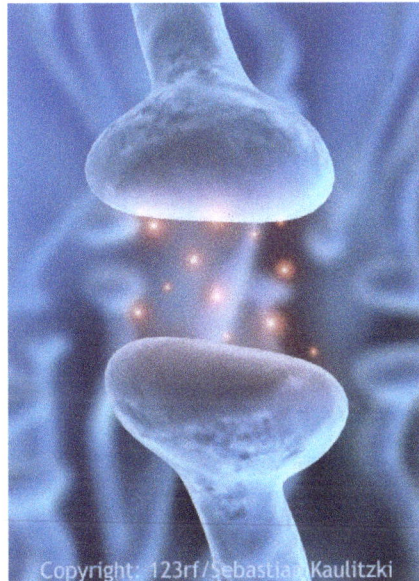
Copyright: 123rf/Sebastian Kaulitzki

- Sensory nerve restrictions would manifest as pain and/or altered sensations (paresthesias).
- Motor nerve restrictions would manifest as muscle weakness which eventually leads to the development of abnormal motion patterns.

These areas of *nerve tethering* or *compression* are no small matter. In some cases, it is not possible to fully resolve Plantar Fasciitis unless these nerves and structures are fully released. (See *Common Nerve Compression Sites for PF on page 87* for more details about this process.)

Fortunately, many of these restrictions can often be dealt with through a process of self-myofascial release, nerve flossing, or some type of soft-tissue therapy (for the more difficult cases).

Decreased Joint Function Can Cause Plantar Fasciitis

Lack of *joint mobility* can cause the development of abnormal motion patterns which then cause subsequent muscle imbalances, that then lead to further compensatory changes in the body.

For example, here are two examples of joints restrictions that we commonly see in cases of Plantar Fasciitis:

Ankle Joint (tibiotalar joint) - The *tibiotalar joint* is located between the shin bone (*tibia*), and the first ankle bone (*talus*). A restriction in this joint will inhibit the ability to flex the foot (both *dorsiflexion* and *plantar flexion*). This will cause a person to compensate by *internally rotating* their foot while walking. [9]

Subtalar Joint - The *subtalar* joint allows for both *inversion* and *eversion* of the foot. Lack of mobility in this joint will affect the normal pronation and supination motions of the feet. There is a very interesting relationship between the *plantar fascia* and *subtalar* joint function. It has been found that even when the *plantar fascia* is severed, the arch of the foot still retains 65% of its structural integrity due to both bone geometry and the joint capsules of the foot. [10]

There are many other joints involved in foot and leg motion that, when they are restricted, can also affect Plantar Fasciitis. Each restricted joint must be released for a full resolution of Plantar Fasciitis.

Repetitive Actions Can Cause Plantar Fasciitis

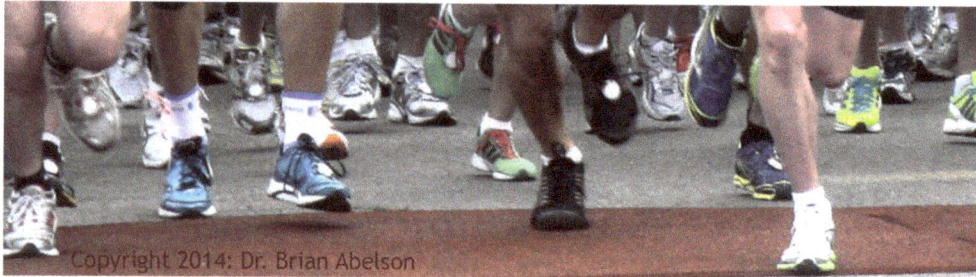

Copyright 2014: Dr. Brian Abelson

Modern lifestyles are full of repetitive actions, from walking and running, to long hours spent standing or sitting each day. Unfortunately there is a cost to pay for all these repetitive motions.

This price is paid by the development of micro-tears within the soft tissues of our body. Basically, the body develops micro-tears in its tissues whenever:

- We exceed the tissue's ability to endure the forces placed upon it.
- We perform repetitive actions for long periods of time.

When enough micro-tears form, the body is no longer able to repair itself, due to its repair systems becoming overwhelmed. At this point, collagen degeneration starts to take place; this degenerative process is very similar to what happens in tendinosis (*chronic necrosis*).

---

9.   Wearing, S. C.; Smeathers, J. E.; Urry, S. R.; Hennig, E.; Hills, A. P., *The pathomechanics of plantar fasciitis.* Sports Medicine 2006, 36 (7), 585-611.

10.   Wright, D. G.; Rennels, D. C., *A study of the elastic properties of plantar fascia.* The Journal of Bone & Joint Surgery 1964, 46-A (3), 482-492

During this degenerative process, several biochemical changes occur, including:[11]

- An increase in *fibroblasts* (the cells that lay down scar tissue).
- An increase in *ground substance* (the matrix of connective tissue).
- A general loss of collagen continuity.

In other areas, a thickening forms between layers of tissues. These thickenings are a hardening of the normal lubricant – *hyaluronic acid* – between muscle layers and between joints. Thickening of *hyaluronic acid* can also cause inflammation, nerve entrapment, and a decrease in circulatory function. These different types of restrictions then cause yet more changes to the normal biomechanics of the body, often leading to yet other injuries.

Injuries caused by repetitive motion can be addressed by:

- Breaking up myofascial restrictions.
- Releasing entrapped nerves.
- Increasing the strength of the weak muscles.
- Stretching short or contracted soft-tissue structures.

Poor Arch Support Can Cause Plantar Fasciitis

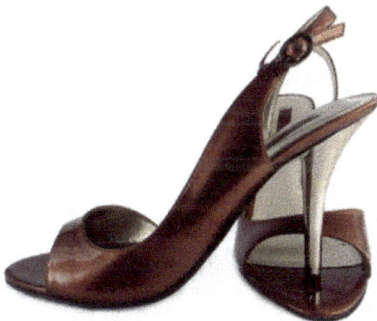

Poor arch support in shoes is a common cause of Plantar Fasciitis. Wearing the wrong shoe is what podiatrists refer to as "*shoe-icide*". Good arch support is an essential tool for reducing the effects of everyday cumulative trauma.

I see my patients spending large amounts of time and money on purchasing just the right car tires, luxury clothes, and expensive nights out, but they give little consideration to the purchase of good shoes. Take my advice – *spend the money to get good shoes*. A good pair of shoes can provide cheap insurance against a host of injuries.

High heels can be the cause of many problems, including Plantar Fasciitis. Yes, they do look lovely, I will admit that. However, high heels place your feet in a position that cancels or negates the shock absorption mechanisms of the foot. You

---

11.   Khan KM, Cook JL, Taunton JE, Bonar F. *Overuse tendinosis, not tendinitis: a new paradigm for a difficult clinical problem (part 1)*. Phys Sportsmed. 2000;28:38–48.

can read more about this in the discussion of the foot's windlass mechanism in *The Workings of the Plantar Fascia - page 39*.

Wearing heels also applies a huge amount of pressure on the balls of the feet (*distal metatarsals*). Too much pressure in this area causes inflammation in the joints and nerves that pass through this area, and in some cases, can even cause the formation of hairline fractures.

On that note, there is another problem that I commonly see when it comes to shoes. This has to do with the *wrong* type of shoe being prescribed for runners. I often treat patients in our clinic who have been prescribed shoes designed for excessive pronation, when they should actually be in a neutral shoe. In addition, I often see the wrong type of *orthotics* being prescribed for the treatment of Plantar Fasciitis.

TIP: If you need orthotics, always make sure they are custom made to avoid future problems. It is also essential to find the right person – with the appropriate training and expertise – to prescribe the orthotics or corrective shoes for your specific needs. So shop around, ask questions, and evaluate the experts you meet to ensure you get the help you need. See the *Wet Foot Test - page 142* for an example of information that can help you to find the right type of shoe.

Case Study - A Runner with Foot Pain

At Kinetic Health (our clinic in Calgary), we commonly conduct a *Biomechanical Gait Analysis* and *Wet Foot Test - page 142* on our patients. Essentially, we have our patients walk up and down the hall, both with and without their shoes. On observation of their gait, we commonly see over-correction caused by the shoes that they are wearing.

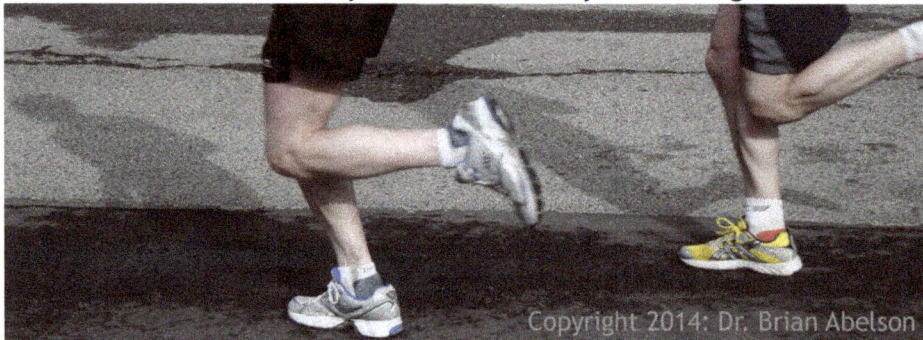

Copyright 2014: Dr. Brian Abelson

Just a short time ago, I treated a runner (Julie) who complained about severe ankle and foot pain. Julie had suffered from the condition for about two months. She became upset when I told her that she was wearing the wrong types of shoe for her particular gait pattern, and that she needed new shoes. She was upset, both because of how much money she had already spent on her shoes, and the fact that it was her shoes that could be part of the problem.

Eventually, I did convince Julie to move into a neutral shoe. Within about a week of doing so, all of her ankle and foot complaints were gone. Sometimes it is just that simple. Bottom line – make sure the person who is prescribing your shoes is adequately trained to make such assessments.

Acute Trauma to the Feet Can Cause Plantar Fasciitis

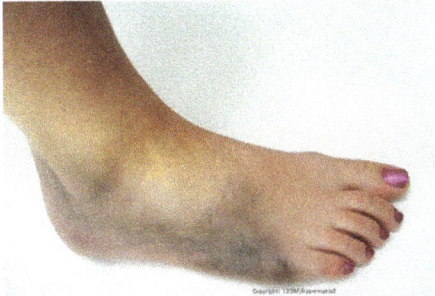

Sprains, strains, or any other type of injury to the feet, ankles, or lower extremity can be a contributing factor in the development of Plantar Fasciitis.

Chronic injuries that occurred years ago can cause numerous biomechanical compensations, followed by corresponding alterations in motion patterns. These changes can eventually lead to the development of Plantar Fasciitis. [12]

It is important to address and treat these biomechanical compensations if you want to achieve long-term resolution of your Plantar Fasciitis.

Poor Hip Stability Can Cause Plantar Fasciitis

Hip stability? What does hip stability have to do with your Plantar Fasciitis? Actually, hip stability has major effects on ALL the structures of the lower body. Research has shown that a lack of hip stability is a major factor in the cause and perpetuation of Plantar Fasciitis. This is why it is essential to determine if your problem is limited to just your foot, or if other structures in the kinetic chain are also involved.[13] [14]

Dr. Reed Ferber, PhD at the University of Calgary, has carried out some remarkable research on the relationship between weak hip muscles and foot stability.[15] [16] Dr. Ferber and his colleagues reviewed 283 studies that researched the correlation between injuries and weak hip-stabilizers and concluded that after an ankle or foot injury:

12.   Bullock-Saxton JE, Janda V and Bullock MI (1994). *The influence of ankle sprain injury on muscle activation during hip extension.* International Journal of Sports Medicine 15: 130-134.
13.   Niemuth P, Johnson RJ, Myers MJ, et al. *Hip Muscle Weakness and Overuse Injuries in Recreational Runners.* Clinical Journal of Sport Medicine 15: 14-21, 2005.
14.   Fredericson M, Cookingham CL, Chaudhari AM, et al. *Hip Abductor Weakness in Distance Runners with Iliotibial Band Syndrome.* Clinical Journal of Sport Medicine 10: 169-175, 2000.
15.   MacKenzie Lobby. *Do Weak Hips Cause Pronation.* Times, Dec 12, 2009. http://times.com/Article.aspx?ArticleID=18359&PageNum=1, Dec 12, 2009.
16.   Reed Ferber PhD, CAT(C) ATC1, Brian Noehren PT PhD2, Joseph Hamill PhD3, Irene Davis PT PhD4. *Competitive Female Runners With a History of Iliotibial Band Syndrome Demonstrate Atypical Hip and Knee Kinematics.* February 2010, Volume 40 #2, Journal of Orthopaedic & Sports Physical Therapy. http://www.mc.uky.edu/healthsciences/research/Pubs_PDFs/Noehren_February2010-RR-Ferber[1].pdf.

- Muscles in the hip (such as the *gluteus maximus*) no longer contract in a normal manner.[17]
- Individuals with weak external hip rotator muscles or weak hip abductor muscles are much more likely to experience injuries such as Plantar Fasciitis.[18]

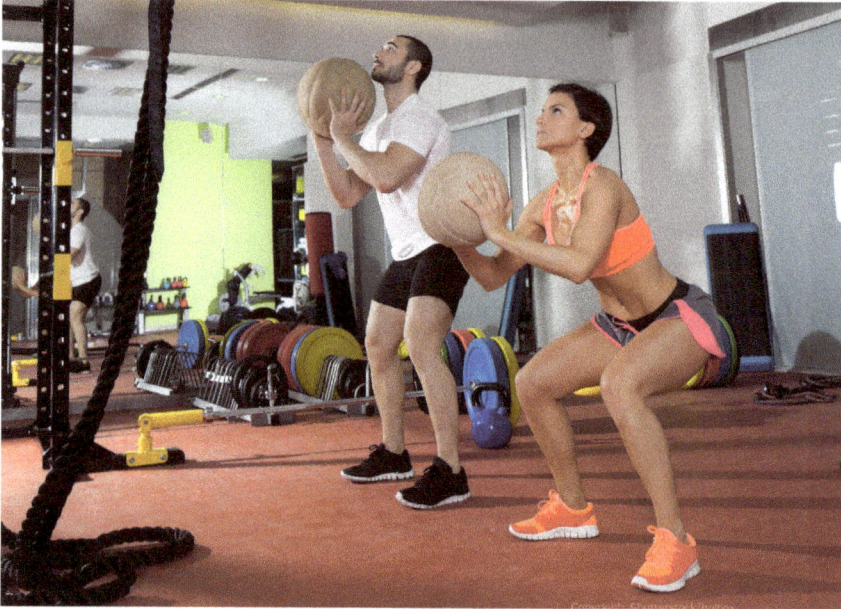

This is why it is essential that you use the self-analysis section (*Phase 2: Finding Problems in Your Kinetic Chain - page 115*) of this book to determine if your hip stabilizers are functioning correctly, and then perform the appropriate exercises and therapy (if required). Only then is it likely that you will obtain a full resolution of your Plantar Fasciitis. See *"Phase 2: Addressing Problems in the PF Kinetic Chain" - page 149*.

Poor Core Stability Can Cause Plantar Fasciitis

Your core is the foundation and source of all your movements, providing a stable base for arm, leg, and body motions. Your ability to maintain good posture is greatly dependent upon your core stability! If you have a stable, balanced, elastic core, then you can easily transfer energy from the center of your body to all your extremities!

---

17. Bullock-Saxton JE, Janda V, Bullock MI. *The influence of ankle sprain injury on muscle activation during hip extension.* Int J Sports Med. 1994;15:330–4.
18. Lehman GJ, Lennon D, Rayfield B, Poschar M, Tressider B. *Muscle recruitment patterns during the prone leg extension test.* BMC Musculo-skeletal Disorders. 2004;5:3. doi: 10.1186/1471-2474-5-3. 10 Feb 2004.

Your body works as a single, coordinated, and functional unit. Good core stability is critical for effective lower-body motions such as walking, running, or standing. A weak or unbalanced core affects every action you perform, from the bottom of your foot right up to the top of your head.

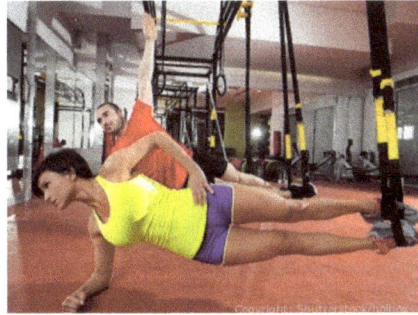

If you have a weak, unbalanced core, you will find that it is difficult to resolve Plantar Fasciitis. You may find that many treatments are able to remove the *symptoms* of Plantar Fasciitis, but in the presence of a weak or unbalanced core, this symptomatic resolution will only last for a short time.

This is why it is essential for you to use the self-analysis section (*Phase 2: Finding Problems in Your Kinetic Chain - page 115*) of this book to determine if a weak core is one of the contributing factors in your Plantar Fasciitis, and then take appropriate actions to resolve this problem.

Environmental and Lifestyle Factors Can Cause PF

Like it or not, there are several lifestyle and environmental factors that may perpetuate or directly lead to Plantar Fasciitis. For example: [19]

- If you are 25-to-50 pounds overweight, you will find that it is much more difficult to resolve your Plantar Fasciitis. I did not say *impossible*, but unless you address your weight issues, it will be much more difficult.

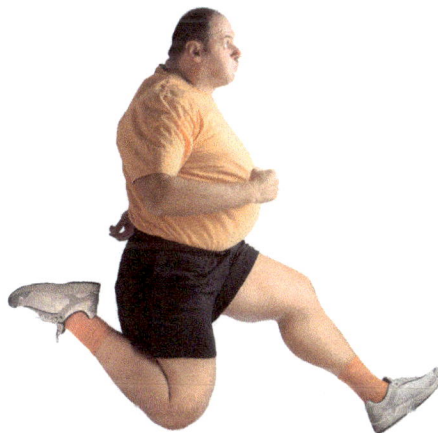

- Good nutrition is a key factor in any successful rehabilitation program. Good dietary practices keep your weight in check, strengthen your immune system, reduce inflammation, and speed injury recovery. When we treat our patients or provide them with exercises, we usually expect to see

---

19.   Rome K, Campbell R, Flint A, Haslock I. *Heel pad thickness - a contributing factor associated with plantar heel pain in young adults.* Foot Ankle Int 2002;23(2):142-147.

good results within a short period of time. If we don't see such results, the most common reason (other than the patient missing appointments or not performing assigned exercises) is usually poor dietary habits.

It is also likely that, as long as your weight remains a contributing factor, your Plantar Fasciitis will eventually return. Remember, Plantar Fasciitis may only be the *first* of a host of problems that you will eventually encounter if you are overweight. People with excess weight also have a tendency to develop degenerative arthritis throughout the body.

■   Smoking cigarettes also reduces your chances of resolving your Plantar Fasciitis. In addition to all the other known side-effects, smoking also reduces the rate at which the body can recover from injuries. For example, it is well established that individuals who smoke and have an injury, will experience more soft-tissue tears. It is a very simple equation, the more you smoke, the slower you heal. The degree of damage is directly related to the number of cigarettes smoked per day – it is a dose-dependant relationship.[20]

TIP: Check out the book – *Choose Health by Dr. Abelson* – and learn how to provide your body with the essential nutrients that it requires, while losing that unwanted weight.

Heel Spurs Do Not Cause Plantar Fasciitis

Heel spurs are:

■   Spike-like projections of new bone that usually do not cause pain and are generally incidental to the cause or resolution of Plantar Fasciitis.
■   Formed *after* the *plantar aponeurosis* becomes inflamed.
■   A by-product of inflammation and soft-tissue adhesions in the foot.

Standard medical literature often misuses the term '*heel spurs*' to describe Plantar Fasciitis. This usage is both confusing and misleading since heel spurs are a secondary effect of tension on the heel bone and are **not** the cause of Plantar Fasciitis. In actuality, increased tension on the *plantar fascia* (or the other tendons attaching to the heel bone) causes a lifting effect across the surface of the heel bone (*periosteum*) causing a bone spur to form.

In most cases, whether or not you still have a heel spur is unimportant in the treatment and resolution of Plantar Fasciitis. Patients often completely resolve their Plantar Fasciitis, become fully functional, suffer no pain, and still have heel

20.   Keith M. Baumgarten, David Gerlach, Leesa M. Galatz, Sharlene A. Teefey, William D. Middleton, Konstantinos Ditsios and Ken Yamaguchi. *Cigarette Smoking Increases the Risk for Rotator Cuff Tears.* CLINICAL ORTHOPAEDICS AND RELATED RESEARCH®, Volume 468, Number 6, 1534-1541, DOI: 10.1007/s11999-009-0781-2.

spurs showing on their X-rays. Heel spurs should be considered more of a secondary effect than the primary problem.[21]

Note: In my opinion, heel surgery (to remove a heel spur) should only be considered after all conservative treatment methods have been tried. Going for the surgical option may not give you the results you need since heel spurs commonly reappear after surgery, especially when the underlying soft tissue problems have not been addressed.

Since Plantar Fasciitis is a soft-tissue condition, it cannot be seen on X-rays. The only reason you would consider getting an X-ray for this condition is to rule out any pathological causes of heel pain. For example, it would make sense to get an X-ray after some type of trauma, or if there were indications of infections, or to determine if degenerative arthritis was a significant factor. In such cases, a medical practitioner would have to decide whether an X-ray or other diagnostic procedures are needed.

What is Needed to Resolve Plantar Fasciitis?

Despite the many different factors that may have caused your Plantar Fasciitis, its long-term resolution typically requires the following:

- **Exercises** to rehabilitate and retrain all the neuro-muscular structures of the affected kinetic chain. See *"Phase 1: Foundational Protocol for Plantar Fasciitis" - page 107* and *Build Your Kinetic Chain Routine for PF on page 154*.
- **Biomechanical analysis** to identify faulty motion patterns throughout your affected kinetic chain. See *"Phase 2: Finding Problems in Your Kinetic Chain" - page 115*.
- **Strengthening exercises** should be selected to appropriately strengthen and reactivate weakened structures. See *"Strengthening Exercises for Plantar Fasciitis" - page 215*.
- **Flexibility exercises** to help restore balance and aid in tissue remodelling during the healing process. See *"Stretching & Myofascial Release Exercises for PF" - page 171*.
- **Myofascial release** to break the soft-tissue restrictions that inhibit the normal gliding action of soft-tissue structures and cause the development of abnormal motion patterns. See *"Stretching & Myofascial Release Exercises for PF" - page 171*.
- **Nerve Flossing Exercises** should be used if you have indications of certain nerves being entrapped. **See** *"Nerve Flossing for Plantar Fasciitis" - page 208*.

---

21.   Singh D, Angel J, Bentley G, Trevino SG. *Plantar fasciitis*. BMJ. 1997;315:172–5.

Keep the 80/20 Effect in Mind

Normally, of all the people who follow this program, 80% of them will see remarkable improvements of their condition within a 4 to 6 week period. However, if after four-to-six weeks of following our Plantar Fasciitis program, you find that you still don't see significant improvement in your symptoms, then you will need to consider what I call the '*The 80/20 Effect on page 94*'.

If you are in this 20%, don't be discouraged. There are seven common reasons why some people fall into the 20% category. We have outlined these reasons in the section about '*Seven Factors Affecting Resolution of Musculoskeletal Conditions on page 95*'.

In most cases all that is needed is a little tweaking of the program, a few lifestyle changes, and you will also experience success. In fact, it is very rare to see someone who does not respond positively after making these additional changes.

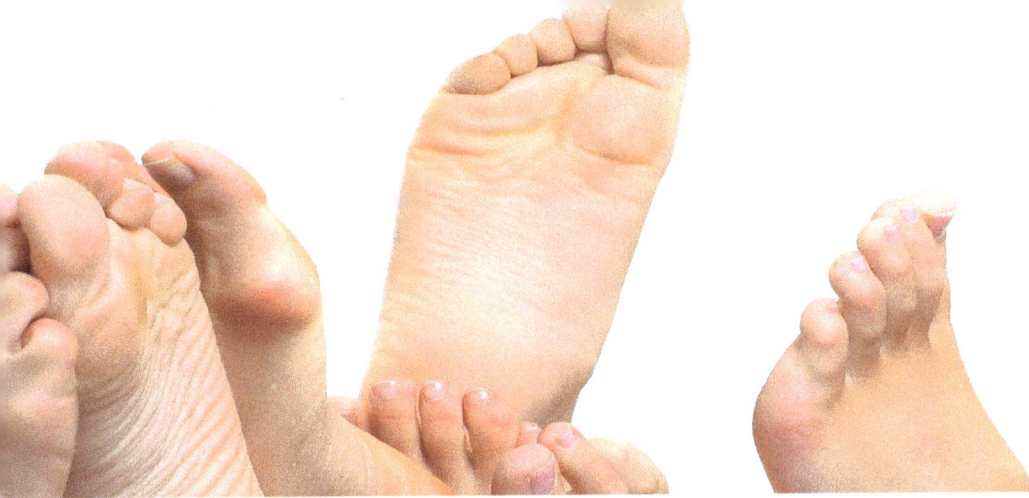

Plantar Fasciitis and the Kinetic Web

In this chapter

Note: This chapter is all about your kinetic web and its involvement in the development of Plantar Fasciitis. If this interests you, then please read on. Or, if you would prefer to get started on the exercises, self-testing, and evaluation, you can jump straight to *Understanding Our Process – The 80/20 Effect on page 91*.

The foot is a truly amazing piece of engineering. When functioning correctly, force and energy are easily transferred and dissipated from the feet and lower extremities, through the core, and even into the upper extremity.

The foot's kinetic chain is composed of a complex series of related structures (muscles, ligaments, tendons, joints, and fascia) that connect the foot to the ankle, knee, hips, core, and upper extremities. As remarkable as these interconnections are, they can also become the root cause of many chronic dysfunctions. That is why it is important to implement exercise routines that focus upon both the *key areas of power transference*, as well as *maintaining whole-body stability*.

Injuries Can Impact Your Kinetic Chain

When a structure in the foot, ankle, knee, or hip is injured or restricted, that structure becomes unable to effectively perform its normal functions (such as pushing off with the foot, bending at the knees, sitting, standing, walking, or running). The body compensates for this inability by using other surrounding muscles to help carry out these actions.

These compensations initially occur within the directly linked muscles, ligaments, tendons, and connective tissue groups. As time goes on, these initial compensations can lead to:

- Reduced nervous system function (due to impingement upon neurological structures).
- Reduced blood flow (circulatory dysfunctions).
- Increased inflammation (due to micro-tears or biochemical changes within the body).
- Collagen degeneration due to repetitive occurrence of micro-tears in the tissue[22].

The body's kinetic chain can be viewed as a synergistic chain of interconnected links. When one part of the link goes down, the whole chain loses the ability to function optimally.

The bottom line – a change in one area of the body can result in a *cascade of changes* throughout the rest of the body, and thus affect all the structures in the body's kinetic chain. In order to achieve a full resolution of Plantar Fasciitis, these kinetic chain relationships must be taken into consideration by any soft-tissue treatment method or exercise protocol.

However, before we get into a discussion of these kinetic chain relationships, we should first come to an understanding of *plantar fascia*, how it works, and its function.

---

22.   Khan KM, Cook JL, Taunton JE, Bonar F. *Overuse Tendinosis, not tendinitis: A New Paradigm for a Difficult Clinical Problem (part 1)*. Pays Sportsmed. 2000; 28:38–48.

The Workings of the Plantar Fascia

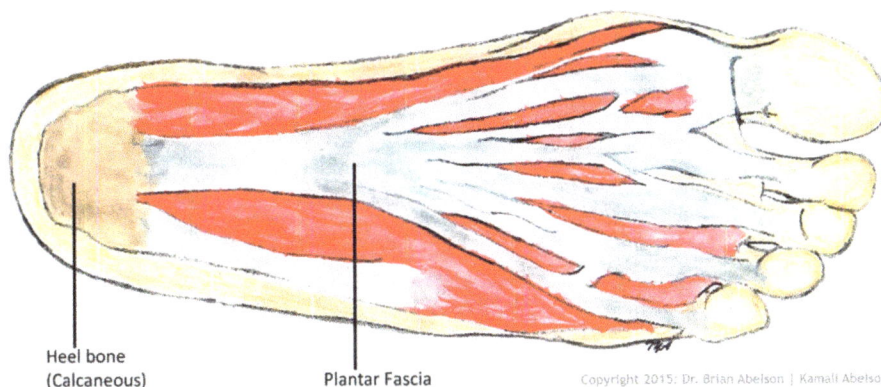

Heel bone
(Calcaneous)   Plantar Fascia

Copyright 2015: Dr. Brian Abelson | Kamali Abelson

Fascia is a type of connective tissue that envelops, passes through, connects, and binds muscles, blood vessels, nerves, and organs. Fascia is the glue that binds all the structures of your body together, it provides the structure and foundation by which all other tissues types connect to each other. It extends in three-dimensions throughout your body, creating a mesh within which all other structures lie, connect, and communicate.

The *plantar fascia* itself is a thin sheet of fibrous connective tissue that runs from the base of the heel bone (*calcaneus*) and fans out to the base of the toes (*proximal phalanges*). The *plantar fascia* is designed to support normal foot motions in its actions of standing, walking, and running. The fiber orientation of this *plantar fascia* is very specific and very important, as it is designed to be extremely functional for both shock absorption and power generation.

The Plantar Fascia's Windlass Mechanism

One of the easiest ways to understand how the *plantar fascia* works is to compare it to a *windlass mechanism* – a very effective device for lifting large loads. [23]

Usually, when we think of a windlass mechanism, we think of a mechanical lifting device that consists of a horizontal cylinder turned by a crank or motor, around which a line or cable is wound. In the foot, the *plantar fascia* simulates the cable in a *windlass mechanism*, with the bones of the foot forming the frame around which the fascia or cable is wrapped.

---

23.   Lori A. Bolga and Terry R. Malone: *Plantar fasciitis and the Windlass Mechanism: A biomechanical link to Clinical Practice*, J. Athl. Train., 2004,77-82.

The Plantar Fascia's Windlass Mechanism

When the Big Toe is Relaxed...

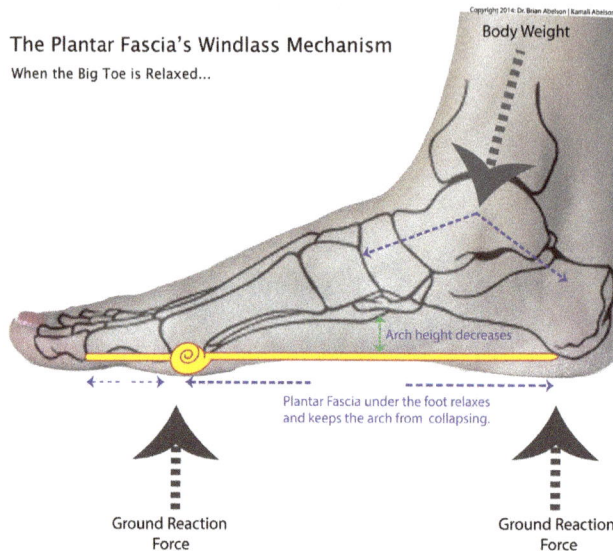

Body Weight

Copyright 2014: Dr. Brian Abelson | Kamali Abelson

Arch height decreases

Plantar Fascia under the foot relaxes
and keeps the arch from collapsing.

Ground Reaction
Force

Ground Reaction
Force

1. The *plantar fascia* loosens and tightens with each change in the weight-bearing forces of the foot.

2. As you push-off with the foot, the *plantar fascia* winds around the forward bones of the foot (heads of the *metatarsals*). This has the effect of reducing the distance between the heel bone (*calcaneus*) and the toes.

The Plantar Fascia's Windlass Mechanism

When the Big Toe Dorsiflexes...

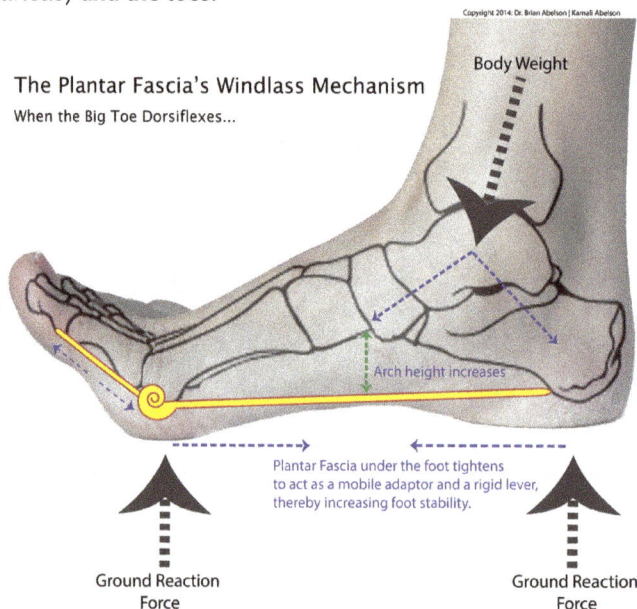

Body Weight

Copyright 2014: Dr. Brian Abelson | Kamali Abelson

Arch height increases

Plantar Fascia under the foot tightens
to act as a mobile adaptor and a rigid lever,
thereby increasing foot stability.

Ground Reaction
Force

Ground Reaction
Force

3. By doing so, the *plantar fascia* elevates the arch of the foot (*medial longitudinal arch*) and prevents the arch of the foot from collapsing, allowing for effective shock absorption, and powering the propulsion mechanism. The Windlass Mechanism packs the bones of the foot together to create a rigid lever for more effective propulsion during push-off.

Fascia and the Kinetic Web

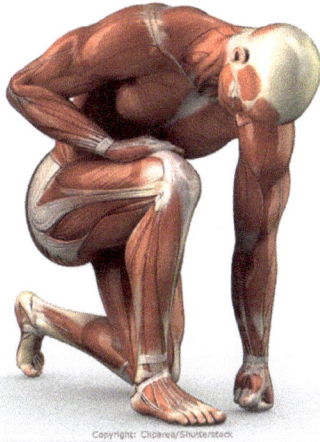

Copyright: Cliparea/Shutterstock

Until now, we have only discussed the *plantar fascia*. But the body's fascia (strong connective tissue) is not limited to just the area under the feet. Fascia is everywhere in the body, weaving through, and connecting every component of the body.[24] Fascia forms a seamless web of connective tissue which *connects, holds*, and *infuses* the tendons, organs, muscles, tissues, and skeletal structures.

Fascia is a key link in the *Myofascial System* – a critical component in the integrated *Kinetic Web*.

Given this degree of connectivity, it is easy to see how restrictions or injury to fascia can propagate to any of the other structures to which the fascia is connected.

The Importance of Fascia

It is important to understand the significance of fascia. New discoveries over the last few decades has shown that fascia plays a much more important role than simply serving as a packing material around muscles and organs.

Fascia is intimately involved in **controlling** both the *movement patterns* and the *neurological control mechanisms* of the entire body, and forms an integral aspect of a body-wide signaling system. In fact, it has been found that fascia is full of neurological receptors.

---

24. Schleip R. *Fascial Plasticity – a New Neurobiological Explanation.* Journal of Bodywork and Movement Therapies 7(1):11-19 and 7(2):104-116: 2003

Fascia and Motion

Standard texts for anatomy and biomechanics teach us that motion is created by the *contraction of muscles*. At the end of these muscles are tendons that insert directly into bone. When a muscle contracts, the two ends of the muscle (origin, insertion) are pulled towards each other to create motion.

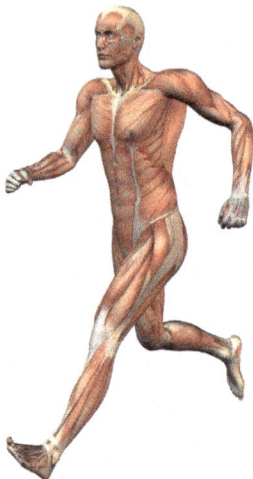

Though this description is quite true, it is also a reductionist perspective on what is really happening in the body.

In 2009, at the *Second International Fascia Congress* in Amsterdam, I had the opportunity to speak to one of the Chancellors of a major European medical school. He explained how most practitioners have learned a "*dumbed-down*" version of anatomy, rather than developing a real understanding of how the body actually works. Basically, it is much easier to teach students by compartmentalizing each group of muscles, and simplifying their functions, rather than thinking about the body as a single, integrated, functional unit – one that works in synergy with all its other components.

Let me explain how an understanding of fascia can help us develop a new, holistic perspective about how the body performs actions. This will give us a better understanding about *why* looking at a bigger anatomical picture can help us to completely resolve cases of Plantar Fasciitis.

First, consider the fact that muscle fibers actually *originate from*, and *insert into*, both *fascial fibers* and *bone*. These *fascial fibers*, in turn, insert into multiple regions of other bones, and even into other adjacent muscles.

These additional points of contact provide muscles with the ability to generate force in multiple directions. This point is very important as we attempt to identify how an injury affects multiple areas of the kinetic chain.[25]

Knowing about these multiple points of fascial attachment – all working across three-dimensions – completely changes our understanding of the biomechanics of muscle action, and also provides us with a much more functional understanding of muscle contraction. Now, when we look at, and analyze muscle contraction, we realize that only *certain sections of the muscle* contract to perform an action (not the entire muscle).

---

25. Jaap van der Wal, MD, PhD. *The Architecture of the Connective Tissue in the Musculoskeletal System - An Often Overlooked Functional Parameter as to Proprioception in the Locomotor Apparatus.* University Maastricht, Faculty of Health, Medicine and Life Sciences, Department of Anatomy and Embryology, Maastricht, Netherlands. Int. J. Ther Massage Bodywork 2009;2(4):9-23.

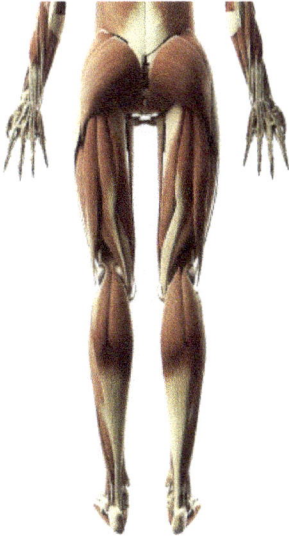

In addition, groups of muscles usually work together as functional units to execute any action. For example, some muscles may act as the *primary movers (agonists)* to perform an action, while other muscles act as *antagonists*; while yet others act as *synergists* and others as *stabilizers*. Fascia is the key link that allow these muscles to work together as functional units by aiding in coordinating actions across multiple joints.

Depending on the degree of motion, and the amount of force that is needed, each muscle will then contract *specific areas* of the muscle, rather than the entire muscle. These very specific motions are largely coordinated by the *neurological receptors embedded in the fascia*, and are not controlled by the brain alone.

Fascial Connections for Plantar Fasciitis

Fascial interconnections are not theoretical entities; they are actual physical structures that have been mapped out. Researchers and clinicians such as Thomas Myers (*Anatomy Trains*)[26] and Luigi, Carla and Antonio Stecco (*Fascial Manipulation*)[27] have spent decades researching these interconnections. During the 2nd and 3rd *International Fascia Research Congresses* in Amsterdam, Netherlands and Vancouver, Canada, I had the privilege of listening to medical experts from around the world confirm this and other related fascial research. (Take a look at these excellent articles for more details.)

■ *Fascia Research II: Second International Fascia Research Congress*
(*http://www.ijtmb.org/index.php/ijtmb/article/view/61/70*)
■ *The Architecture of Connective Tissue in the Musculoskeletal System*
(*http://www.fasciacongress.org/2009/articles/IJTMB_vanderWal_62-436-4-PB%5B1%5D_Pre-Pub.pdf*)

---

26. Thomas W. Meyers, Churchill Livingstone. *Anatomy Trains, 2nd Edition, Myofascial Meridians for Manual and Movement Therapists.* Kinesis Inc, Copyright: 2009.
27. Luigi Stecco, Carla Stecco, and Antonio Stecco, *Fascial Manipulation*, Copyright 2009.

The Superficial Back Line and Plantar Fasciitis

It is truly quite amazing how these fascial interconnections run throughout the body, connecting one group of structures to the next. With Plantar Fasciitis, some of the key fascial connections that should be considered lie along what Thomas Myers (*Anatomy Trains*) calls the *Superficial Back Line*.[28]

The following short summary describes the *Superficial Back Line* as described in *Anatomy Trains*. As you read this, consider how the fascia on the bottom of the foot connects directly into the calf muscles, hamstrings, low back, into the neck, and even to the top of the head.

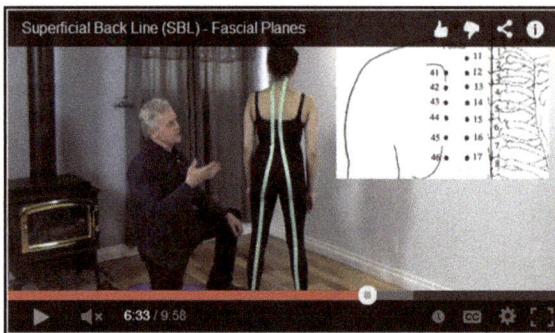

Watch our YouTube Video about the Fascial Planes of the Superficial Back Line. YouTube Address: http://youtu.be/1DMqul3CzhU

The *Superficial Back Line*:

- Begins at the bottom of the foot with the *plantar fascia*, passes over the heel (*calcaneus*) and inserts into the *Achilles tendon*.
- The Achilles tendon is formed from the bottom end of the calf muscles (*gastrocnemius* and *soleus*) and has a direct fascial connection into the hamstrings.
- From the hamstrings (*semitendinosus, semimembranosus* and *biceps femoris*), the fascia connects into the *sacral ligaments*, which then runs into the low back's connective tissue (*lumbosacral fascia*).
- Connections from the *lumbosacral fascia* run directly into the back muscles (*erector spinae*), up to the mid-back (*thoracic spine*), and then into the neck (*splenius capitus* and *semispinalis capitus*).
- These fascial connections then continue up the neck to the fascia on the skull (*nucal line*), and continue along the scalp's fascia to the forehead, ending just above the eyes[29].

---

28. Thomas W. Meyers, Churchill Livingstone. *Anatomy Trains, 2nd Edition, Myofascial Meridians for Manual and Movement Therapists.* Kinesis Inc, Copyright: 2009.

29. Thomas W. Meyers, Churchill Livingstone. *Anatomy Trains, 2nd Edition, Myofascial Meridians for Manual and Movement Therapists.* Kinesis Inc, Copyright: 2009.

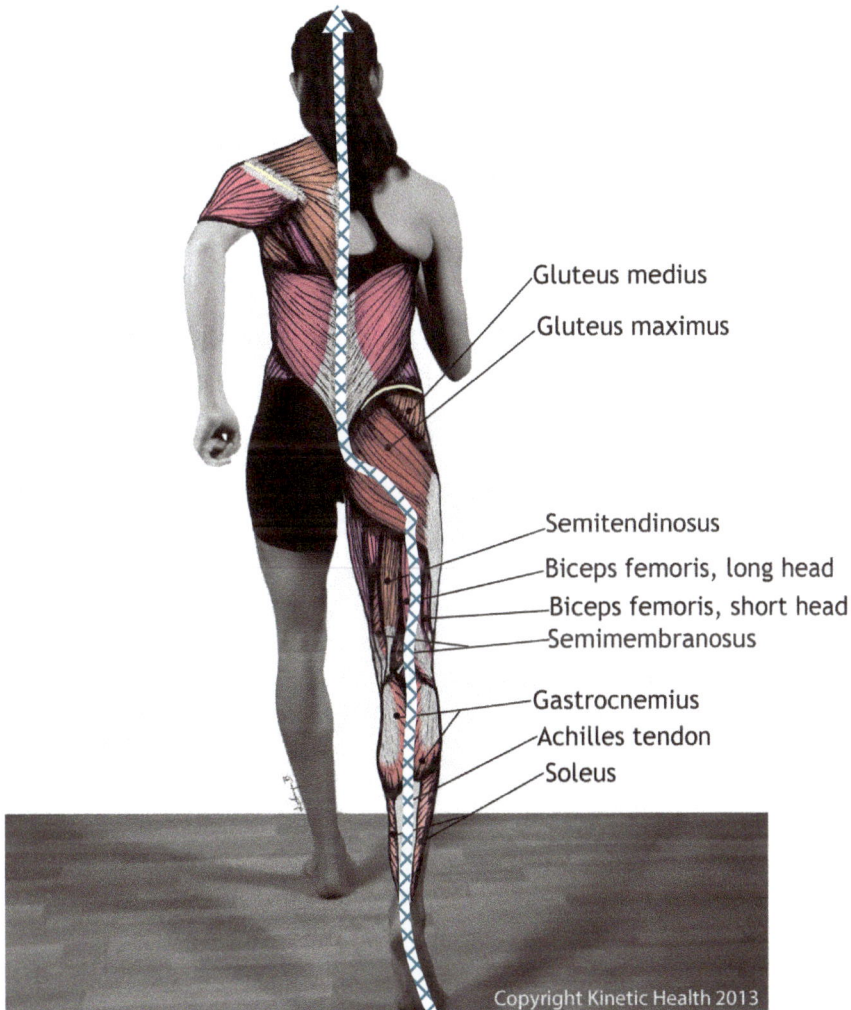

Gluteus medius

Gluteus maximus

Semitendinosus

Biceps femoris, long head

Biceps femoris, short head

Semimembranosus

Gastrocnemius

Achilles tendon

Soleus

Copyright Kinetic Health 2013

Fig 2.1: Structures along the Superficial Back Line.

When one considers these direct inter-fascial connections, it is easy to see how a single area of dysfunction in one area can lead to problems in a multitude of other areas along the kinetic chain, even in structures that lie far from the area of pain.

What starts out as a foot problem can soon cascade into a hip issue; and vice versa; a hip issue can easily cause problems in the lower extremity, leading to altered motion patterns, which eventually cause stress and pain on the *plantar fascia*.

Tibialis Anterior - A Kinetic Chain Example

As we discussed earlier, the body's kinetic chain can be viewed as a synergistic chain of interconnected links. When one part of the link goes down, the whole chain loses the ability to function optimally. This can affect the biomechanics of your body.

DEFINITION: Biomechanics is best described as an interface between the *muscular* and *neurological* activities of the body.[30]When these two aspects work well together, your movement system runs efficiently and smoothly. But when there is an interruption or dysfunction in either of these two aspects, then your movement system becomes disrupted.

Although foot stability and ankle mobility are important aspects in the treatment and prevention of Plantar Fasciitis, it is equally critical that we address core stability and hip strength, since both of these affect the foot's ability to function.

Although it is beyond the scope of this book to discuss all the structures of the foot's kinetic chain, we think it is important to understand just how inter-related all these structures actually are. To do this, we have selected just one key structure – the *tibialis anterior* muscle – as an example.

Foot Function and the Tibialis Anterior

To better understand this principle, as it relates to Plantar Fasciitis, let us consider just one link in this kinetic chain — the *tibialis anterior* (shin) muscle — and how it affects the other structures of the foot. In general, the *tibialis anterior* serves as a dorsiflexor that helps to control the deceleration of the foot as it impacts down on the ground during running or walking.

- The *tibialis anterior* muscle originates from the upper two-thirds of the lateral side of the shin (*tibia*) and inserts into the medial side of the foot (*medial cuneiform* and the base of the first *metatarsal bone*).
- Normally, the *tibialis anterior* acts to flex the foot upwards (dorsiflexes) and to roll the foot outwards (inverts the foot).
- The *tibialis anterior* acts to stabilize the foot as it makes contact with the ground during walking or running (eccentric contraction or elongation of tissue under load).
- The *tibialis anterior* also helps you to lift the foot clear of the ground during the swing phase of gait (concentric contraction).

---

30.   Sahrmann SA. *Movement System Impairment Syndromes of the Extremities.* Cervical and Thoracic Spines. St. Louis, MO: Mosby; 2011.

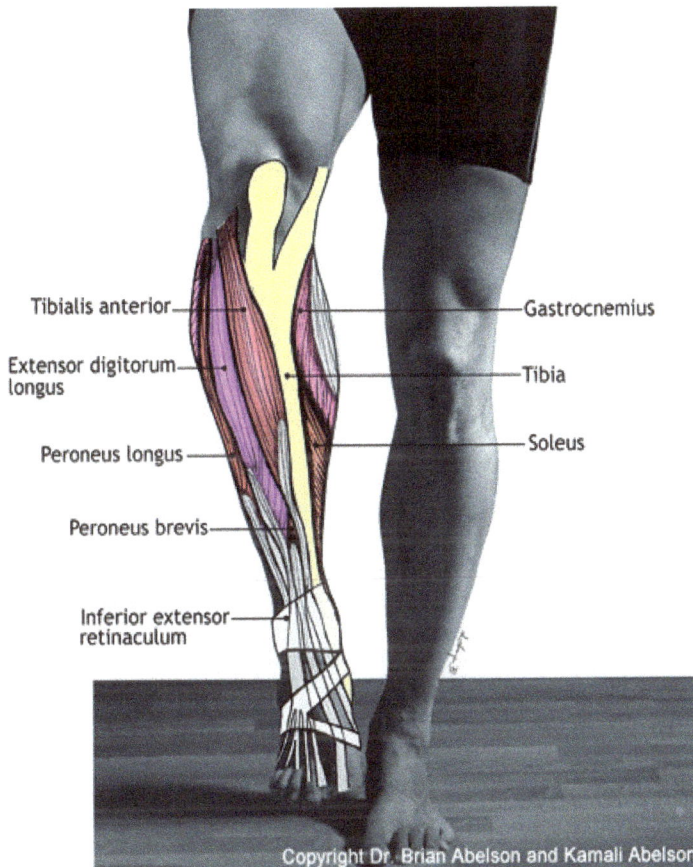

Tibialis anterior
Extensor digitorum longus
Peroneus longus
Peroneus brevis
Inferior extensor retinaculum
Gastrocnemius
Tibia
Soleus

Copyright Dr. Brian Abelson and Kamali Abelson

Fig 2.2: Kinetic Chain of the Tibialis Anterior

When dorsiflexors (such as the *tibialis anterior*) become weak or restricted, numerous structures of the lower extremity will soon become unstable, and your feet will experience increased shock.

Weakness of just this single muscle could lead to increased incidences of Plantar Fasciitis. The *tibialis anterior* muscle is a good example of how a fascial restriction in any part of the kinetic chain can directly affect the biomechanics of the foot. Again, Thomas Meyers of *Anatomy Trains*[31] does a great job of explaining this relationship when he describes the body's *Spiral Line*. (It is important to note that these lines are based upon precise anatomical dissections, and are NOT conjecture.)

---

31.   Thomas W. Meyers, Churchill Livingstone. *Anatomy Trains, 2nd Edition, Myofascial Meridians for Manual and Movement Therapists.* Kinesis Inc, Copyright: 2009.

In describing the lower part of the *Spiral Line*, Meyers explains how direct fascial connections run from a muscle on the outer hip (*tensor fascia latae*), connect into the IT band (*iliotibial band*) and the *tibialis anterior* muscle. At this point, the *tibialis anterior* wraps under the inside of the foot to connect with the *peroneus longus* muscle. The function of this connection is very similar to that of a stirrup supporting the bottom of the foot. The *peroneus longus* muscle then goes up the side of the ankle to the knee where it connects into the hamstring muscle (*biceps femoris*) on the outside of the leg.

The location where the symptoms manifest is directly dependant upon where the most tension is experienced. By understanding these fascial connections, it is easy to see how tension or restriction at any point along the *Spiral Line* can directly affect the function of the *tibialis anterior*. It is rather like pulling on one-end of an outstretched rope; whatever force is directed down the rope is felt at the other end of the rope. In this case, tension or abnormal motion patterns anywhere along the *Spiral Line* will affect the motion patterns of the *tibialis anterior*, thus making it an essential muscle that must be addressed for a full resolution of Plantar Fasciitis.

This is just one example that demonstrates how damage or restrictions to a single structure can easily affect the larger kinetic chain. Each structure in your foot and leg has a similar effect on its kinetic chain,. For more information about *Balancing Fascial Lines*, read the following article about Tensegrity – *http:// www.anatomytrains.com/fascia/tensegrity/*.

TIP: Learn how to evaluate the strength and flexibility of your foot in *Functional Tests for Joint Mobility on page 123*.

In Conclusion...

When evaluating a case of Plantar Fasciitis, it is important to take into consideration the fascial and muscular inter-connections between the various structures that are involved in performing and coordinating motion. This approach ensures that we are looking at the big picture, and addressing all the many muscles, working across multiple joints, which are all interconnected to each other by fascia.

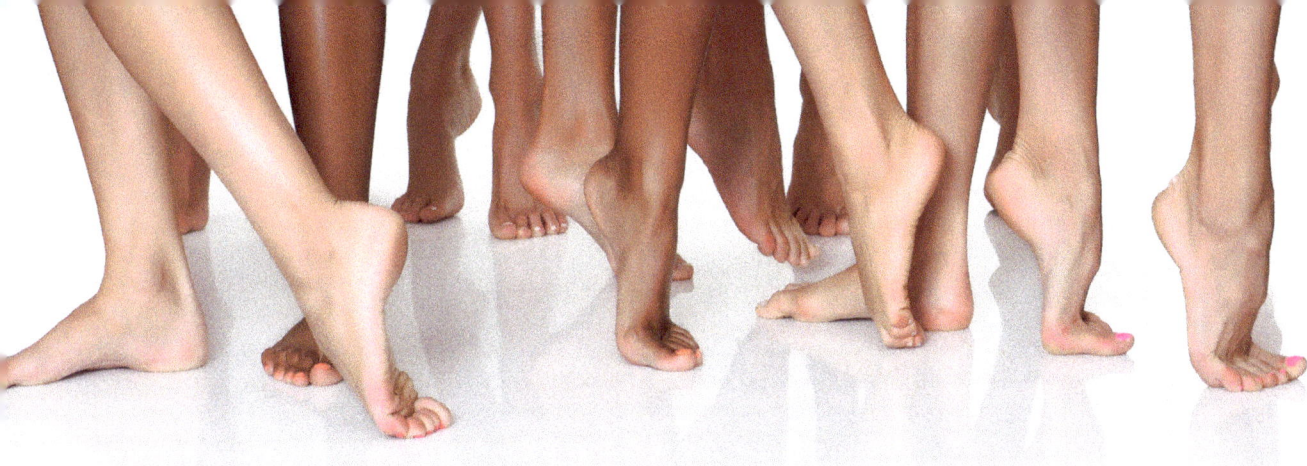

The Anatomy Behind Plantar Fasciitis

Chapter

3

In this Chapter

Note: This chapter is all about how your body's anatomy affects foot motion, and about the kinetic chain relationships between the structures that are often involved in the development of Plantar Fasciitis. If this interests you, then please read on. Or, if you would prefer to get started on the exercises, self-testing, and evaluation, you can jump straight to *Understanding Our Process – The 80/20 Effect on page 91*.

Our feet are much more complex than most people imagine. There are many layers of muscle that lie directly under the superficial layer of the *plantar fascia*. Within each layer, each muscle performs a specific task. Many of these muscles also connect into other structures that are located far above the foot, and often perform synergistic roles with these other anatomical structures. A restriction or injury to any one of these muscles or joints can result in the development of abnormal motion patterns in the foot, which may increase stress, cause a loss of stability, and eventually cause Plantar Fasciitis. See *"Plantar Fasciitis and the Kinetic Web" - page 37* for more details about this inter-relationship.

Think of each of these structures as the wheels on a car. When one wheel is out-of-alignment, the entire vehicle is affected. In the same way, it only takes one injured muscle, ligament, tendon, joint, or damaged connective tissue to significantly alter normal movement patterns, which in turn can eventually result to the development of Plantar Fasciitis.

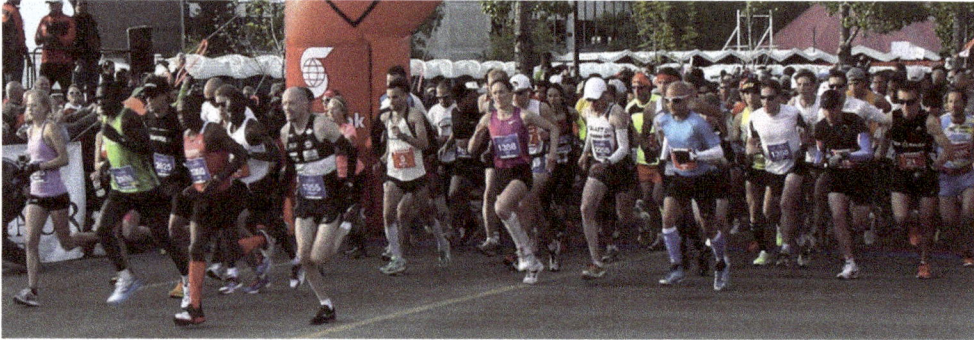

About Your Anatomy and Plantar Fasciitis

It is far beyond the scope of this book to discuss all of the varied structures of the foot, and each of their individual biomechanical impacts on other structures. However, for the balance of this chapter, we will take the time to quickly review some of the key structures that are typically involved in cases of Plantar Fasciitis, and discuss some of these inter-relationships.

The Role of Your Foot Bones in PF

When discussing anatomy and its effect upon the development of Plantar Fasciitis, it makes sense to start with the osseous (bony) structures of your feet. The skeletal structures of your foot provide the framework and support system for all the soft-tissues around them, and thus greatly affect the development (and resolution) of Plantar Fasciitis.

When any of the joints of the feet become restricted in their movement, abnormal motion patterns are soon created that could eventually lead to the development of Plantar Fasciitis. When these joint restrictions are not properly addressed and released, they could also lead to the reoccurrence of PF.

Skeletal Anatomy of the Foot

The foot has a complex skeletal structure with 26 bones, and 33 joints. Any restriction in any of these foot joints will greatly impact the foot's function, and can easily become a cause of Plantar Fasciitis.

Anatomically, the foot is divided into 3-sections, the *Forefoot, Midfoot*, and *Hind Foot*, with each section playing key roles in the support of your gait, balance, and shock absorption.

The Bones of the Forefoot

The forefoot consists of five toes (comprised of 14 *phalangeal* bones) and the five longer *metatarsal bones* in your foot.

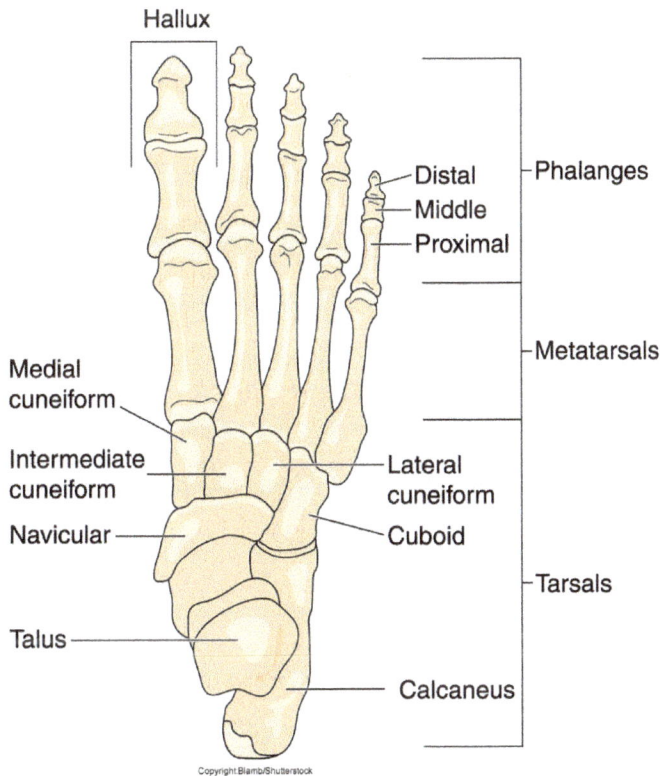

Fig 3.1: Bones of the Foot

The Phalanges (The Toes of Your Foot)

- The 14 *phalangeal* bones of your foot, and especially those of your big toe (*hallux*), play a vital role in both shock absorption and propulsion when walking and running.
- The *phalangeal* bones of the big toe also play an essential role in arch stabilization during mid-stance and during the *take-off phase* of the *Normal Gait Cycle*. Without this stabilization, the foot would have limited, to no, shock absorption capability, and very limited propulsive force.

In order for this stabilization to occur effectively, the big toe must be properly aligned with its surrounding and supporting structures. This requires both good **joint mobility** as well as a **balanced synchronization of action** with the structures that attach to the big toe. Otherwise key muscles such as the *flexor hallucis longus* and *flexor hallucis brevis* will not be able to perform their function of foot stabilization.

Misalignment of the big toe is known as *Hallux Valgus*, and often occurs in individuals who wear high heels or shoes with a pointed toe box. Both of these shoe types causes increased foot pronation. This abnormal foot pronation greatly affects big toe stability and affects the functional anatomy of your big toe. For example:

- Along the underside of the big toe are two *sesamoid bones*. These are floating bones that are embedded into the tendons that surround the big toe. These *sesamoid* bones slide around with each change in position of the big toe.
- When the big toe is in its ideal position, these *sesamoid* bones slide into two grooves (within the *first metatarsal*), giving them the ideal position for providing foot stability.
- When the big toe is misaligned, these *sesamoid bones* slide towards the inside of the big toe into a position where attaching muscles (*flexor hallucis*) cannot provide the required stability.

Thus, you can see how a simple misalignment of the big toe can cause a decrease in foot stability.

The Metatarsals

- There are five *metatarsal bones*, with the first metatarsal (which leads to the big toe) being the widest and shortest of the *metatarsal bones*.
- The second *metatarsal* is the longest of the five metatarsal bones.
- Excessive pronation often causes hypermobility of the mid metatarsal area. The instability caused by this hypermobility can lead to increased stress upon the *plantar fascia*.

It is common to have restrictions form between the *metatarsals*. These restricted areas are a common cause for the development of abnormal motion patterns throughout the foot and lower extremities.

The Midfoot

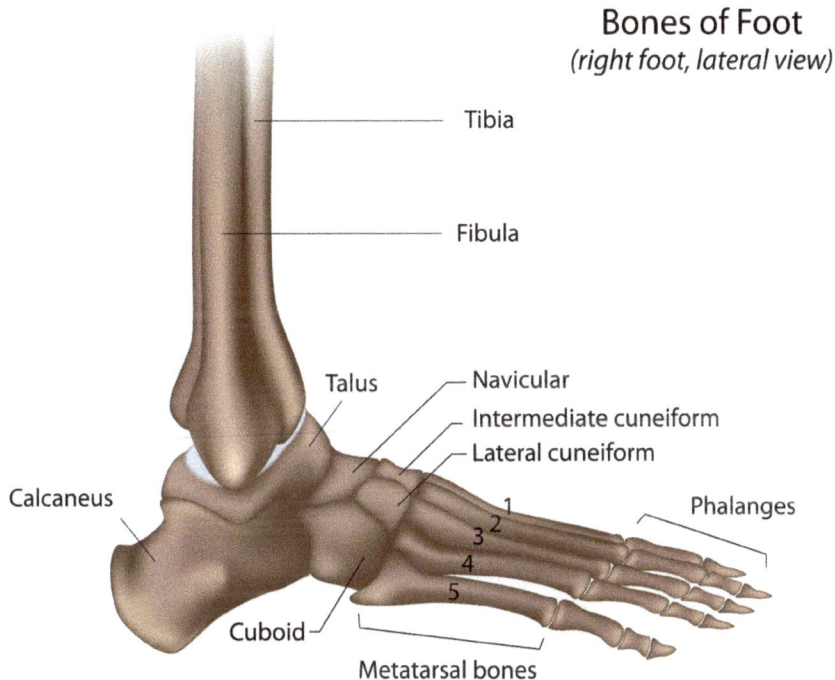

Fig 3.2: Bones of the Foot: Lateral View of the Right Foot

The midfoot contains five bones that forms the arch of the foot. These are the three *cuneiform bones,* the *cuboid bone,* and the *navicular bone.*

Cuneiform Bones

- The three *cuneiform bones* are named for their location: *medial cuneiform, intermediate cuneiform,* and *lateral cuneiform.*
- The positioning of the three *cuneiform bones* forms a keystone effects that Increases stability of the midfoot.

Cuboid Bone

- The *cuboid bone* is located on the lateral side of the foot just in front of the heel bone (*calcaneus*), and just behind the 4th and 5th *metatarsals.*
- The *cuboid bone* articulates with four different bones (*calcaneus, 3rd cuneiform, 4th metatarsal,* and the *5th metatarsal*).

Navicular Bone

- This boat-shaped bone is located in the midfoot, between the three *cuneiform* bones on the front, and the *talus* posteriorly.
- Anatomists often referred to this bone as the *keystone* for the uppermost portion of the medial longitudinal arch of the foot.
- Excessive pronation of the foot causes the *navicular* bone to move more medially in the foot. The joint of this bone are often restricted in cases of Plantar Fasciitis.

The Hind Foot

The hind foot consists of two bones that together form the ankle and heel. These are the *talus* and the *calcaneus* bones.

The Ankle Joint of the Right Foot

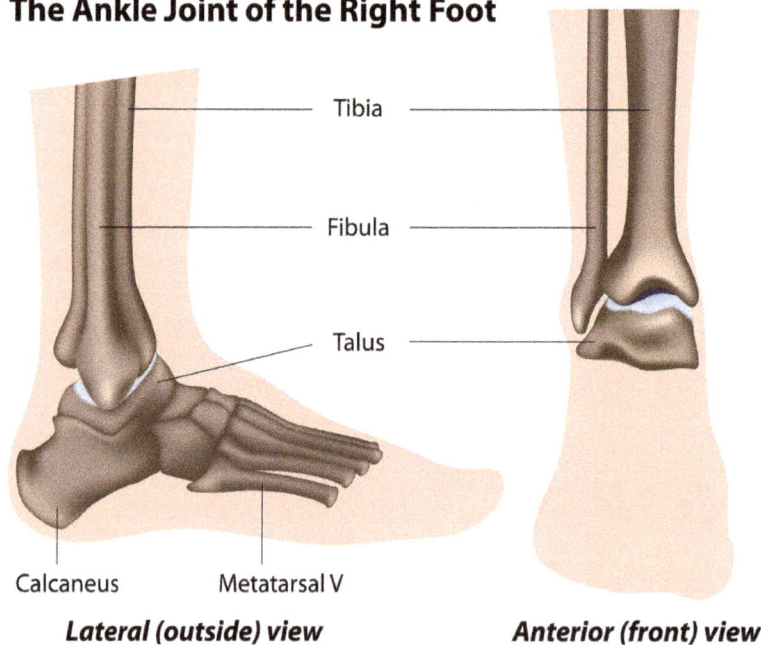

Tibia

Fibula

Talus

Calcaneus   Metatarsal V

Lateral (outside) view   *Anterior (front) view*

Copyright: Alta Medical Media/Shutterstock

Fig 3.3: Ankle Joint of the Right Foot - Lateral and Anterior Views

Talus

- The *talus* is unique in that no tendons or muscles insert into, or originate from, this bone.
- The *talus* sits on top of the heel bone (*calcaneus*), which is the largest bone in your foot.
- The *talus* articulates with the heel bone (*calcaneus*) below, with the *navicular* in front, and with the two long bones of your shin (*tibia* and *fibula*).
- The bones of your lower leg, the *tibia* and *fibula*, rest on the top of the *talus*, to form the ankle.

Calcaneus (Heel Bone)

- The *calcaneus* is the largest bone of the foot and works to support the *talus*.
- The *subtalar joint* is formed between the ankle (*talus*) and the *calcaneus*.
- The *calcaneal-cuboid joint* is formed between the calcaneus and the *cuboid bone*.
- The *plantar fascia* originates from the *calcaneus* and extends towards the toes, where it splits into five segments at the *metatarsal bones*.
- The *calcaneus* has a prominent projection on its medial side that is known as the *sustentaculum tali*, which serves as a key attachment point for a number of ligaments and tendons.
- The joint between the *talus* and *calcaneus* is the *subtalar joint*. Pronation and supination of the foot take place at the *subtalar joint*.

Conditions of the Hind Foot

The bones of the hind foot play important roles in maintaining the stability of the foot, and controlling the gait-cycle. Restrictions in the joints in this area can have a number of adverse effects, leading to conditions such as *Plantar Fasciitis*.

For a full resolution of Plantar Fasciitis, it is critical to address any restrictions in these joints. Our routines have several exercises that are specially designed to address joint issues in the foot. Severe, or long standing cases of Plantar Fasciitis may also need manipulation of these joints by a qualified health care professional.

The Soft-Tissue Structures of the Feet

In the following section, we will explore each layer of the foot, consider how these bones, joints, muscles, and other structures directly, or indirectly, affect motion within the foot, and how changes to the function of these structures can contribute to the development of Plantar Fasciitis.

The Plantar Fascia

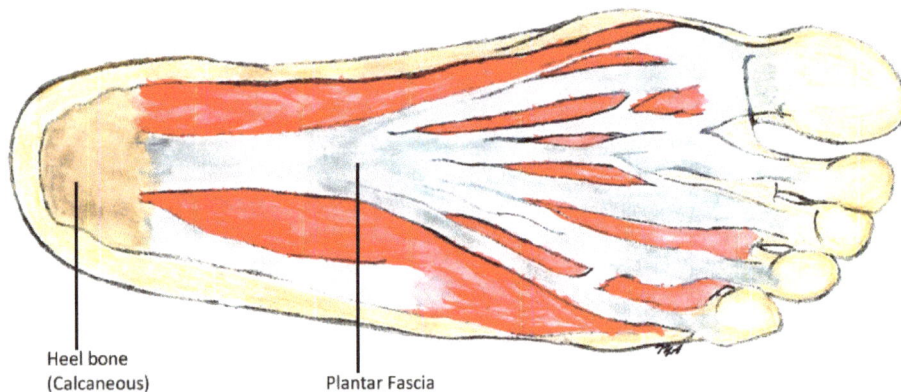

Heel bone
(Calcaneous)

Plantar Fascia

The *plantar fascia* is a tough, strong layer of fibrous material that lies along the bottom of your feet (along the plantar surface). It inserts at the *Achilles tendon* and at the heel bone (*calcaneus*) along the underside of the foot, and fans out to attach at the base of each toe.

- The central area of the fascia (*plantar aponeurosis*) is very thick, while the medial and lateral portions are much thinner.
- The *plantar aponeurosis* plays an important role in transmitting force experienced by the *Achilles tendon* (during the end of the Stance Phase) to the forefoot.[32]

---

32. Ahmet Erdemir, PhD; Andrew J. Hamel, PhD; Andrew R. Fauth, MSc; Stephen J. Piazza, PhD; Neil A. Sharkey, PhD, "Dynamic Loading of the Plantar Aponeurosis in Walking", *The Journal of Bone and Joint Surgery*. 2004 Mar;86-A(3):546-552, http://jbjs.org/article.aspx?articleid=26410

- The *plantar fascia* stabilizes the arch of the foot and prevents the arch from collapsing (by lifting the arch in preparation for the take-off phase). Read *The Plantar Fascia's Windlass Mechanism - page 39* for a detailed description of how this works.
- The *plantar fascia* supports shock absorption by acting as a mobile adaptor, stabilizes the *metatarsal* joints, and aids in propulsion when walking and running by becoming a rigid lever.

In most cases, when I palpate the *plantar fascia* of a patient's foot, I find that there is only minimal, to no tenderness; often it is the deeper structures in the foot that are causing them pain.

The *plantar fascia* experiences sudden lengthening and shortening during the *landing phase* of a running stride. When the *plantar fascia* is strong and supple, it is able to do this easily. But if it has poor elasticity, it may cause over-pronation, which further stresses and tensions the fascia.

Increased stress in the *Achilles tendon*, hamstrings, hips, lower leg, or foot will result in the *plantar fascia* having to do more than its fair share of the work. For example, during impact with the ground, a tight *Achilles tendon* will tend to throw the foot forward – thus causing increased stress on the *plantar fascia*.

TIP: Read more about this inter-relationship in *The Plantar Fascia's Windlass Mechanism on page 39*.

First Superficial Layer: Muscles of the Foot

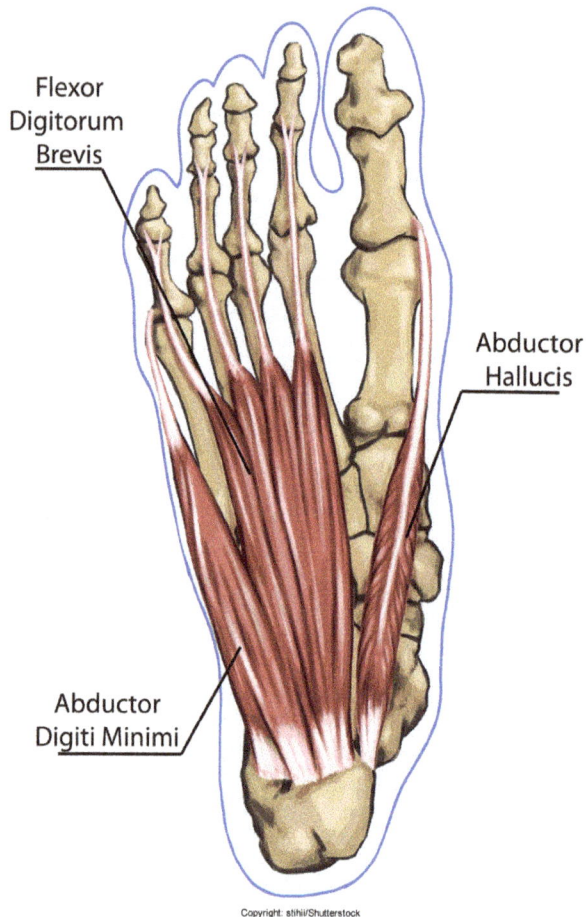

Flexor
Digitorum
Brevis

Abductor
Hallucis

Abductor
Digiti Minimi

Copyright: stihii/Shutterstock

Fig 3.4: Muscles of the Foot: First Superficial Layers

The first superficial layer of the foot contains four structures that are often involved in causing pain which appears to originate from the *plantar fascia*. They are the:

- *The Plantar Fascia - page 56.*
- *Flexor Digitorum Brevis Muscle - page 59.*
- *Abductor Hallucis Muscle - page 59.*
- *Abductor Digiti Minimi Muscle - page 59.*

Flexor Digitorum Brevis Muscle

- The *flexor digitorum brevis* muscle flexes the toe joints of toes two (2) to five (5).
- This muscle originates from both the heel bone (*calcaneus*) and the *plantar fascia*, and inserts into the tendons of the toes.
- Restrictions in the *flexor digitorum brevis* are often responsible for causing a condition known as "*claw foot*".

Abductor Hallucis Muscle

- The *abductor hallucis* muscle moves the big toe (*hallucis*) away from the second toe (*abduction*) and assists in flexing the big toe.
- The *abductor hallucis* originates from both the heel bone (medial process of the tuberosity of the *calcaneus*) and the *plantar fascia*.

Abductor Digiti Minimi Muscle

- The *abductor digiti minimi* moves the little toe away (*abduction*) from the fourth toe and assists in flexing the little toe.
- This muscle also originates from both the heel (*calcaneus*) and the *plantar fascia*.

Since all three of the above muscles insert into the heel bone (*calcaneus*) and into the *plantar fascia*, it is often very difficult to determine if the pain in your foot is caused by injuries to the actual *plantar fascia*, or caused by injuries to one of these other structures. However, strengthening of these structures can reduce the incidence of Plantar Fasciitis and help to stabilize the arch of the foot. See *"Muscles of the Foot: First Superficial Layers"* - *page 58* for an image of these structures.

Secondary Layer: Muscles of the Foot

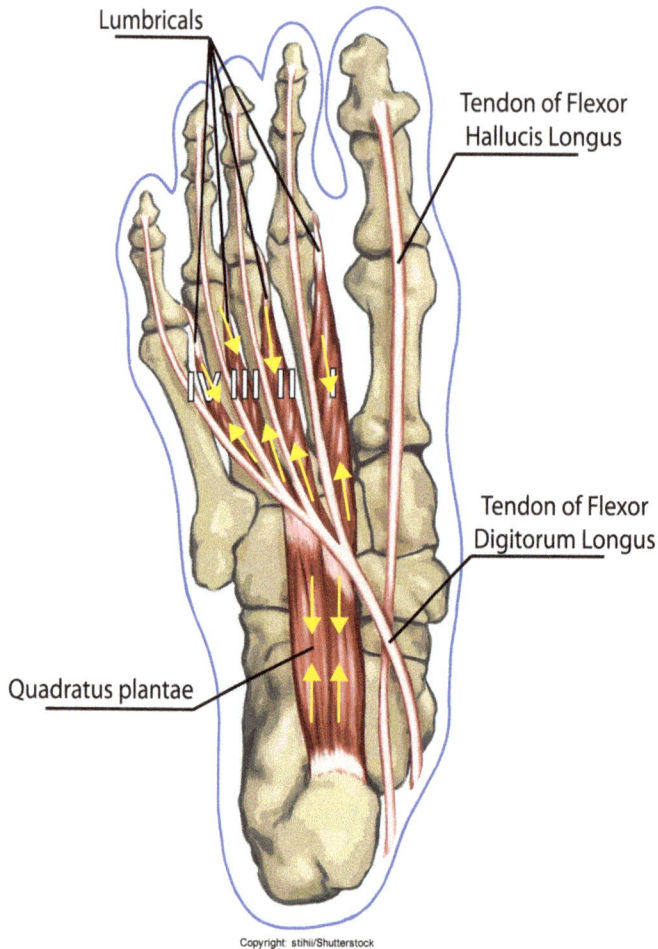

Lumbricals

Tendon of Flexor Hallucis Longus

Tendon of Flexor Digitorum Longus

Quadratus plantae

Copyright: stihii/Shutterstock

Fig 3.5: Muscles of the Foot - Secondary Layer

The yellow arrows show the lines of force during muscle contraction of the *quadratus plantae* and the *lumbricals*.

Many of these deeper muscles in the second layer of the foot provide stability during propulsion. These muscles have to work extremely hard to provide this stability, especially if you tend to pronate excessively.

- *Quadratus Plantae (QP) Muscle - page 61*.
- *Lumbrical Muscles - page 61*.

Quadratus Plantae (QP) Muscle

- The *quadratus plantae* muscle assists with flexion of the four smaller toes.
- This interesting muscle attaches to the tendon of the *flexor digitorum longus (FDL)* muscle which originates under the calf muscles. The *tendons* of the FDL go all the way down to insert under the foot onto the four smaller toes.
- The *quadratus plantae* works with the *flexor digitorum longus* to increase the strength of contraction and creates a direct line-of-pull for the FDL.
- A tight FDL directly affects the function of the *quadratus plantae*.
  The FDL-QP relationship shows how tension in a distant and deep muscle (lying under the calf muscles) can result in the creation of abnormal motion patterns far down in the foot.

Lumbrical Muscles

- The four small *lumbricals* help to extend and flex the toes two through five.
- The *lumbricals* work in coordination with the *interosseous* muscles to provide stability to the forefoot.
- These four small muscles attach directly to the tendons of the *flexor digitorum longus (FDL)* and *extensor digitorum longus* (EDL) through the *dorsal digital expansion.*

Within any joint, a fine balance must be maintained between the tensions exerted by the muscles performing flexion and extension movements. The functionality of the *lumbrical* muscles is directly affected by any tension in either the FDL or EDL.

Thus, in this case, the quality of foot motion is directly affected by the balance of tension between the shin muscles *(extensor digitorum longus)* and the deep muscles of the calf *(flexor digitorum longus).*

Any restrictions in the FDL or the EDL muscles will result in the development of abnormal motion patterns, which then forces the opposing muscle to work even harder in compensation. This abnormal motion pattern will eventually be transferred into the foot, ultimately leading to increased tension and pain on the underside of the foot.

TIP: See *"Muscles of the Foot - Secondary Layer" - page 60* for an image of these structures.

Tertiary Layer: Muscles of the Foot

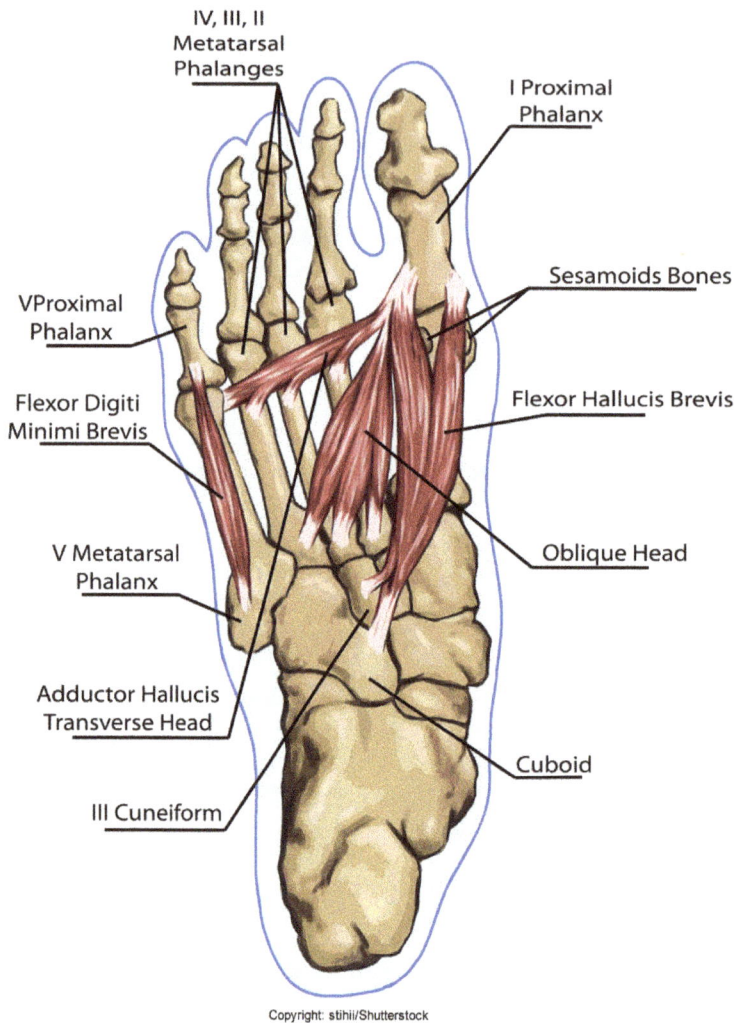

IV, III, II
Metatarsal
Phalanges

I Proximal
Phalanx

Sesamoids Bones

VProximal
Phalanx

Flexor Digiti
Minimi Brevis

Flexor Hallucis Brevis

V Metatarsal
Phalanx

Oblique Head

Adductor Hallucis
Transverse Head

Cuboid

III Cuneiform

Copyright: stihii/Shutterstock

Fig 3.6: Muscles of the Foot - Tertiary Layer

The Tertiary (third layer) of muscles controls the action of the big and little toes, and act synergistically with structures in the foot's kinetic chain to stabilize and propel the body forward. The key structures here include:

- *Flexor Hallucis Brevis Muscle - page 63*.
- *Adductor Hallucis Muscle - page 63*.
- *Flexor Digiti Minimi Brevis Muscle - page 63*.

Flexor Hallucis Brevis Muscle

- The *flexor hallucis brevis* flexes the big toe (MP joint) and helps to prevent "*clawing*" of the big toe.
- This muscle acts synergistically with the *flexor hallucis longus* (FDL).

Synergistic muscles are groups of muscles that contract together to accomplish the same body movement.

When the *flexor hallucis brevis* is not functioning correctly, more force will be directed into the FDL muscle (located deep within the calf muscles on the lateral side of the leg). The increased force exerted on the FDL can result in the development of abnormal motion patterns in the lower extremity, eventually leading to the development of Plantar Fasciitis.

Adductor Hallucis Muscle

- The two-headed *adductor hallucis* muscle moves the big toe inward towards the second toe (*adduction*). The *adductor hallucis* also participates in flexion of the big toe and in maintaining stability.
- The oblique head of this muscle originates from the second, third and fourth *metatarsal bones*, and from the sheath of the *peroneus longus*. It inserts into the base of the big toe with the *flexor hallucis brevis*.
- The transverse head originates from the plantar (*metatarsophalangeal*) ligaments of the third, fourth, and fifth toes, in addition to the transverse ligaments of the *metatarsals*. It also inserts into the lateral base of the big toe (*first phalanx*).

The *adductor hallucis* muscle is often involved in cases of bunions, foot instability, and altered foot-motion patterns. See *"Muscles of the Foot - Tertiary Layer" - page 62* for an image of these structures.

Flexor Digiti Minimi Brevis Muscle

- The *flexor digiti minimi brevis* muscle flexes the little toe (MP joint).
- This muscle arises from both the fifth metatarsal bone and from the fascia which connects to the sheath of the *peroneus longus* (a muscle on the outside of the leg).

See *"Muscles of the Foot - Tertiary Layer" - page 62* for an image of these structures.

Fourth Layer: Muscles of the Foot

This deep layer of muscles is active in stabilizing foot motion. The primary structures in the fourth layer are the *dorsal interossei* and *plantar interossei* muscles.

Dorsal Interossei Muscles

- The four *dorsal interossei* muscles aid in the outward motion (*abduction*) of the second to fourth toes.
- These muscles originate from the sides of adjacent *metatarsal* bones (proximal half). It then inserts into the base of the second, third, and fourth toes (*proximal phalanges*) and the tendon of the *extensor digitorum longus*.
- These muscles also act as stabilizers of the forefoot (as did the *lumbricals* in the second layer of the foot).

Plantar Interossei Muscles

- The *plantar interossei* muscles originate in the *metatarsals* and insert into toes three (3) to five (5).
- Their principle action is to plantar flex the *proximal phalanges*.
- The *plantar interossei* also act to adduct toes three to five.

The Role of the Shins & Calves in Plantar Fasciitis

Having strong, flexible, un-restricted shin and calf muscles is critical for the resolution of any case of Plantar Fasciitis. Your foot and ankle's range-of-motion is affected by the strength and flexibility of the shin and calf muscles, as well as by the ligaments and soft-tissue structures of the ankle.

Any muscle imbalances between the shin and calf muscles, or a difference in the range-of-motion between the two legs, can cause the development of abnormal motion patterns which are often directly related to an increased incidence of Plantar Fasciitis. See the following for more information:

- *The Function of Your Shin Muscles on page 65.*
- *The Function of Your Calf Muscles on page 67.*

Note: Muscles in your body typically work as pairs (agonist and antagonist), and are usually located on the opposite side of a bone or joint. The antagonist works in opposition to the agonist, and is responsible for returning the limbs to their initial position. In this case, the shin (agonist) and calf (antagonist) work as pair.

The Function of Your Shin Muscles

It is very important to maintain the strength and flexibility of your shin muscles since these structures control how your foot hits the ground with each foot-strike (*eccentric contraction*). The muscles of the shins also help your foot to clear the ground during the **Swing Phase** (*concentric contraction*) of your stride, and absorb much of the shock from impact during running.

The most important of these dorsi-flexors (the muscles that control how your foot strikes the ground) are the:

■ *Tibialis Anterior (TA) on page 66.*
■ *Extensor Hallucis Longus (EHL) on page 67.*
■ *Extensor Digitorum Longus (EDL) on page 67.*
■ *Peroneus Tertius on page 67.*

Most people are surprised to discover just how weak their shin muscles have become. Shin muscles are responsible for:

■ Absorbing shock during running and walking.
■ Inverting and stabilizing the ankle (to cushion against sprains).
■ Controlling how the foot strikes the ground (*during **eccentric** contraction*).
■ Helping your foot clear the ground during the Swing Phase of a stride.
■ Locking of the ankle, such as occurs when toe-kicking a ball, during which time the shin muscles are held in an **isometric** contraction.

See *"Shin Muscles - Working together to dorsiflex the foot." - page 66* for an image showing these structures. Restrictions, pain, tightness in these and their related kinetic chain structures can aggravate and increase your tendency to get Plantar Fasciitis.

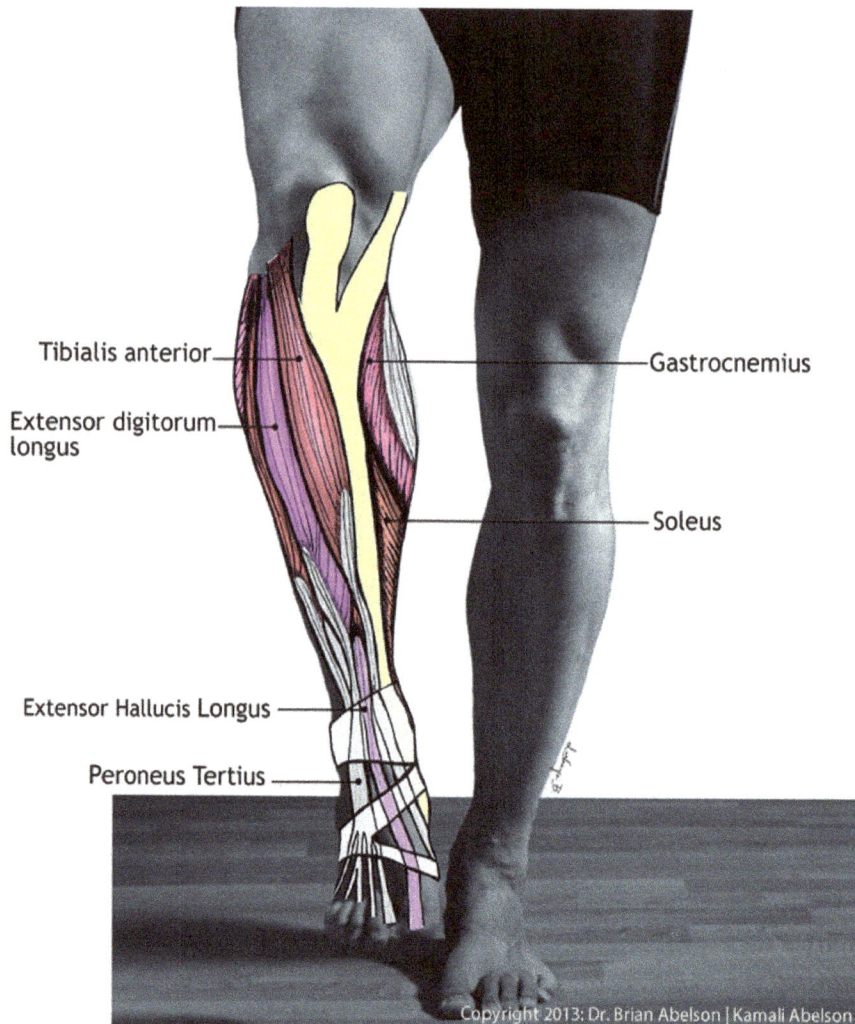

Fig 3.7: Shin Muscles - Working together to dorsiflex the foot.

Tibialis Anterior (TA)

- The *tibialis anterior* originates at the *lateral condyle* and the *superior lateral shelf of the tibia*. It then passes through the *extensor retinaculum* and inserts into the base of the first *metatarsal*.
- The *tibialis anterior* acts to dorsiflex and invert the foot.

Extensor Hallucis Longus (EHL)

- The *extensor hallucis longus* originates in the middle of the *anterior fibula* (*interosseus membrane*). It inserts into the dorsal surface of the big toe at the base of the *distal phalanx*.
- The EHL is involved in the extension of the big toe, dorsiflexion of the foot, eversion of the foot (through the *subtalar joint*), and lifting of the medial edge of the foot.

Extensor Digitorum Longus (EDL)

- The *extensor digitorum longus* originates from the *tibia* (*lateral condyle*) and the *fibula* (along the *anterior fibular shaft* and the *interosseus membrane*).
- It inserts into toes two(2) through (5), also known as the middle phalanges or PIP joints.
- The *extensor digitorum longus* stabilizes the ankle and subtalar joints. It also supports extension of the toes, dorsiflexion of the ankle, and foot eversion.

Peroneus Tertius

- The *peroneus tertius* originates from the distal, anterior portion of the *fibula* and from the *interosseous membrane*. It inserts into the dorsal surface of the fifth metatarsal bone. This muscle is absent in some people.
- The *peroneus tertius* is an extension of the EDL and may be missing in some people.
- It is involved in the eversion and dorsiflexion of the ankle and the foot.

The Function of Your Calf Muscles

Having strong calf muscles is crucial in the support of your lower body's kinetic chain. Your calf muscles (*gastrocnemius* and *soleus*) help you to push off by bringing your heel up (induce plantar flexion) and stabilize your ankle along the transverse plane. As we mentioned previously, there are many direct fascial connections between the *plantar fascia* and the muscles of the calf.

Your calf muscles are your foot's plantar-flexors and act to propel you forward. Any type of restrictions in the calf muscles will directly reduce the efficiency of the shins (their antagonists).

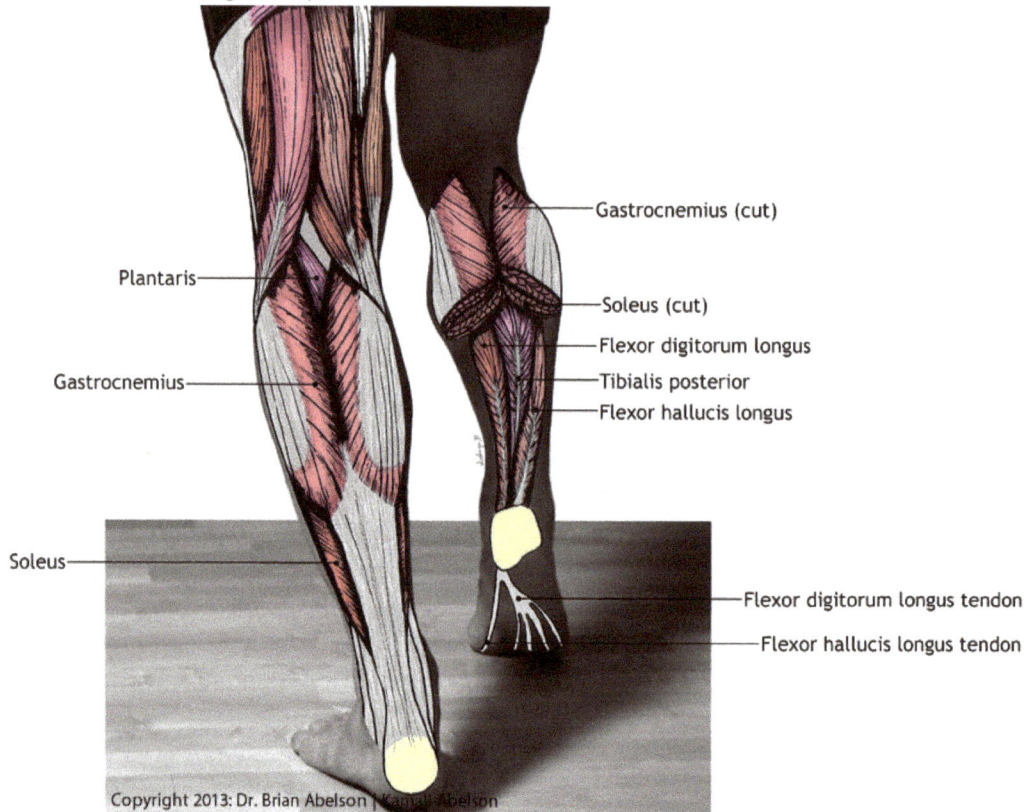

Fig 3.8: Calf Muscles - Many of these muscles participate in the plantar flexion of the foot.

The plantar-flexion muscles of the calves include:

- *Superficial gastrocnemius.*
- *Soleus.*

In addition, there are three other muscles that are involved in plantar flexion of the foot. These are often known (in anatomy classes) as *Tom (tibialis posterior), Dick (flexor digitorum longus),* and *Harry (flexor hallucis longus).*

The *tibialis posterior, flexor digitorum longus,* and *flexor hallucis longus* pass under the superficial calf muscles within the *deep posterior compartment.* As these three muscles run down the lower leg, their tendons combine and interact with each other in a similar pattern. All three tendons run behind (posterior and distally) the *medial ankle bone* (*medial malleolus*). This causes all three of these structures to perform the same function – inversion and plantar flexion of the foot.

Calf muscles act like strong cables on a suspension bridge. During impact with the ground, all the structures of the calf tense up, and counteract the bending forces that strain or deform the tibia. Thus the stronger the calf muscles, the less strain there is on the *tibia*.

Weak, inflexible calf muscles can commonly lead to the development of abnormal motion patterns which eventually result in Plantar Fasciitis.

TIP: Every muscle (*agonist*) in your body has a balancing *antagonist* muscle. These two sets of muscles must work in coordination with each other, and remain balanced in terms of strength, flexibility, and action. In this case, the antagonists to your shins are the calf muscles.

Gastrocnemius or Superficial Calf Muscle

- The *gastrocnemius* originates from the posterior leg (*femur*), above the knee joint (*medial* and *lateral femoral condyles*). It inserts into the heel bone (*calcaneus*) via the *Achilles tendon*.
- The *gastrocnemius* primarily acts as a plantar flexor, but is also involved in knee flexion and foot inversion.

Soleus or Deep Calf Muscle

- The *soleus* lies deep to the *gastrocnemius*. It originates on the *posterior tibia* and *fibula,* and inserts into the heel bone (*calcaneus*) via the *Achilles tendon*. It does not cross the knee joint.
- The *soleus* makes up the bulk of your calf muscle and is much wider than the *gastrocnemius*.
- The *soleus* is primarily involved in plantar flexion of the foot and in foot inversion.

Tibialis Posterior (Tom)

- The *tibialls posterior* originates on the posterior *tibia* and *fibula*, and inserts into several areas of the foot (*navicular, cuneiformus, cuboid*, and 2nd, 3rd, and 4th *metatarsals*).
- Its primary insertion point is the *navicular* (along the *medial tubercle*).
- It is the deepest calf muscle and is primarily involved in plantar flexion of the foot, as well as in foot inversion.
- Posterior shin splints are often caused by a tight or painful *tibialis posterior*.

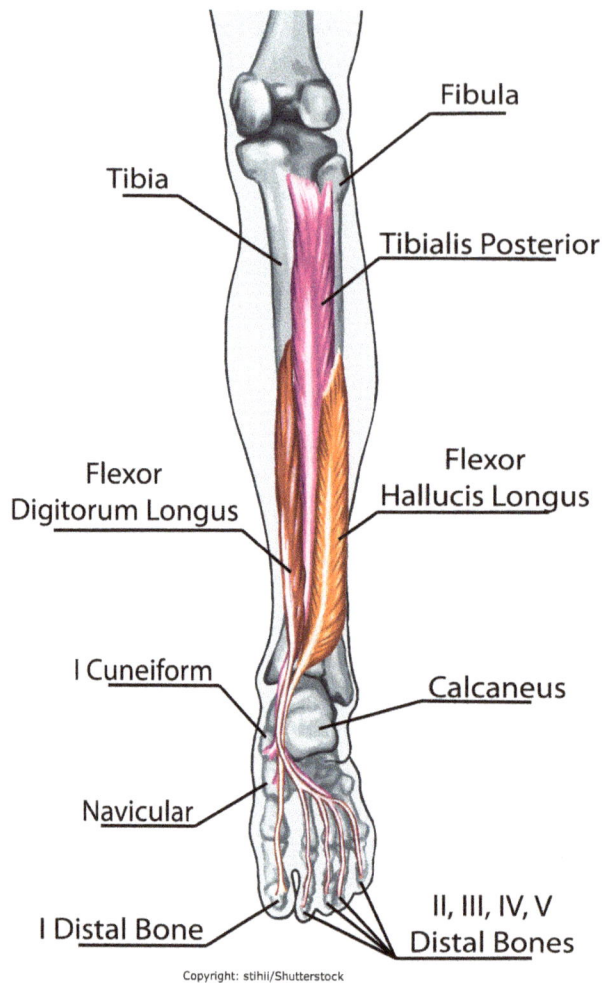

Fibula

Tibia

Tibialis Posterior

Flexor
Digitorum Longus

Flexor
Hallucis Longus

I Cuneiform

Calcaneus

Navicular

I Distal Bone

II, III, IV, V
Distal Bones

Copyright: stihii/Shutterstock

Fig 3.9: Calf Muscles - Tom, Dick, and Harry

Flexor Digitorum Longus (Dick)

- The *flexor digitorum longus* (FDL) originates from the middle, posterior tibia and the fascia that covers the tibia. Its tendons insert into the 2nd to 5th toes along their plantar surface. See *"Muscles of the Foot - Secondary Layer" - page 60* for an image of this structure.
- The FDL is primarily involved in plantar flexion of toes two(2) through five (5), as well in the inversion of the foot.

Flexor Hallucis Longus (Harry)

■ The *flexor hallucis longus* (FHL) originates along the lower part of the fibula (along the distal, posterior aspect). The FHL tendons inserts into the big toe along the plantar surface. See *"Muscles of the Foot - Secondary Layer" - page 60* for an image of this structure.

■ The FHL is involved in the plantar flexion of the big toe, plantar flexion of the foot at the ankle, as well as the inversion and support of the medial arch of the foot.

■ The FHL plays an important role in the propulsive phase of walking or running.

The Role of the Lateral Leg Muscles in PF

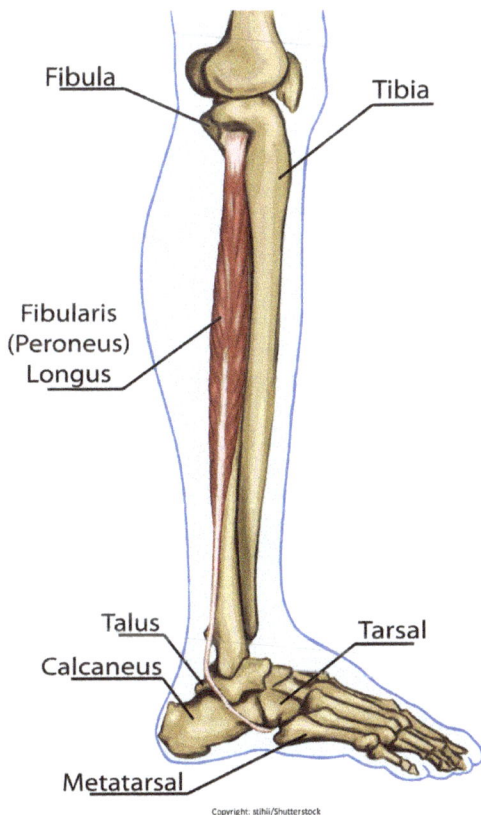

Fibula
Tibia
Fibularis (Peroneus) Longus
Talus
Calcaneus
Tarsal
Metatarsal

Copyright: sūhii/Shutterstock

Fig 3.10: Lateral Leg Muscles

The lateral leg muscles run along the sides of your legs. These include the *peroneus longus, peroneus brevis*, and *peroneus tertius*. (These three muscles are also known respectively as the *fibularis longus, fibularis brevis*, and *fibularis tertius*).

All three of these muscles are involved in the eversion of the foot at the *subtalar joint*. The *peroneus tertius* also participates in the dorsiflexion of the ankle and foot. See *"Peroneus Tertius" - page 67* for more information.

From a kinetic chain perspective, the *peroneus longus* has direct fascial connections to the lateral hamstrings (*biceps femoris*). This means that any tension in the lateral hamstrings will be transferred into the *peroneus longus*, which will then directly affect foot motion, especially foot eversion.

Peroneus Longus or Fibularis Longus

- The *peroneus longus muscle* (also known as *fibularis longus*) originates at the proximal end of the *lateral fibula* (at the fibular head).
- It inserts into the plantar side of the foot at the 1st and 2nd *metatarsals*, and at the *medial cuneiform bone.*
- The *peroneus longus muscle* is located within the *lateral compartment* of the lower leg.
- The *peroneus longus muscle* is involved in foot eversion, ankle plantar flexion, and support of the *transverse arches* of the foot. The tendons of the *peroneus longus* and *tibialis anterior* (*page 66*) form a sling under the middle part of the foot. Together, this *sling* supports the arch of the foot.

Peroneus Brevis or Fibularis Brevis

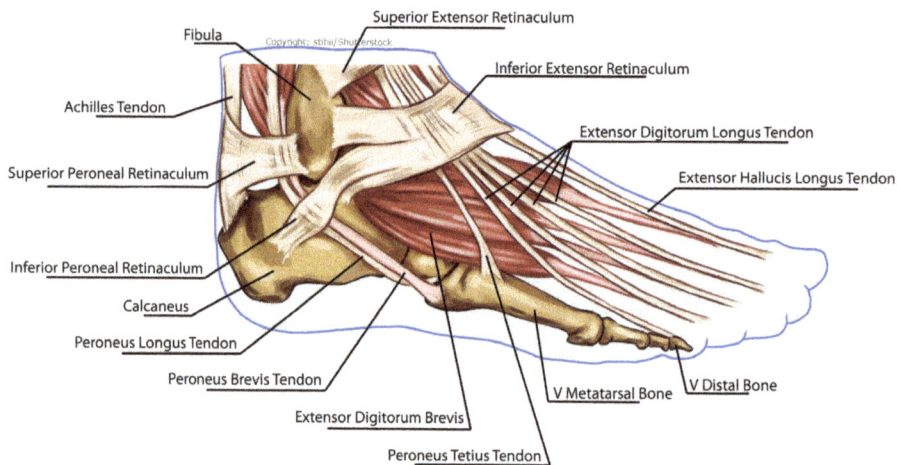

Fig 3.11: Muscles and Tendons of the Foot - Lateral View

- The *peroneus brevis* originates at the distal end of the *lateral fibula.* It lies deep to the *peroneus longus*, and is located within the *lateral compartment* of the lower leg.
- The *peroneus brevis* inserts into the tuberosity on the lateral surface of the foot's *5th metatarsal.*
- The *peroneus brevis* participates in the plantar flexion and eversion of the foot.
- Both the *peroneus longus* and the *peroneus brevis* help to support the lateral arch of the foot, and to support the ankle.

The Role of the Hamstrings and Quadriceps in PF

It often surprises our patients to discover that their hamstrings and quadriceps are often involved in their Plantar Fasciitis. In fact, due to the importance of these structures, we are going to spend some time discussing their inter-relationships, their impact on the kinetic chain, and the consequences of damage to these muscles.

TIP: For those of you who are interested in understanding this key relationship, *keep reading*. However, if you are keen to find out if YOUR hamstrings and quadriceps are involved, we recommend that you jump ahead to *Functional Tests for the Legs and Hips on page 129.*

Both the *hamstrings* and *quadriceps* are composed of multiple muscle groups, each interacting closely with the other to perform their required functions. You can find information about these key structures in the following sections of the book:

Hamstring Structures	Quadricep Structures
■ *Semimembranosus (SM) on page 77.*	■ *Rectus Femoris on page 79.*
■ *Semitendinosus (ST) on page 77.*	■ *Vastus Lateralis on page 79.*
■ *Biceps Femoris (BF) on page 78.*	■ *Vastus Medialis on page 79.*
	■ *Vastus Intermedius on page 79.*

Learn how to evaluate the strength of your hamstrings and quadriceps with the *Functional Tests for the Legs and Hips - page 129.*

Antagonists and Agonists - Hamstrings and Quadriceps

The *hamstrings* are primarily involved in both hip extension and knee flexion. In contrast, the *quadriceps* are primarily involved in hip flexion and knee extension. In other words, they play opposite roles to each other. Depending on the action being performed, when one structure is the *agonist* (primary mover), the other plays the role of the *antagonist* (primary counter-acting force).

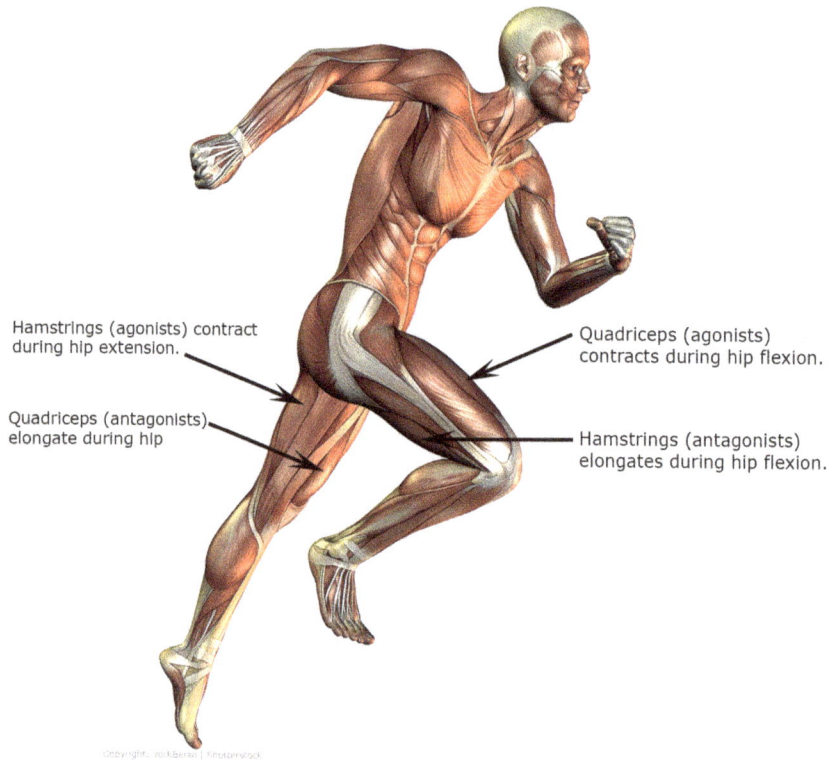

Hamstrings (agonists) contract during hip extension.

Quadriceps (antagonists) elongate during hip

Quadriceps (agonists) contracts during hip flexion.

Hamstrings (antagonists) elongates during hip flexion.

For example:

- Hip Extension: When the *hamstrings (agonists)* contract to cause hip extension, the *quadriceps (antagonists)* elongate to support this action.
- Hip Flexion: When the *quadriceps (agonists)* contract to cause hip flexion, the *hamstrings (antagonists)* elongate to balance this action.

For optimum performance, both the oppositional muscles must be in balance, for both strength and flexibility. When they are out of balance, the body develops abnormal motion patterns that can eventually lead to a host of problems, including Plantar Fasciitis.

Take a look at what happens when the hamstrings become tight:

- *Causes of Tight Hamstrings - page 75.*
- *Consequences of Tight Hamstrings - page 75.*

Causes of Tight Hamstrings

The *Anterior Pelvis Syndrome* is one of the most common causes of tight hamstrings. Ideally, your pelvis should be in a neutral position, not tilted forward or back, and level from side-to-side. *Anterior Pelvis Syndrome* occurs when your *quadriceps* muscles (*rectus femoris*) tighten up. This pulls the front of the pelvis down, tensioning the hamstrings along the back of the leg (thereby increasing the distance between the origin and insertion of the hamstrings) and destabilizing the pelvis. Lack of pelvic stability can also be caused by a lack of core stability.

Hamstring Weakness Causes Imbalances

In the *hamstrings–quadriceps* inter-relationship, we often find that our patient's *hamstrings* are weak and overstretched, while their *quadriceps* are tight, overactive, and considerably stronger than the *hamstrings*. The tight *quadriceps* tend to neurologically inhibit the *hamstrings* (reciprocal inhibition), making them even weaker. This imbalance in strength and flexibility has a number of adverse effects.

Consequences of Tight Hamstrings

Tight hamstrings can result in ripple effects along the entire kinetic chain. Tension in the hamstrings causes tight calf muscles, which in turn limit dorsiflexion of the foot. Decreased dorsiflexion of the foot is directly related to increased stress on the *plantar fascia*. In addition, the increased calf tension (through reciprocal inhibition) also increases tension and weakens the shin muscles. This in turn causes increased foot instability.

Tight hamstrings also prevent effective *terminal knee extension*. Terminal knee extension is the ability of your knee to fully straighten and lock during the **Stance Phase** of the gait-cycle. During the Stance Phase of the gait-cycle, your knee must extend fully into a locked position. The inability to do this causes you to spend more time on your forefoot which then has the effect of tightening up the *plantar fascia*, and results in the development of Plantar Fasciitis.

See *The Role of the Hamstrings and Quadriceps in PF - page 73* and *Anatomy and Function of the Hamstrings - page 76* for a more in-depth discussion about the role of hamstrings in Plantar Fasciitis.

Anatomy and Function of the Hamstrings

The hamstring muscles cross two joints, once at the knee and once at the hip joints. This means they can perform two key actions, *knee flexion and hip extension*. There are three hamstring muscles, the *semimembranosus (SM)*, *semitendinosus (ST)*, and the *biceps femoris (BF)*. The SM and ST form the *medial hamstring*, while the two headed BF forms the *lateral hamstring*.

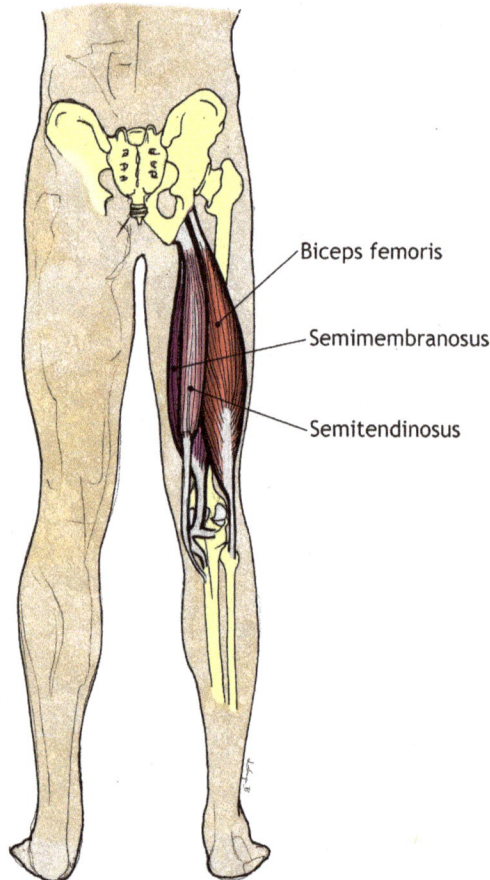

Biceps femoris

Semimembranosus

Semitendinosus

Copyright 2013: Dr. Brian Abelson | Kamali Abelson

Fig 3.12: Hamstrings - Posterior View

The SM, ST, and long head of the BF all originate at the pelvis (*ischial tuberosity*). The short head of the BF originates at the lower posterior *femur* (*linea aspera*). All of these muscles work together to stabilize the pelvis, hip, thigh, and knee joint.

The Hamstring Group

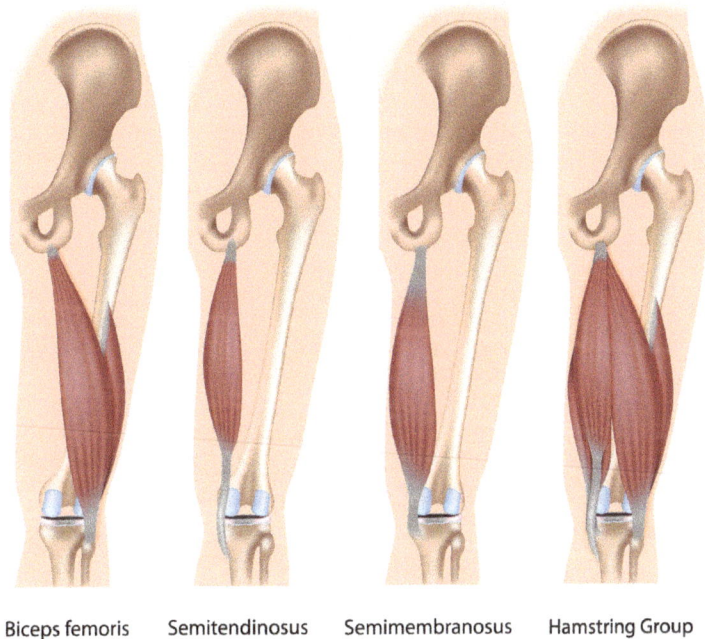

Biceps femoris   Semitendinosus   Semimembranosus   Hamstring Group

Copyright: Alila Medical Media/Shutterstock

Fig 3.13: Hamstring Group - Biceps Femoris, Semitendinosus, and Semimembranosus

Semimembranosus (SM)

- The *semimembranosus* is the largest of the hamstring muscles.
- The *semimembranosus* originates at the *ischial tuberosity* of the pelvis and inserts into the *medial tibia (medial condyle)*. It also inserts into the *medial meniscus,* which helps to prevent entrapment of the *meniscus* between the *tibia* and *femur.*
- The *semimembranosus* extends the thigh at the hip, flexes the leg at the knee, and medially rotates the leg when the knee is flexed.

Semitendinosus (ST)

- The *semitendinosus* originates at the *ischial tuberosity of* the pelvis and inserts into the *anterior medial tibia (pes anserinus)*. This is a very sensitive area as the gracilis and *sartoris muscles* also attach into this structure.

- This is the most superficial of the medial hamstring muscles.
- The *semitendinosus* acts to extend the thigh at the hip, flexes the knee at the knee, and medially rotates the leg when the knee is flexed.

Biceps Femoris (BF)

- The *biceps femoris* has two heads. The long head arises from the inner impression of the *ischial tuberosity* of the pelvis, and inserts into the top of the lateral head of the *fibula*. The short head arises from the lower part of the *femur*, and inserts into the head of the *fibula*.
- The *biceps femoris* has direct fascial connections to the *peroneus longus*.
- It acts to flex the leg at the knee, and to laterally rotate the leg while the knee is flexed.

The Quadriceps

The *quadriceps* are made up of four muscles that cover the anterior (front) thigh. They are the *rectus femoris, vastus lateralis, vastus medialis,* and *vastus intermedius.* All of these muscles have a common insertion point on the *tibial tuberosity* via the knee cap (*patellar ligament*).

The *quadriceps* are often tight, restricted, and overactive. This is because most people tend to over-use their *quadriceps* and *adductors* to perform lower extremity motions, when they should actually be using their *gluteals* and *hamstrings*. This results in the development of muscle imbalances (strong *quadriceps* and weak *hamstrings*).

These muscle imbalances have two effects. Firstly, as the *quadriceps* become stronger, they neurologically inhibit *hamstring* activation. Secondly, this inhibition of *hamstring* activation leads to the development of **abnormal motion patterns** throughout the lower extremity. These abnormal motion patterns have a direct impact on both the initial development, and eventual resolution of Plantar Fasciitis.

TIP: When an agonist (the muscle causing the movement) contracts, there is a neurological inhibition of its antagonist (opposite) muscle. This reduction in the neurological activity of the antagonist muscle is known as *reciprocal inhibition*. Reciprocal inhibition describes how muscles on one side of a joint relax to allow the agonist to contract. When the agonist becomes considerably stronger, more contracted, and more active than the antagonist, then this neurological inhibition can make the antagonist muscle much weaker.

Rectus Femoris

- The *rectus femoris* originates from two tendons, in the front from the *anterior inferior iliac spine*, and from the back at the rim of the *acetabulum*. It inserts into the base of the *patella* (knee cap).
- When the knee is extended, since it's muscle fibers are already shortened, it acts as both a weak hip flexor and a weak knee extensor.
- Its primary action is to extend the leg at the knee, and to act as a weak hip flexor.
- The *rectus femoris* is the direct antagonist to the hamstrings.

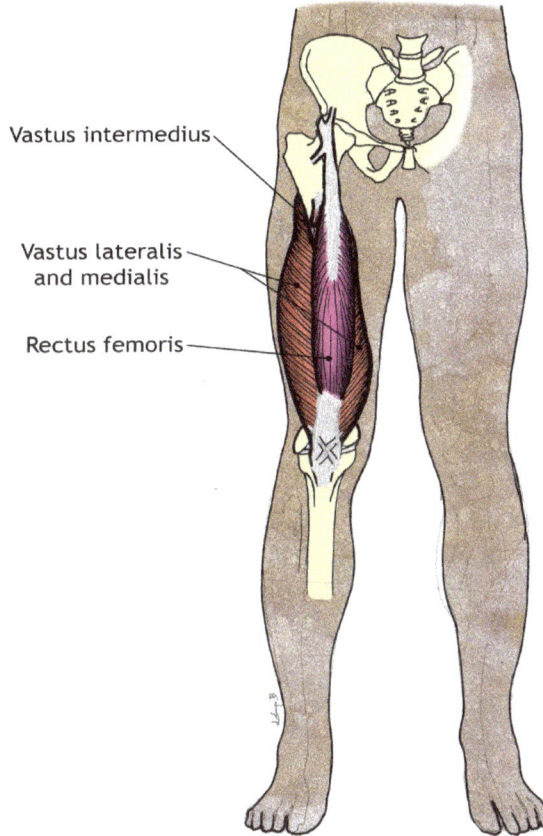

Vastus Lateralis

- The *vastus lateralis* originates on a ridge on the posterior surface of the *femur (linea aspera)*. It inserts into the base of the knee (*patella*) and onto the *tibial tuberosity* via the *patellar ligament*.
- The *vastus lateralis* works to extend the knee.

Vastus intermedius

Vastus lateralis and medialis

Rectus femoris

Copyright 2013: Dr. Brian Abelson | Kamali Abelson

Fig 3.14: Quadriceps - Anterior View

Vastus Medialis

- This muscle originates on the posterior surface of the femur (*linea aspera*).
- The lower section of the *vastus medialis* is referred to as the VMO (*vastus medialis oblique*) due to its muscle fiber orientation.

Vastus Intermedius

- The *vastus intermedius* originates on the anterior femur (*anterior linea aspera*).

The Role of the Adductor Group in PF

The *adductor group* is made up of five muscles: the *adductor magnus, adductor brevis, adductor longus, gracilis,* and *pectineus.*

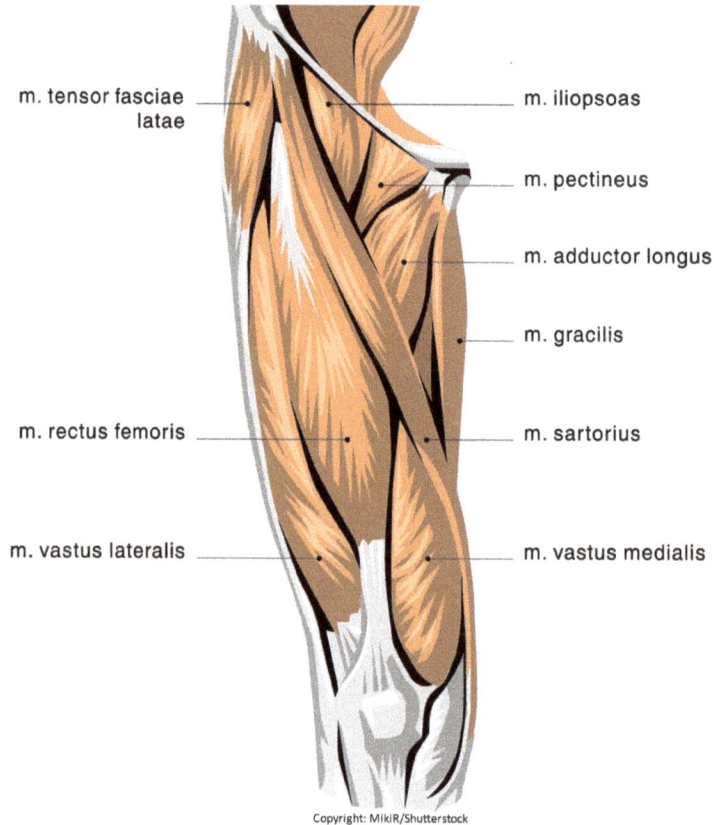

m. tensor fasciae latae — m. iliopsoas

m. pectineus

m. adductor longus

m. gracilis

m. rectus femoris — m. sartorius

m. vastus lateralis — m. vastus medialis

Copyright: MikiR/Shutterstock

Fig 3.15: Adductor Group

These are the muscles that make up the *groin (medial compartment* of your thigh). The primary function of these muscles is the adduction of the leg (moving the leg towards the midline of the body). Depending on the degree of hip flexion, this adductor group can also participate in hip flexion and internal rotation of the hip.

When practitioners think of an adductor strain, they are usually thinking about a groin strain or a knee problem (*Patellofemoral Syndrome*). On the other hand, restrictions or weakness in the *adductors* can cause several other problems. The hip's adductor muscles are the antagonists to the *gluteus medius* muscle. The function of the gluteus medius is to pull your thigh out to the side (abduction) as well as rotation of the leg.

When the *adductors* become short and contracted, they will neurologically inhibit the *gluteus medius* muscle. This will cause your thigh to move inwards and rotate into an abnormal motion pattern. This abnormal motion pattern will affect both knee and ankle motion patterns, and could lead to problems on the bottom of the foot, such as Plantar Fasciitis. A common muscle pattern that we see at our clinic is short restricted *adductors* (which need myofascial work and stretching) and a weak *gluteus medius* (which needs strengthening).

Adductor Magnus

- The *adductor magnus* originates on your lower pelvis (*ischial* and *pelvic rami*, and the *ischial tuberosity*).
- It inserts in to the femur (*linea aspera, medial supracondylar line*, and *adductor tubercle*).

Adductor Brevis

- The *adductor brevis* originates on your lower pelvis (body and *inferior ramus of pubis*).
- It inserts in to the *femur* (*linea aspera*).

Adductor Longus

- The *adductor longus* originates on your lower pelvis (*pubis*).
- It inserts in to the femur (*linea aspera, posterior aspect of femur*).

Gracilis

- The *gracilis* originates on your lower pelvis (*inferior ramus or pubis*).
- It inserts into the *tibia* (*pes anserinus*).

Pectineus

- The *pectineus* originates on your lower pelvis (*pectineal line of pubis*).
- It inserts into the *femur* (*pectineal line of femur*).

The Role of the Hip Flexors in PF

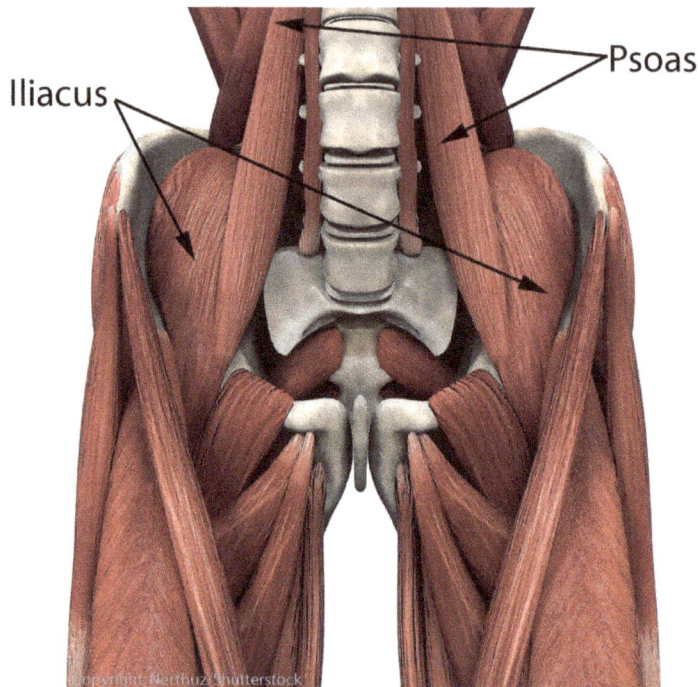

Fig 3.16: Hip Flexors

Hip flexors are among the strongest muscle groups in your body, and when they do not work properly, they can cause numerous problems throughout the kinetic chain. The hip flexors are located on the front (anterior) of the hip joint. They work to flex your thigh bone (*femur*), connect your legs to your pelvis, and act to pull the knee upwards.

Individuals who lead a sedentary life style, sit for long periods of time, spend a lot of time driving, or are involved in sports such as triathlon, cycling, or kicking activities (soccer, football, rugby) often develop tight hip flexors.

There are many major and minor structures that make up the hip flexors. Some of the key structures include:

- Inner hip muscles (*psoas major, psoas minor,* and *iliacus* muscles).
- Front of the thigh (*rectus femoris* and *sartorius*).
- Middle of the thigh (*pectineus, adductor longus, adductor brevis,* and *gracilis*).

Hip flexors also play an important role as *antagonists* to the external hip extensors (the *gluteal* muscles). As discussed earlier in this book, good gluteal function is essential for proper lower extremity stabilization, and for the prevention of Plantar Fasciitis.

Problems Caused by Tight Hip Flexors

People are often surprised to learn that pain, restrictions, injuries, or changes to movement patterns in the *hips* and *legs* are directly related to their Plantar Fasciitis. Extremely tight or contracted hip flexors can:

- *Neurologically inhibit* the function of the gluteal muscles (their antagonists).
- Cause the gluteals to lengthen and become weaker.
- Cause postural issues such as excessive arching of the lower back, which in turn creates numerous compensations and abnormal motion patterns.
- Cause instability in your feet, ankles, and knees.

So when you want to visualize the *direct* connection between your hip flexors and the bottom of your feet, just follow this path; a tight hip flexor can **turn off** (through reciprocal inhibition) your gluteal muscles, which then causes **instability** in your ankle and foot, and eventually lead to the **formation** of your Plantar Fasciitis. Learn how to evaluate the strength of your hip flexors in *Functional Tests for the Legs and Hips on page 129*.

Primary Hip Flexors - Iliopsoas

The *iliacus* and *psoas* muscles make up your primary hip flexors. Although these two muscles originate at different locations, they eventually fuse together and share a common insertion point at the *lesser trochanter* of the *femur*. Sitting for long periods of time can cause your *iliopsoas* to become tight and restricted. This important issue must be addressed (for several reasons) if you want to fully resolve your Plantar Fasciitis, for it has far reaching implications on your kinetic chain.

- Firstly, your *iliopsoas* is the main antagonist for your *gluteals* – major participants in maintaining the stability of the lower extremity. A tight *iliopsoas* inhibits and decreases normal gluteal function, which results in increased instability, and hence, decreases foot stability - leading to increased occurrence of Plantar Fasciitis.
- Secondly, a tight *iliopsoas* can cause your pelvis to tilt forward (anteriorly), which then causes your hamstrings to tighten, which in turn puts stress on your calf muscles – which have a direct fascial connection to your plantar fascia. Again causing increased stress and trauma to the structures of your foot.

Psoas Muscle

- The *psoas* muscle originates on the anterior, lateral side of the lumbar spine. Once it joins the *iliacus*, it inserts into the *lesser trochanter* of the femur.
- It acts to flex and externally rotate the hip joint, as well as to lift the upper leg towards the body (when the body is fixed), or pull the body towards the leg (when the leg is fixed in location).
- Rotation of the spine will cause the psoas to stretch.

Iliacus Muscle

- The *iliacus* is a flat triangular muscle that originates on the inside of the pelvis (*internal ilium*).Once it joins the *psoas*, it inserts into the *lesser trochanter* of the *femur*.
- It acts to bend the trunk forward, lift the trunk from a lying down position (sit-ups), lift the upper leg towards the body (when the body is fixed), or pull the body towards the leg (when the leg is fixed in location).

The Role of the Gluteals in PF

The *gluteals* are made up of three muscles: the *gluteus maximus, gluteus medius,* and *gluteus minimus.* These muscles are the antagonists to the *iliopsoas* muscle group, and need to stay strong and flexible in order to provide stability to the lower extremities. Maintaining this strength and flexibility is a critical factor in resolving any case of Plantar Fasciitis.

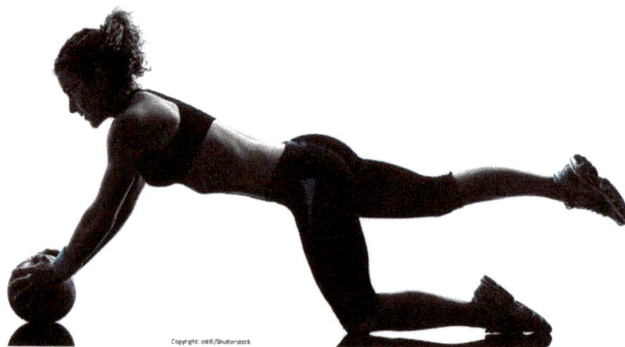

Copyright: m88./Shutterstock

The *gluteals* play an extremely important role in resolving any injury or condition of the lower extremity. This group of muscles:

- Stabilizes the hip (by offsetting what is known as *gravity's hip adduction torque*).
- Preserves proper leg position (by eccentrically controlling internal rotation and adduction of the leg).
- Play an important role in pelvic and spinal stabilization.

From an evolutionary perspective, the *gluteal* muscles evolved to stabilize the trunk of the body when in a standing position. This is the main reason that our *gluteals* are so large (in humans) as compared to other animals – so that we can have stability in the trunk of our body when we stand on two legs instead of four.

Problems Caused by Weak Gluteal Muscles

In today's increasing sedentary world, biomechanical specialists talk about '*gluteal amnesia*'! Gluteal amnesia is what occurs when we spend *too much time sitting*. Excessive sitting causes our hip flexors to become short and contracted. Since these hip flexors (*page 83*) are the natural antagonists to the gluteals, when they tighten, they neurologically inhibit gluteal function. Inhibition of gluteal function decreases lower body stability and is the cause of numerous lower extremity injuries – including Plantar Fasciitis.

In addition, weak gluteal muscles have a cascading series of effects from the hips to the feet. Weak gluteal muscles will cause internal rotation of the leg (*femur*), which then causes the knee to move inward (*knee valgus*), and the foot to pronate excessively. This pronation then places stress upon the *plantar fascia* and other deep structures of the foot.

Gluteus Maximus

- The *gluteus maximus* originates from multiple locations on your pelvis (*ilium, sacrum, coccyx, and sacrotubular ligaments*). It inserts into the *illiotibial tract* of the *fascia lata* and into the *gluteal tuberosity* of the *femur*.
- The *gluteus maximus* is the largest and strongest of the three gluteal muscles, with a quadrilateral shape.
- The *gluteus maximus* Is involved in extension, external rotation, abduction and adduction of the hip. It also acts as a stabilizer for the knee.
- The lower part of the *gluteus maximus* is an adductor and external rotator of the leg.
- The upper part of this muscle act as an abductor and internal rotator for the hip joint.

Gluteus Medius and Gluteus Minimus

- The *gluteus medius and gluteus minimus* originate from the outer surface of the *ilium* of the pelvis.
- Both of these muscles insert into the lateral surface of the *greater trochanter* of the femur.
- Both of these muscles are involved in abduction, internal rotation, external rotation, and extension of the hip.

The Role of the Core in PF

I could easily write an entire book about the importance of *core stability*. Obviously, covering all of the anatomy and biomechanics of the core is far beyond the scope of a book about Plantar Fasciitis. But it is important that you understand that good core stability is a fundamental requirement for the full resolution of Plantar Fasciitis.

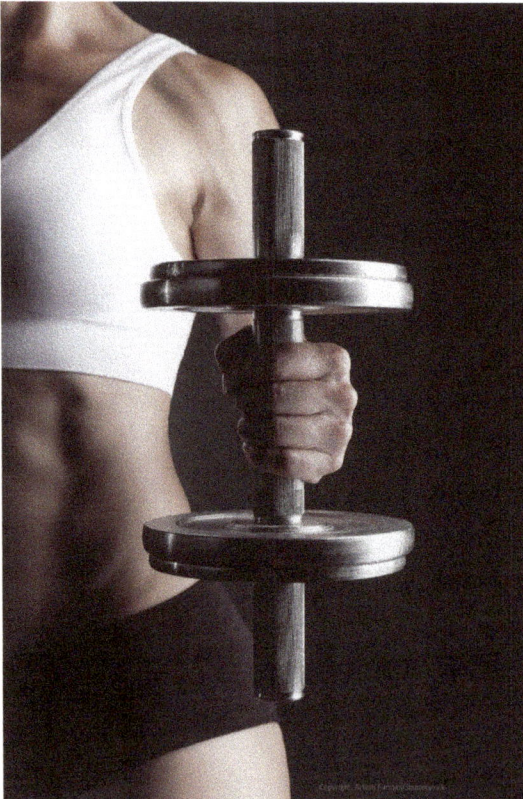

Let me **briefly** explain why a strong, flexible, unrestricted core is such an essential factor in resolving Plantar Fasciitis.

What is Your Core

To start with, your core in NOT just your abdominal region. Your core is made up of all of your central body (excluding the extremities). Your core consists of your hips, pelvis, abdominals, lumbar, thoracic, and shoulder regions. This area is where all movement begins, and is the center of gravity for your body. The core provides a stable base from which your arms and legs can generate efficient movement and power.

A strong stable core is critical for maintaining your center of gravity, for controlling the movements of your lower extremities, and for providing good mobility and stability. Poor core stability can affect the biomechanics of your stride from your hips down to your feet.

The Core as the Foundation of Movement

Your core is the foundation and source of all your movements, and provides a stable base for all lower body actions. When you have a strong, stable, balanced, elastic core, you can easily transfer energy from the center of your body to all your extremities, and dissipate force from your extremities to other parts of the body.

Before you take a single step, the structures of your core are activated to stabilize your actions. It does not matter how strong your legs, ankles, and feet are – if your core is weak, you will lack the stabilization needed to develop efficient movement patterns in the extremities.

In the case of Plantar Fasciitis, a lack of core stability can easily lead to the development of abnormal motion patterns in the hips, knees, ankles, and feet. For example, if the muscles of the hip (*gluteus medius*) are weak and unable to control the internal rotation of the leg (*femur, tibia,* and *fibula*), then excessive pronation of the foot can occur. This excessive pronation would cause tensioning of the *plantar fascia*, eventually causing Plantar Fasciitis [33].

Bottom line, a strong stable core equals efficient movement patterns in your lower extremities, which leads to a faster, more effective resolution of your condition.

Common Nerve Compression Sites for PF

Nerve Compression Syndrome (compression neuropathy) is not a factor that is commonly considered when treating Plantar Fasciitis. But nerve compression can play a significant role in inhibiting the resolution of Plantar Fasciitis. For example, some of the most common symptoms of nerve compression include *Paresthesia* (altered sensation) and *Hyperalgesia* (increased sensitivity to stimuli).

TIP: Parasthesia is a change in feeling (*tingling, pins and needles, prickling, burning, ticklIng, or pricking sensations*) in a specific area of the body. It is typically caused by compression of a single nerve that passes through that portion of the body. In cases of Plantar Fasciitis, patients may experience parasthesia in various parts of their lower body, commonly caused by compression of the *tibial nerve.*

---

33.   Shirley Saurman. *Diagnosis and Treatmetn of Movement Impairment Syndromes.* Philadelphia:Mosby; Sept. 2002

Nerve compression, especially of the *tibial nerve,* can imitate many of the symptoms presented by Plantar Fasciitis.

The *tibial nerve* (which is a branch of the *sciatic nerve*) travels down the back of the calf muscles (through the *popliteal fossa)*, branches into the *gastrocnemius, popliteus, soleus, plantaris, tibialis posterior, flexor digitorum longus,* and *flexor hallucis longus* muscles, to the inside of the ankle (*tarsal tunnel*), and then bifurcates into two nerves – the *medial plantar nerve* and *lateral plantar nerve.*

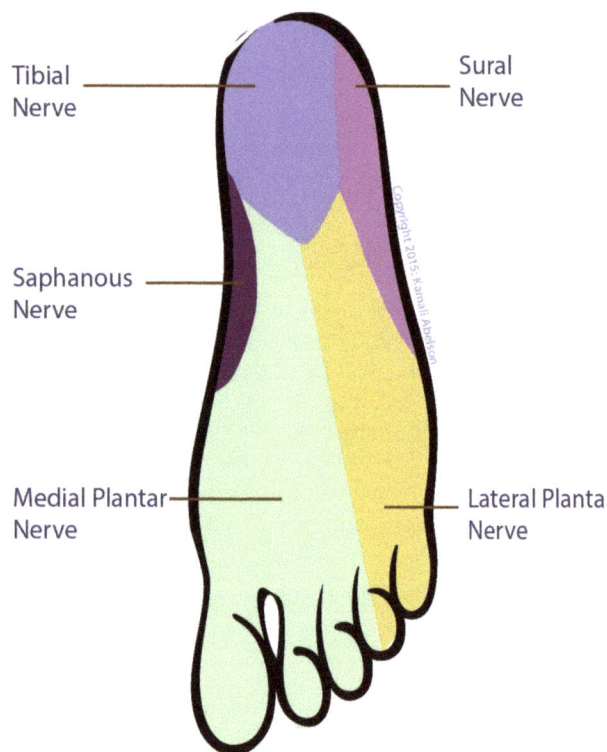

Fig 3.17: Nerve innervation zones of the foot

Adhesions and restrictions in any of these structures can compress this nerve and cause pain, altered sensation, and/or abnormal motion patterns to develop. All of which can lead to cases that mimic Plantar Fasciitis.

It is important to realize that when the *tibial nerve* is injured or compressed anywhere along its pathway, it can mimic many of the characteristic symptoms of Plantar Fasciitis.

Fortunately, we can apply specific tests that can tell us when the *tibial nerve* is involved. In addition, by comparing the common pain patterns of Plantar Fasciitis with the pain that arises from nerve compression, we can further clarify the cause of this occurrence of Plantar Fasciitis.

Inflammation and restrictions in any of the these structures can compress this nerve and cause parasthesia to manifest at the skin's surface. If you are wondering if you have nerve compression, then take a few minutes to check your symptoms against the following chart.

Comparing Pain Caused by Tibial Nerve Compression vs. Common PF

Common Plantar Fasciitis Pain	Pain Caused by Tibial Nerve Compression
■ Pain is worse upon rising in the morning. ■ Medial heel pain (slow onset at the *medial tubercle* of the *calcaneus*). ■ Arch pain which is most noticeable when pushing off with your foot.	■ Pain is felt in the medial ankle *(tarsal tunnel)*. ■ Pain is felt with palpation of the *tibial nerve's* area of distribution (see Nerve innervation zones of the foot ------ page 88). ■ Pain, upon palpation, may radiate into the ankle, up the calf, or down the foot. ■ Palpation may elicit altered sensation (*tingling, burning,* or *sharp shooting pain* emanating out from the point of palpation).

In addition, you can learn how to test for nerve entrapment with *Functional Test for Tibial Nerve Impingement on page 146*.

In Conclusion

When running or walking, each portion of your body's shock absorption and support system (from the bottom of your feet, up into the legs, hips, and core) are all responsible for controlling, absorbing, and dissipating a portion of the force. Insufficient strength, flexibility, or neurological control in any of these structures can cause problems.

Each of these anatomical structures have their own unique kinetic chain, which can be adversely affected by damage to any link in that chain. Once you understand the concepts behind the kinetic chain inter-relationships, it quickly becomes obvious why the exercise recommendations for your condition must focus beyond the simple strengthening or stretching of isolated muscle groups.

Note: It is beyond the scope of this book to discuss each of the foot's kinetic chain relationships. Take a look at Dr. Abelson`s blogs and his other books for more information about the various structures and their kinetic chain involvements.

Understanding Our Process - The 80/20 Effect

Chapter

4

In this chapter

Understanding Our Process

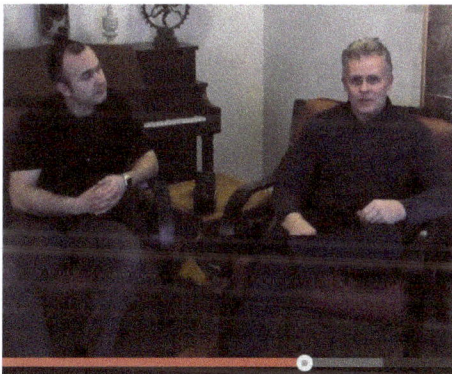

YouTube Address: http://youtu.be/jkLR_BpCGEM

Before starting this *rehabilitative process*, I believe it is very important to set realistic expectations about exactly what is possible, and not possible, to achieve through our program. I use the word '**process**' because that is exactly what you will be experiencing. Our rehabilitative program is a *process* that takes you from a state of simply *living* with your current condition, to as close to a *full resolution* of your condition as is possible.

For about 80% of cases, following our program is a very straightforward progression that generates excellent results. For the remaining 20%, it may be necessary to do a little tweaking, and implement a variety of other strategies to achieve full resolution.

Fortunately, we have a strategy that you can use to exponentially increase your success rate. However, before getting into the details of this strategy, let us first discuss what I call *The 80/20 Effect'*© and the use of the '*Scientific Method*'.

What is the Scientific Method (Trial and Error)?

Some time ago, I watched a great TED lecture presented by *Tim Harford* (an Economics writer). It was called "*Trial, Error, and the God Complex*"[34]. During this lecture, Tim Harford demonstrated how, with complex systems, the most successful solutions for problems were inevitably derived through the process of trial and error. Well, when it comes to complex systems, we can count the human body as being among the most intricate and complex!

Here is how Kinetic Health uses the *Scientific Method* (commonly known as the *Trial and Error Method*) concept to improve our treatment success rate. First, we have to come up with a list of the most common reasons why 20% of patients **don't** respond effectively to the treatment process. Then we need to consider which of these common reasons applies to each individual. And finally, we need to implement a new, perhaps more complex strategy, to see if we can improve our results.

Trial and Error is a fundamental scientific method of problem-solving, process-tuning, and obtaining knowledge. This experimental approach uses a variety of means or methods, and eliminates those that do not work.

Thus, at our clinic, by using this methodology, our process for healing your injury would be to:

- Conduct a comprehensive physical examination of our patient.
- Develop a working diagnosis and treatment protocol.
- Implement the treatment protocol.
- Prescribe an appropriate and carefully selected exercise routine.
- Follow-up with the patient to see if the patient has complied with, and followed all recommendations by the practitioner.
- Evaluate the success or failure of the treatment.

---

34.   http://www.ted.com/talks/tim_harford

Applying the Scientific Method to Resolving Conditions

Copyright 2014: Dr. Brian Abelson and Kamali Abelson

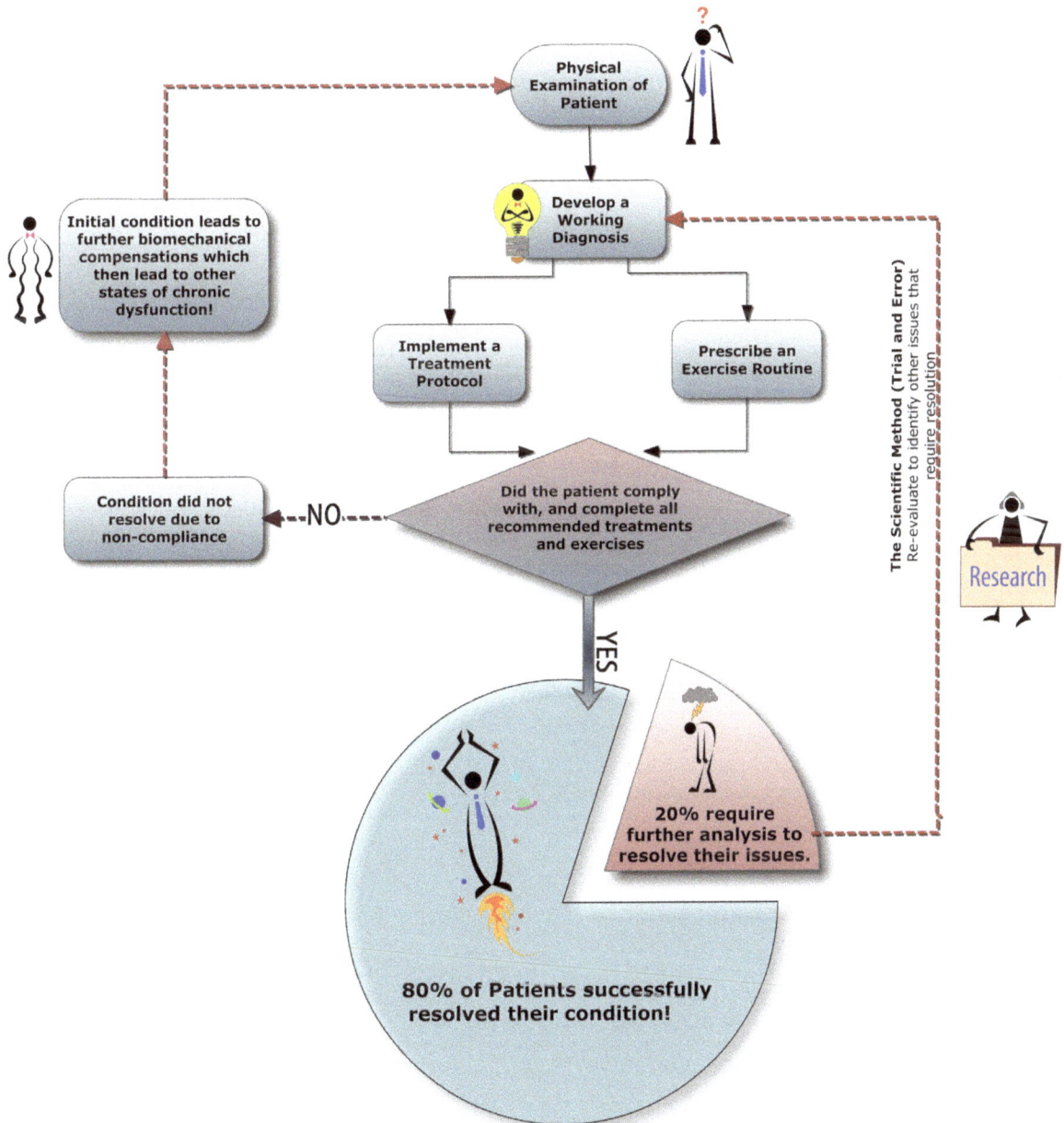

Physical Examination of Patient

Develop a Working Diagnosis

Implement a Treatment Protocol

Prescribe an Exercise Routine

Did the patient comply with, and complete all recommended treatments and exercises

Initial condition leads to further biomechanical compensations which then lead to other states of chronic dysfunction!

Condition did not resolve due to non-compliance

NO

YES

The Scientific Method (Trial and Error) Re-evaluate to identify other issues that require resolution

Research

20% require further analysis to resolve their issues.

80% of Patients successfully resolved their condition!

If the treatment did not achieve the results we wanted, we would re-evaluate the condition and:

- Determine if it was the lack of patient compliance that caused the problem.
- Determine if some other problem is preventing the resolution of the condition. If this is the case, we would repeat the process until we were able to resolve the condition.

TIP: This scientific process of *'Trial and Error'* works remarkably well. It can be used with both the self-care recommendations in this book and by your health-care practitioner. Yes, it requires patience, but the results are well worth it.

The 80/20 Effect

The *80/20 Effect©* is based on following a very logical process that uses analysis, the formation of a *working diagnosis*, and the implementation of *appropriate therapy and exercise* to resolve the condition. Basically, it postulates that if we come up with a sound working diagnosis (based on examination), and if appropriate therapy and exercises are implemented correctly, then we should achieve an 80% success rate in treating this musculoskeletal condition.

In the world of medicine, 80% is considered to be a **very high** success rate. Nonetheless, in my opinion, this is not good enough. When I hear these statistics, the first thing I think is, "*What about the other 20%, why do they have to keep suffering?*" Fortunately, there is a well-known process that can be used to increase our success rate, and it is the *Scientific Method (Trial and Error)* that we just discussed.

Seven Factors Affecting Resolution of Musculoskeletal Conditions

80/20 Effect
Understanding the Factors that Impact Your Treatment Success

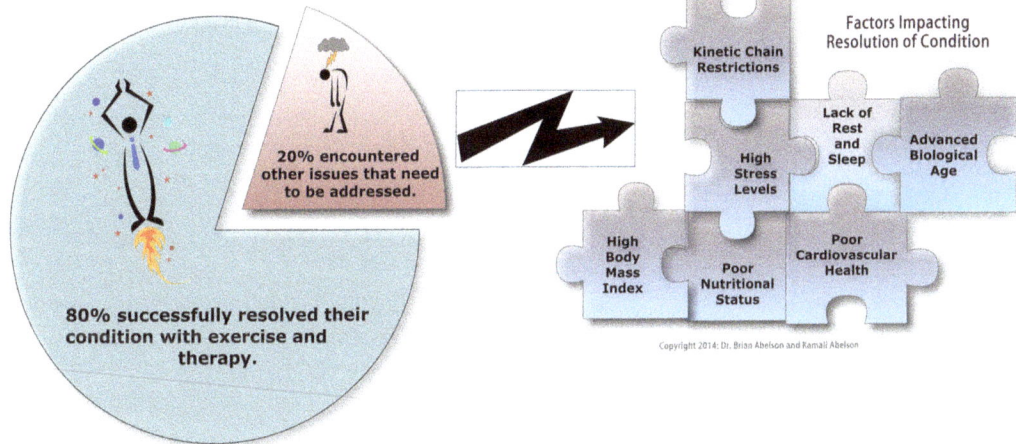

20% encountered other issues that need to be addressed.

80% successfully resolved their condition with exercise and therapy.

Factors Impacting Resolution of Condition

- Kinetic Chain Restrictions
- Lack of Rest and Sleep
- Advanced Biological Age
- High Stress Levels
- Poor Cardiovascular Health
- High Body Mass Index
- Poor Nutritional Status

Copyright 2014: Dr. Brian Abelson and Kamali Abelson

In the case of musculoskeletal conditions, there are seven (7) common factors that can stop you from achieving optimum results. In fact, the presence of even one of the following factors can stop you from achieving a full resolution of your injury:

- *1. Impact of Kinetic Chain Restrictions on page 96.*
- *2. Importance of Cardiovascular Health on page 97.*
- *3. Importance of Nutritional Status and Diet on page 98.*
- *4. Dealing with the Issue of Weight on page 99.*
- *5. Stress Levels and Healing on page 100.*
- *6. Rest and Sleep on page 101.*
- *7. Reverse Your Biological Age on page 103.*

The Importance of an Honest Self-Assessment

Self-assessment is all about being *honest with yourself.* Our program will work extremely well for 80% of all cases, but, if you have identified any of the '*7-factors*' in your own body, then it is critical to properly address and resolve these in order to achieve full resolution of your condition.

Let us take a look at **each** of these seven factors. Don't be discouraged if you suffer from one (or more) of these factors in this 20% group, because now there is a good chance to fully resolve your condition simply by addressing those issues. Now is the time to make those changes.

1. Impact of Kinetic Chain Restrictions

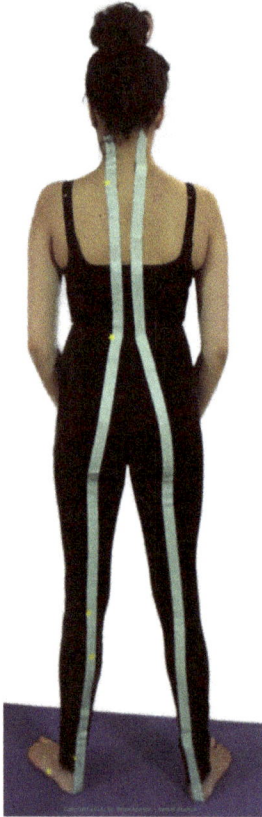

Every structure in your body is connected to, interacts with, and affects all the other structures (muscles, tendons, bones, nerves, etc.) around it. This inter-relationship is known as a kinetic chain.

Think of your body as being comprised of a series of small kinetic chains, each linked to other kinetic chains to form a complex body-encompassing *Kinetic Web*! Tension, weakness, or injury to any part of a kinetic chain immediately affects the function of all its interlinked components.

From a kinetic chain perspective, this means that other areas of your body (other than the part that is manifesting pain) may be the actual cause of your dysfunction, rather than the most common one that is usually addressed by most treatment protocols.

For example, it has been well established that weak hip muscles are directly related to an increase in abnormal foot pronation. Abnormal pronation, in turn, has been shown to be directly related to the development of Plantar Fasciitis. In such a case, until you strengthen your hips, you will not be able to reach a full resolution of your condition (Plantar Fasciitis).

This is just one example of just how interlinked the structures of the body are. For every condition or problem, there are several such areas that should be evaluated, especially if you are in the 20% category discussed under the *The 80/20 Effect on page 94*.

What You Can Do!

Don't be discouraged! In addition to having your practitioner conduct a more comprehensive biomechanical examination, we also provide an entire playlist of videos about **Biomechanical Assessment** on our *Kinetic Health YouTube Channel*. These videos can be a great resource in helping you to assess other possible problems in areas of the kinetic chain that you may not normally consider. The information derived from these evaluations is often invaluable to any practitioner who is aiding you in the treatment of your condition.

2. Importance of Cardiovascular Health

Good cardiovascular health is essential for effective injury repair. Individuals who do not exercise, who work in polluted environments, or who smoke tend to heal at a much slower rate.

Aerobic exercise (walking, cycling, running, and swimming) is the fastest way to increase the strength and function of your cardiovascular system. The problem is, most people never work their cardiovascular system hard enough to actually experience these changes. You must work within your aerobic zone to achieve these benefits.

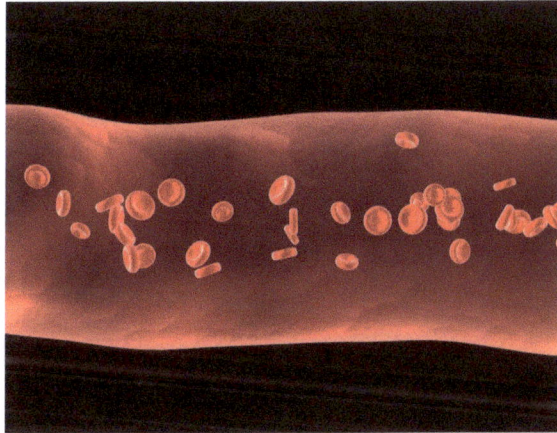

The Importance of Aerobic Exercise

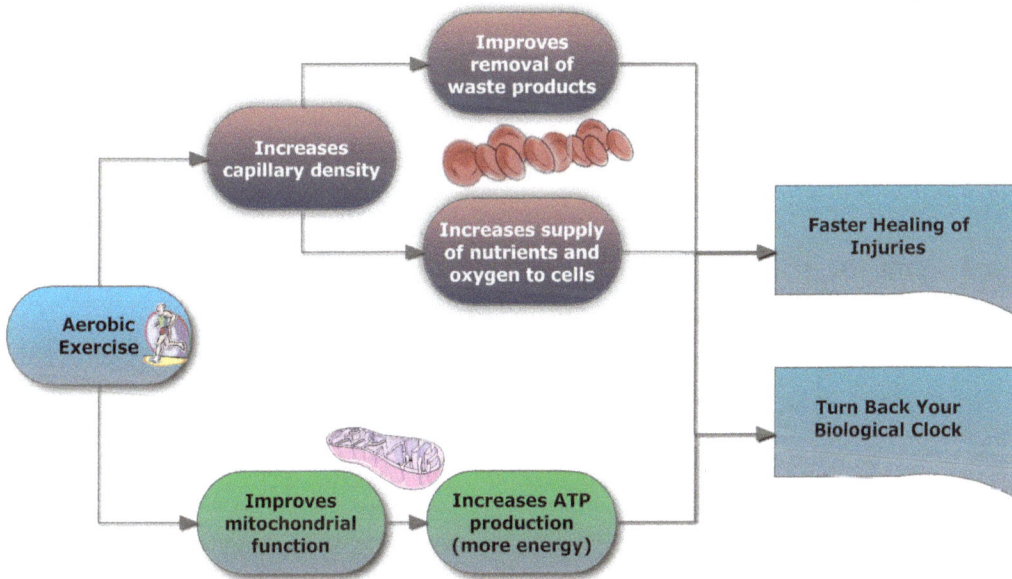

Copyright 2014: Dr. Brian Abelson®

By increasing the capillary density, you are able to get more nutrients and oxygen into your soft-tissues (muscle, ligaments, tendons, and connective tissue), thereby helping them to heal at a much faster rate. The increased capillary density also means that you are better able to eliminate the waste by-products produced during healing (or with normal cell metabolism) again allowing them to perform more efficiently

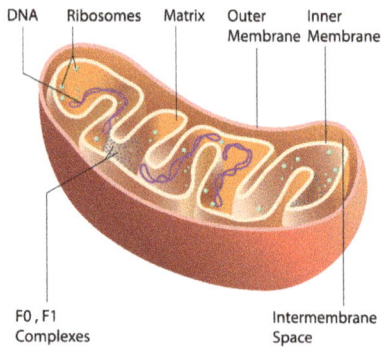

DNA   Ribosomes   Matrix   Outer Membrane   Inner Membrane

F0, F1 Complexes   Intermembrane Space

Aerobic exercise also increases the function of mitochondria in your cells. This increased mitochondrial function immediately boosts your body's ability to generate power and energy since your mitochondria are the principal energy generators for your cells. Mitochondria convert existing nutrients into ATP (adenosine triphosphate), a form of energy that is readily usable by all the cells in your body. Your body uses this energy to perform all of its functions - from healing existing injuries, to eliminating waste, and powering your muscles when you walk, talk, or perform any action.

As we age, or when we injure ourselves, our ability to produce ATP decreases. Exercise is one of the few factors that will *naturally increase ATP production* to give you increased energy. Increased ATP production is one very significant way in which exercise can help turn back your biological clock.

3. Importance of Nutritional Status and Diet

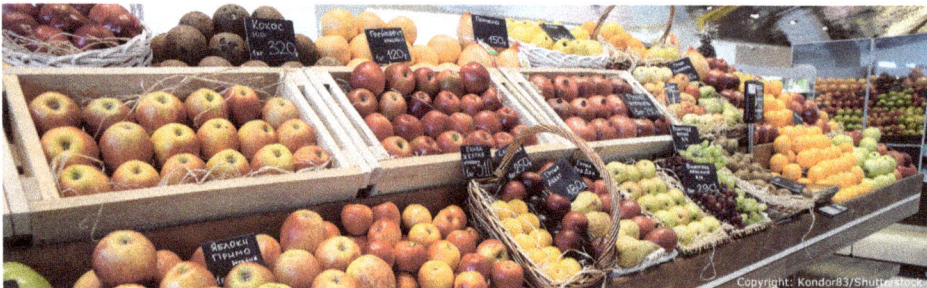

When we treat our patients and provide them with exercises, we expect to see positive results within a short period of time. When we do not see these positive results, the most common culprit (other than the patient missing appointments or not doing their exercises) is **diet**. For some reason, many of us think that we can keep our bodies dehydrated, stuffed full of fast foods and processed junk, and still somehow *not* have to pay the price.

We can give you some great suggestions to improve your nutritional status. Take a look at the nutritional guidelines in our book *Choose Health*. This book can help you to speed the healing process, and make **long-term sustainable changes** to your health.

4. Dealing with the Issue of Weight

You can't get away from the fact that being overweight causes major damage to the joints and soft-tissue structures of the body. It does this by increasing the mechanical stress on your body, and by causing an increase in the levels of pro-inflammatory chemicals stored by your body. The saying '*You Are What You Eat*' was never truer than when it comes to the fats you store in your body. Eat good fat, you store good fats; if you eat bad fats, you become a reservoir of inflammatory chemicals.

Consider the 'Fat Equation'

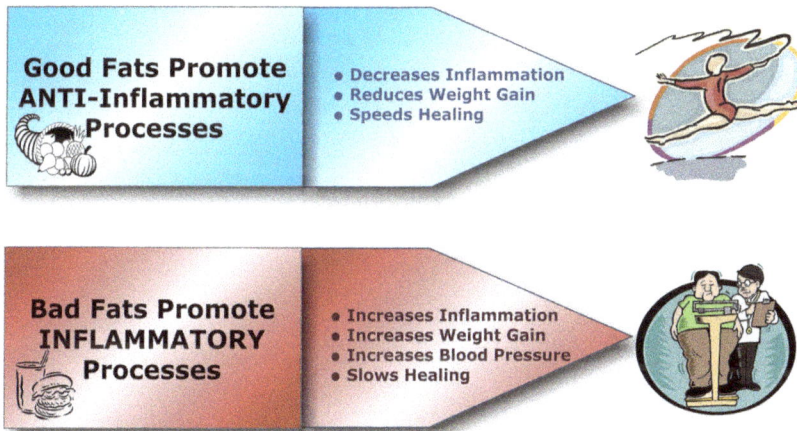

The **Fat Equation** is really quite simple. Good fats promote anti-inflammatory activity in your body; bad fats promote destructive inflammatory processes.

The Fat Equation

Good Fats Promote ANTI-Inflammatory Processes
- Decreases Inflammation
- Reduces Weight Gain
- Speeds Healing

Bad Fats Promote INFLAMMATORY Processes
- Increases Inflammation
- Increases Weight Gain
- Increases Blood Pressure
- Slows Healing

Copyright 2014: Dr. Brian Abelson®

The Relationship between Inflammation and Fats

Inflammation is part of the natural immune response, and is triggered by injury, allergens, disease, or poisonous chemicals. During this natural immune response, fatty acids are released from your cell membranes. These fatty acids are then transformed into substances called *Eicosanoids*.

There are both good and bad *Eicosanoids*, some will reduce inflammation and encourage healing, while others will create states of destructive inflammation. *Eicosanoids* also help to control other bodily functions such as blood pressure and immune functions (including inflammatory responses).

The behaviour of the *Eicosanoids* is dependent on the types of certain fats stored in your cell membranes. If your cell membranes have stored healthy Omega-3-fatty acids (obtained through good dietary habits), then your body will heal faster and cope with any aggressive inflammatory states.

If you have a history of consuming high levels of Omega-6-fatty acids (bad oils), then the destructive Eicosanoids will be released and your body will have to deal with increased aggressive inflammatory states. It is important to maintain an optimal balance of Omega-6 to Omega-3 fatty acids in your body.

If weight is an issue that needs to be addressed, then we suggest you take a look at our eBook *Choose Health*. In it, you will find lots of great ideas that really work about how to lose weight, reduce inflammation, and how to stay healthy.

5. Stress Levels and Healing

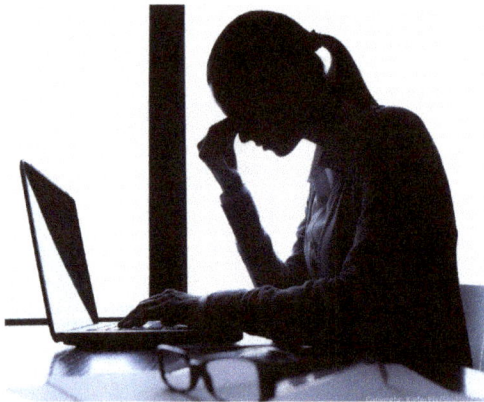

In our clinic's *Patient Admittance Form*, there is a section where we ask our patients to perform a self-evaluation of their stress levels. Basically, patients are asked to indicate their level of stress on a scale from zero (none) to five (high). Most patients mark down zero to two, indicating that they believe they are under minimal stress.

Yet these same people often work 10 - 12 hours per day, for 6 days per week, don't exercise, have poor eating habits, sleep only 4-5 hours a night, and have major deadlines on a continual basis. Yet, they really believe they are not stressed!

In truth, not only are they **stressed**, they are in major denial of this fact. Adrenaline and Cortisol (stress hormones) are roaring through their bloodstream. These high hormone levels are great to have when a lion is chasing you, but the last time I looked, we didn't have too many lions chasing us down our streets.

Stress is accompanied by significant physiological problems. Having continually high levels of these stress hormones in your body can have some very serious consequences, such as:

- Suppressed thyroid function.
- Imbalances in blood sugar.
- Decreased muscle and bone density.
- Slowed rates of healing.
- Increased abdominal fat.
- Increased hypertension.

Reduce Your Stress!

Bottom line, anything you can do to **decrease your stress levels** will help. Some of the best ways to decrease stress and lower the levels of those destructive stress hormones are by performing:

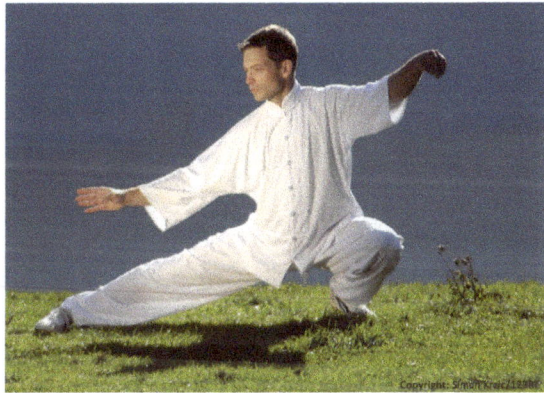

- Regular physical activity, especially aerobic exercise such as walking, cycling, or swimming.
- Meditation, Tai Chi, or Yoga. Over the past few decades, there have been some remarkable research results revealing the positive effects of Tai Chi, and how it can reduce cortisol levels. The same has been shown for Meditation and Yoga.

6. Rest and Sleep

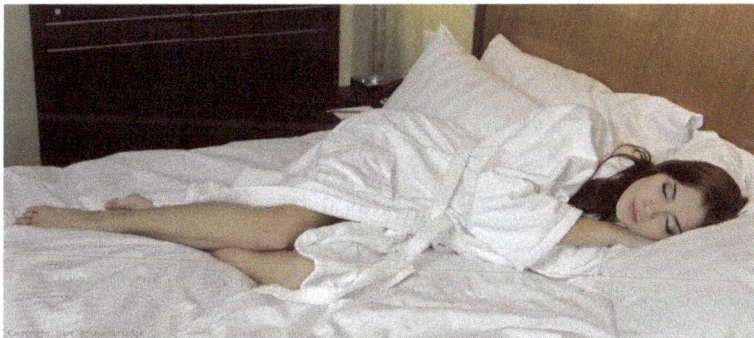

Rest, in our busy world, is becoming an increasingly rare commodity. But it is an essential component for healing the body.

Your body needs rest and sleep in order to function properly and to repair itself. While you sleep, your body performs much of its maintenance and renewal functions. If you have any type of soft-tissue injury (caused by sports, career, home life, or just daily activities), then you must **rest** that area to give your body a chance to recover properly. **Lack of sleep can sabotage everything!**

Lack of sleep results in decreased immune function, increased potential for disease (heart disease, stroke, cancer), decreased hormone production (human growth hormone), decreased tissue repair, decreased cognitive function, decreased fat metabolism, increased depression, increased inflammation, and even decreased life span.

Some very interesting research has come out of the *National Academy of Science* about the effects of sleep deprivation. Sleep deprivation causes an elevated level of the stress hormone, *corticosterone*. Increased levels of this hormone cause a reduction in the function of brain cells. This, in turn, has been directly related to problems in concentration and other possible cognitive issues. A little sad, but lack of sleep may even reduce cognitive function so much that you don't even realize there is a problem.

We have found that for many of our patients, a lack of rest and sleep is one of the primary reasons for a slow or delayed recovery from an injury.

How much sleep you require will vary based on several factors, including your diet (good diet, bad diet), environmental factors (smoking, drinking), quality of sleep, genetics, and current injuries. Even the quality of light that you are exposed to will affect the amount of sleep you need (spending a long time in front of the computer disrupts your circadian rhythm). In general terms we recommend at least 7 to 8 hours of sleep per night.

Reducing sleep by as little as one-and-a-half hours, for just one night, reduces daytime alertness by about one-third. Bottom line: without proper sleep, your body will not repair itself, you decrease the overall quality of your life, and you may even decrease your life span.

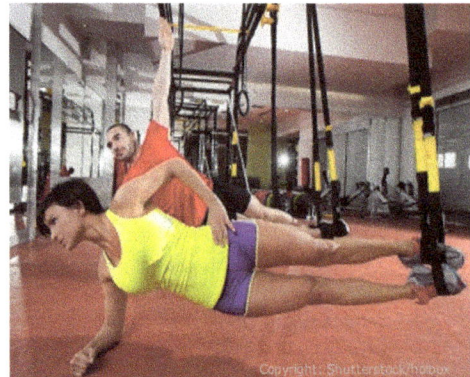
Copyright: Shutterstock/hotbox

So, immediately after an acute injury:

- Reduce the activity performed by that structure.
- Do not perform weight-bearing exercises that can stress that area.
- Rest that structure.
- Keep it elevated to reduce inflammation.

Avoid over-using an injured area before it has recovered as that can cause further injury, more inflammation, and increased healing time.

By doing these simple steps, you provide your body with a critical element needed for self-healing...**REST**!

7. Reverse Your Biological Age

You probably noticed, I said *biological age*, not *chronological age*. Your chronological age is merely your age in years. Your biological age is your age at a cellular level. Sorry, there is nothing you can do about your chronological age. But there is a tremendous amount you can do about your biological age.

Every day in our practice we hear people say, *"I guess the reason I have this condition is my age."* My answer is most often, *"Nonsense! You really are not that old, your chronological age is not important, and there is a tremendous amount you can do to turn back your biological clock."*

Remember, the choices **you** make on a daily basis will either quicken or slow down your biological aging process. Good nutrition, exercise, supplementation, and effective stress reduction are all techniques that can literally help **to turn back your biological age**. All of these factors are under your control and can greatly influence your ability to heal.

TIP: If you would like to learn some great ideas for turning back your biological clock, take a look at our eBook – *Choose Health*.

So, make the right choices; make the good choices!

Plantar Fasciitis

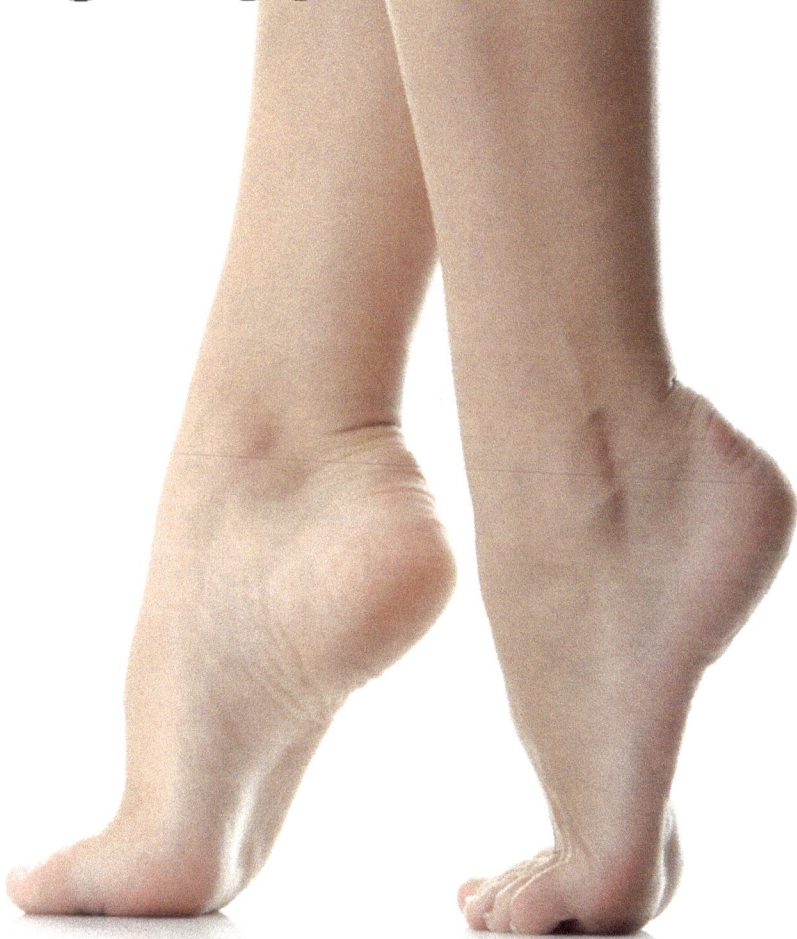

Our Program

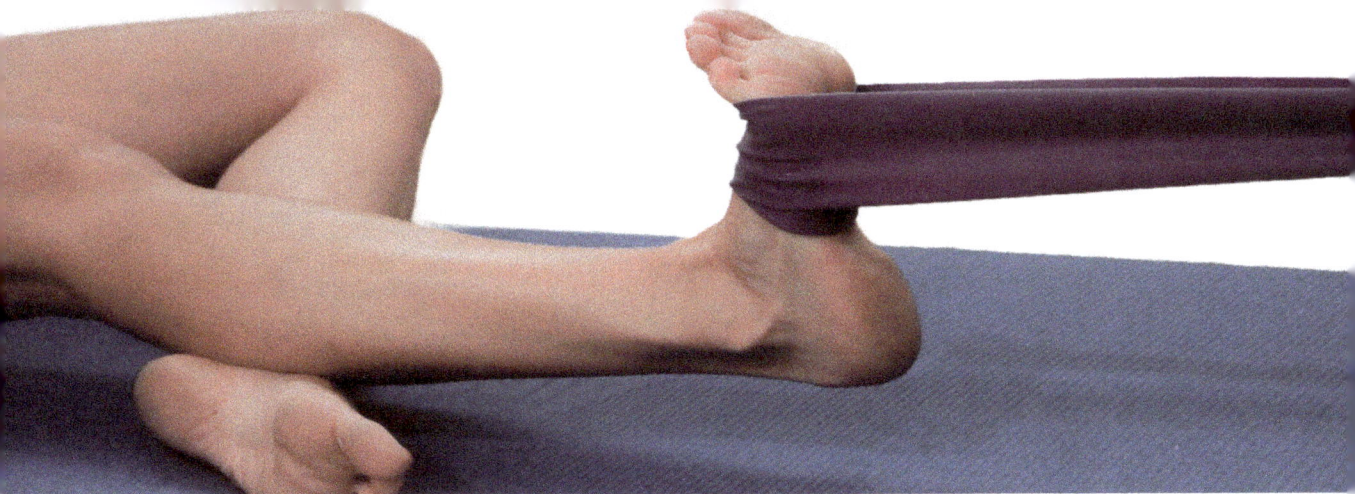

Phase I: Foundational Protocol for Plantar Fasciitis

In this Chapter

Well, you are probably reading this book because you already know (or suspect) that you have Plantar Fasciitis, and are looking for a long-term, workable solution to this problem. For a complete resolution of Plantar Fasciitis, it is important to use the RIGHT combination of exercises; otherwise you increase the probability of this condition returning. There are four important areas that must be addressed when developing exercise routines for Plantar Fasciitis: stretching, myofascial release, strengthening, and balance.

In the following chapters we will be guiding you through a three-phase series of tests and exercises to help you resolve your Plantar Fasciitis. Take a few minutes to review and familiarize yourself with the process you will be following (as shown in the illustration on the next page). It will help to clarify and set your expectations for the time frame required for resolving your Plantar Fasciitis.

In this first phase, you will start by addressing common issues that affect most Plantar Fasciitis patients, and first address the *local* structures of the foot and *plantar fascia*.

Your Healing Process

The following diagram illustrates the path you will be following to resolve your case of Plantar Fasciitis.

Plantar Fasciitis - The Healing Process

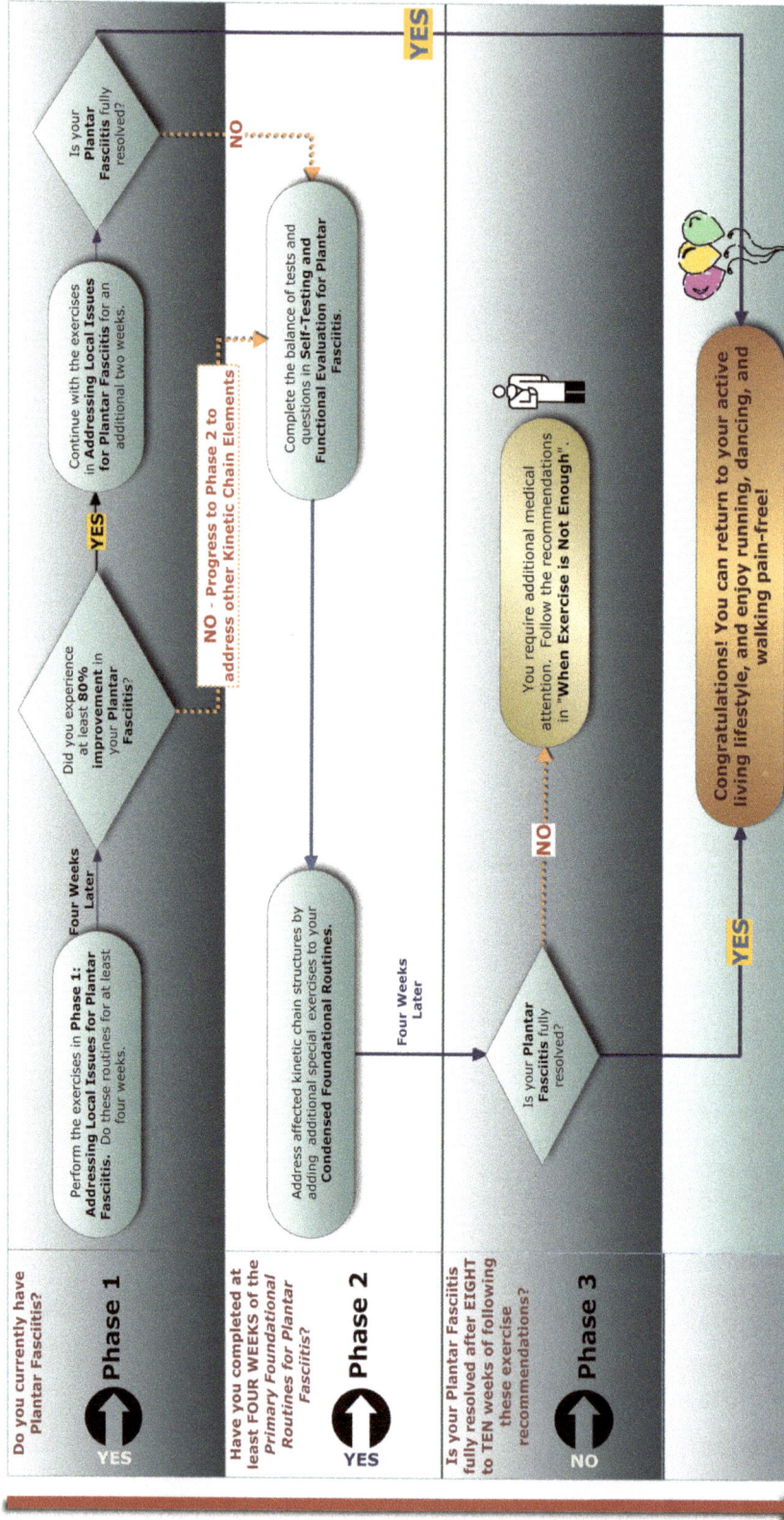

Phase 1

Do you currently have Plantar Fasciitis?

YES

Perform the exercises in **Phase 1: Addressing Local Issues for Plantar Fasciitis.** Do these routines for at least four weeks.

Four Weeks Later

Did you experience at least **80% improvement** in your **Plantar Fasciitis?**

YES — Continue with the exercises in **Addressing Local Issues for Plantar Fasciitis** for an additional two weeks.

Is your **Plantar Fasciitis** fully resolved?

NO — Complete the balance of tests and questions in **Self-Testing and Functional Evaluation for Plantar Fasciitis.**

YES

NO - Progress to Phase 2 to address other Kinetic Chain Elements

Phase 2

Have you completed at least FOUR WEEKS of the *Primary Foundational Routines for Plantar Fasciitis?*

YES

Address affected kinetic chain structures by adding additional special exercises to your **Condensed Foundational Routines.**

Four Weeks Later

Phase 3

Is your **Plantar Fasciitis** fully resolved after EIGHT to TEN weeks of following these exercise recommendations?

NO

Is your **Plantar Fasciitis** fully resolved?

NO — You require additional medical attention. Follow the recommendations in "**When Exercise is Not Enough".**

YES

Congratulations! You can return to your active living lifestyle, and enjoy running, dancing, and walking pain-free!

Start with the first lane, and progress through the rest. If, after four weeks of strengthening the local structures, you find that your Plantar Fasciitis is still not fully resolved, then you should move on to identify other kinetic chain elements that may be affecting or causing your Plantar Fasciitis (*Phase 2: Finding Problems in Your Kinetic Chain on page 115*). Continue performing these exercises on an occasional basis to prevent the return of this condition.

Checking for Red Flags

Before we get into the exercises and self-evaluation sections, you need to first verify that you are only dealing with a simple case of Plantar Fasciitis, and do not have some other type of condition that may require immediate attention by a physician.

Be sure to see a physician immediately if you:

- Have swelling of the feet with severe pain. This needs to be addressed if the swelling does not decrease after two or three days.
- Have severe foot pain occurring after physical trauma. You must rule out possible fractures that may be causing foot pain.
- Have symptoms of severe nerve compression such as muscle atrophy, or pain that does not change with increased rest or changes in body position.
- Have indications of an infection (fever over 38°C (100°F), with tenderness, warmth, and redness of the foot).
- Are unable to walk or put any weight on your feet, even after the day progresses.

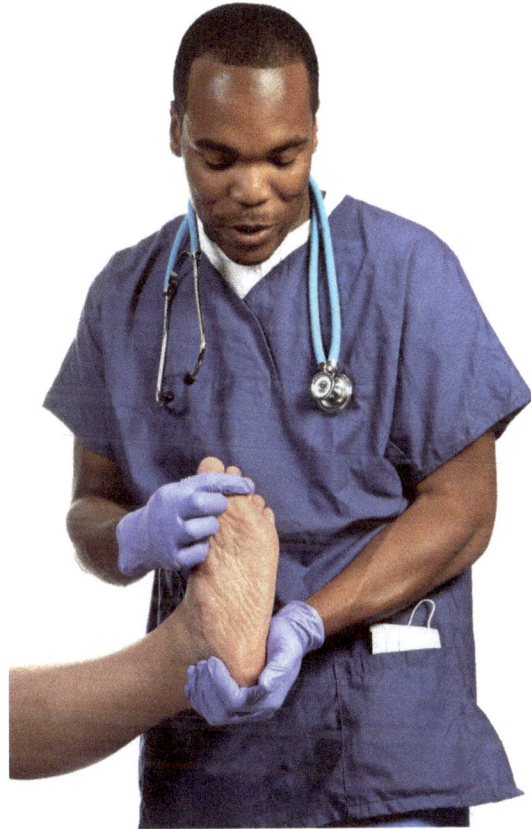

Caution: In most cases, the pain caused by Plantar Fasciitis is musculoskeletal in nature. However, if there are indications of something more serious, you should see your physician immediately before using any of the exercise routines or tests in this book.

Phase 1: Addressing Local Issues for PF

We begin your healing process by performing specifically selected exercises that address the *most **common** local causes of Plantar Fasciitis*, as shown in the following diagram.

Primary Foundational Exercise Protocol for Plantar Fasciitis

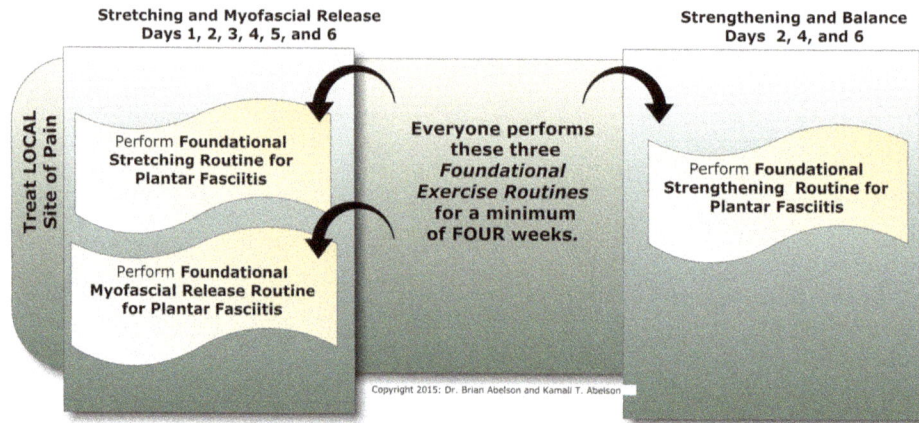

Stretching and Myofascial Release
Days 1, 2, 3, 4, 5, and 6

Strengthening and Balance
Days 2, 4, and 6

Treat LOCAL Site of Pain

Perform **Foundational Stretching Routine for Plantar Fasciitis**

Everyone performs these three *Foundational Exercise Routines* for a minimum of FOUR weeks.

Perform **Foundational Strengthening Routine for Plantar Fasciitis**

Perform **Foundational Myofascial Release Routine for Plantar Fasciitis**

Copyright 2015: Dr. Brian Abelson and Kamali T. Abelson

Anyone with Plantar Fasciitis should perform this recommended **Primary Foundational Routine for Plantar Fasciitis**, for a **minimum period of FOUR weeks**. During this four-week period, you can expect to see substantial improvements in your condition.

These carefully selected exercises address the key **local areas** that are typically involved in causing Plantar Fasciitis, and help to prepare your body for more extensive and difficult exercise routines. Your *Foundational Routine for Plantar Fasciitis* is comprised of three main sets of exercises, with each set to be performed on specific days, as described in the following sections:

- *Scheduling Your Exercise Routines on page 111.*
- *Foundational Stretching Routine for PF on page 112.*
  (Days 1, 2, 3, 4, 5, and 6).
- *Foundational Myofascial Release Routine for PF on page 113.*
  (Days 1, 2, 3, 4, 5, and 6).
- *Foundational Strengthening Routine for PF on page 114.*
  (Days 2, 4, and 6).

If, at the end of this four-week period, you do not see substantial improvement, or feel that your progress has plateaued, then you will need to progress to the next part of our program - *Phase 2: Addressing Problems in the PF Kinetic Chain on page 149.*

Scheduling Your Exercise Routines

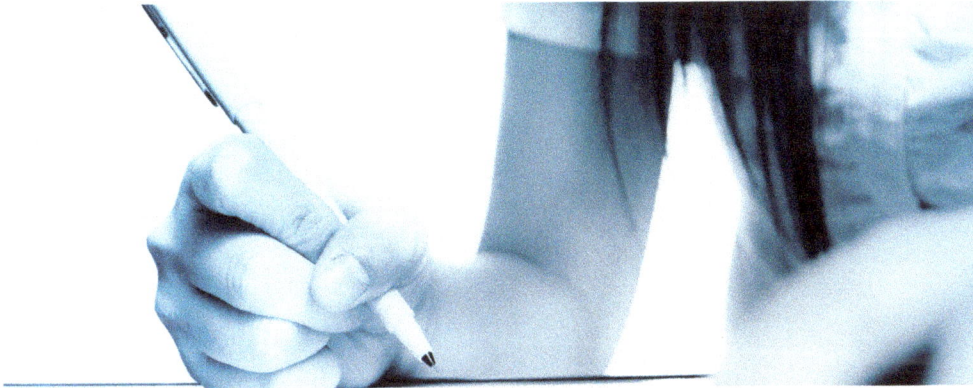

You must perform your customized exercise routine for *at least four weeks.* It is important to monitor your results during this period of time.

Don't expect too many changes for the first week. In fact, you may even notice an overall *increase* in your symptoms. On the other hand, by the end of the four-week period, you should expect to see a considerable improvement in your symptoms. In many cases, our patients find that they are completely pain-free.

To reduce your time commitment (and hopefully increase your compliance) we have divided the exercises as follows:

- Ice massage the affected areas at least once a day (or as needed) until the pain has reduced. (See *Cold Therapy - page 241* for more information.) Once the pain has substantially decreased, you can start using heat therapy. (See *Heat Therapy - page 245* for more information.)
- During days 1-to-6, perform all the recommended stretches and myofascial releases. Depending on your condition, this section can take between 10 to 20 minutes to complete.
- During days 2, 4, and 6, add the strengthening and osseous release exercises. Depending on your condition, this section can take between 5 to 25 minutes to complete.On these days, you may choose to perform the stretching and myofascial routines in the morning, and the strengthening exercises in the evening.
- During the seventh day of this program – REST.

Foundational Stretching Routine for PF

During the regenerative or repair phase of an injury, the body creates and lays down collagen to repair the injured area. When the injured person performs the correct stretching exercises, the majority of this new tissue will be laid down in the same direction as the tissue that is being repaired, thereby allowing this tissue to properly perform its function.

Caution: To prevent injuries, be sure to perform 10 - 20 minutes of cardiovascular exercise to warm-up these structures BEFORE stretching. It is very important to perform this full stretching routine on each of days 1, 2, 3, 4, 5, and 6.

Perform the following *stretching exercises on days 1, 2, 3, 4, 5, and 6.*

Table 5. 1: Foundational Stretching Routine for Plantar Fasciitis

	Follow-Along Foundational Foot Stretching Routine For detailed instructions on how to do each exercise, see *Foundational Foot Stretching Routine - page 176.*
	Stretching the Tibialis Anterior - page 190.
	Peroneal Stretch - page 193.
	Stretching the Calf Muscles - page 196.

Caution: Do **NOT** 'pick and choose' your stretching exercises. All these exercises are essential and play an important role in your healing and resolution process.

Foundational Myofascial Release Routine for PF

Self-myofascial release exercises can be used to break down soft-tissue restrictions or adhesions that form after an injury. These exercises can be performed in conjunction with stretching exercises in order to help release restricted areas and increase relative motion between the soft-tissue layers.

Perform the following *myofascial release exercises* on *days 1, 2, 3, 4, 5, and 6.*

Table 5. 2: Foundational Myofascial Release for Plantar Fasciitis

	Follow-Along Foundational Myofascial Release of the Foot For detailed instructions on how to do each exercise, see *Foundational Myofascial Release of the Foot - page 185.*
	Myofascial Release of the Shins - page 191.
	Myofascial Release of the Calf - page 198.
	Myofascial Release of the Peroneals - page 194.

Caution: Do **NOT** 'pick and choose' your myofascial exercises. All these exercises are important and play an essential role in your healing and resolution process.

Foundational Strengthening Routine for PF

Every time you injure yourself, your body lays down new tissue to repair itself. The new tissue is initially very fragile, thin, and easily torn or re-injured. Strength or weight training places stress upon these new tissues, causing them to go through a remodeling process. In this process, the new tissue literally converts from one type of collagen to a different type which is up to 10 times thicker and 10 times stronger. However, this collagen conversion only occurs when you apply continued stress upon the tissue, as you do when you perform weight and strength training exercises.

Perform the following *strengthening routine on days 2, 4, and 6.*

Table 5. 3: Foundational Strengthening Routine for Plantar Fasciitis

	Theraband Strengthening of the Foot Routine on page 218.
	Salsa Towel Crunch on page 220.
	Pen and Loonie Exercise on page 221.
	Shin Strengthening Advancing to Dynamic Pulses on page 222.
	Eccentric Calf Raises on page 223.

Caution: Do **NOT** 'pick and choose' your strengthening exercises. All these exercises are essential and play an important role in your healing and resolution process.

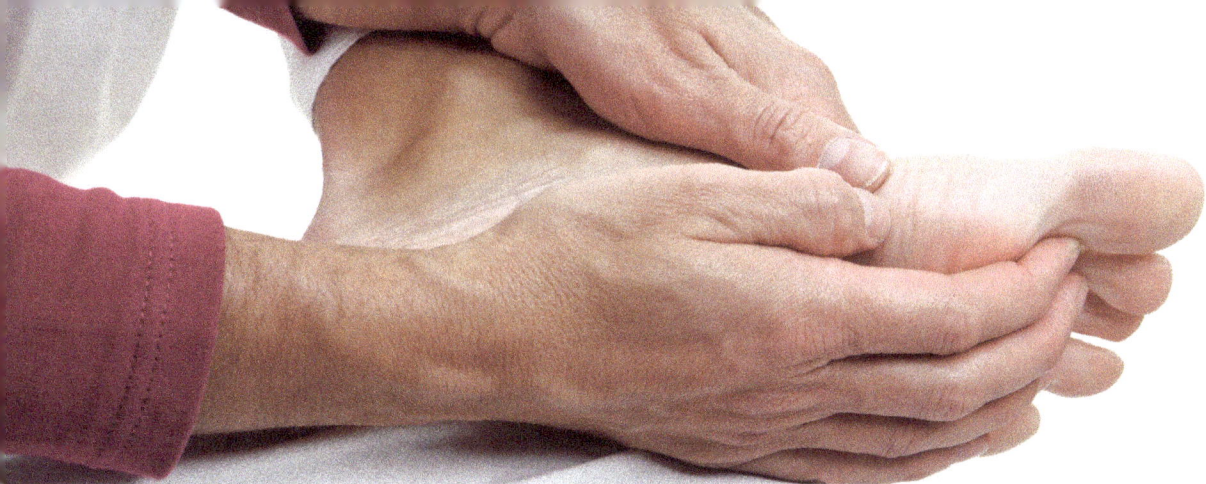

Phase 2: Finding Problems in Your Kinetic Chain

Chapter

6

In this Chapter

Do not become discouraged if the *Foundational Exercise Program* did not fully resolve your Plantar Fasciitis. Complete success is often only achieved by addressing any weak links in your kinetic chain.

In this chapter, we provide some *simple functional tests* that can help you to identify the weak links in *your* particular kinetic chain. The information derived from these tests is invaluable for the resolution of Plantar Fasciitis, as they can help to determine just which areas of your body need treatment and exercise.

Obviously, it is far beyond the scope of this book to provide training in gait analysis, anatomical palpation, or the many other standard orthopedic tests performed by medical professionals. However, we believe that you do not have to become an expert in biomechanics in order to locate many of the weak links in your body's kinetic chain, especially the ones that have lead to Plantar Fasciitis.

The functional self-evaluation tests in this chapter assess your body and help you to identify any abnormal motion patterns or stability issues. These tests, combined with the results of a self-examination, can help to identify exactly which areas of *your* kinetic chain need to be addressed in order to achieve a full resolution of your Plantar Fasciitis.

Caution: Do NOT progress to *Phase 2: Addressing Problems in the Kinetic Chain* until you have completed at least four weeks of the *Phase 1: Foundational Protocol for Plantar Fasciitis on page 107*. You need to give your body sufficient time to adapt, heal, and strengthen past the acute injury phase.

When to Start Phase 2 of Your Treatment Protocols

How will you know if you are ready for *Phase 2: Finding Problems in Your Kinetic Chain on page 115*?

If, after performing the *Phase 1: Foundational Protocol for Plantar Fasciitis - page 107* for at least **four weeks**, you find that you are still manifesting symptoms related to your Plantar Fasciitis, or if you feel that your progress has plateaued, then you will need to complete the questions and tests in this chapter.

These questions and tests will help you to determine which other areas of your kinetic chain are affecting or causing your Plantar Fasciitis. If you find you have a problem in any area, or if you fail a test, then you will need to add specific exercise to your routine.

About the Self-Evaluation Process

It is important to carefully follow the instructions we have provided for your self-evaluation and testing. The following illustration details how to prepare for these tests, and the order in which to perform each set of activities. Please take a few minutes to carefully review this process, and refer back to it whenever you need.

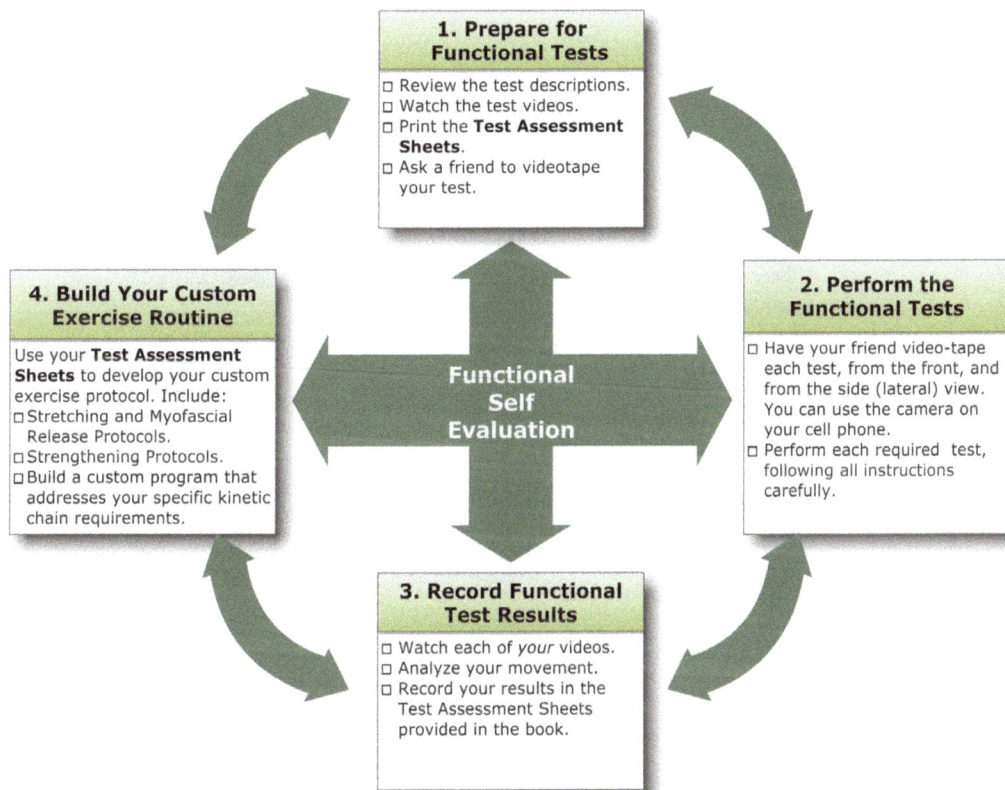

1. Prepare for Functional Tests
- Review the test descriptions.
- Watch the test videos.
- Print the **Test Assessment Sheets**.
- Ask a friend to videotape your test.

Functional Self Evaluation

2. Perform the Functional Tests
- Have your friend video-tape each test, from the front, and from the side (lateral) view. You can use the camera on your cell phone.
- Perform each required test, following all instructions carefully.

3. Record Functional Test Results
- Watch each of *your* videos.
- Analyze your movement.
- Record your results in the Test Assessment Sheets provided in the book.

4. Build Your Custom Exercise Routine
Use your **Test Assessment Sheets** to develop your custom exercise protocol. Include:
- Stretching and Myofascial Release Protocols.
- Strengthening Protocols.
- Build a custom program that addresses your specific kinetic chain requirements.

Copyright 2015: Dr. Brian Abelson and Kamali T. Abelson

We start by testing the feet and ankles, progress to testing your shins, calves, and hips, and end with a basic assessment of your core stability. We will also test to identify possible areas of nerve entrapment (identified by neurological pain, numbness, tingling, or burning sensations).

We have provided eight (8) self-evaluation tests for you to perform, with the last test for core stability consisting of three sections. It will take you about 25-to-45 minutes to complete all these tests. As you complete each test, write down your assessments in the space provided (you may want to print these assessment pages). You will be using these results in subsequent chapters to build a personalized custom exercise program for resolving your specific case of Plantar Fasciitis. See *"Phase 2: Addressing Problems in the PF Kinetic Chain" - page 149*.

Throughout this process, keep in mind that your body operates as one, *very integrated*, kinetic web. A problem in one area can easily cascade into problems across multiple regions. All of these linked areas must be addressed to achieve a complete resolution of your Plantar Fasciitis.

Accessing the YouTube Videos for the Tests

To make it easy for you, we have videotaped each of these tests and placed them on our YouTube site (*http://www.youtube.com/kinetichealthonline*). Once at this site, you will need to search for the **Plantar Fasciitis - Functional Testing Play List.** Click on the link or the video icon shown on the left side of the page.

- To access these videos, you will need internet connections and YouTube compatibility from your e-reader device or computer.
- For our eBook users, if your e-reader device supports internet and video viewing, you can simply click the video icon beside each test, and learn how to perform each functional test.
- For our hard-copy book readers, simply type in the YouTube address that we have provided into your internet browser, and view these tests as needed.

Recording your Functional Test Results

Print pages 119-223 and record your test results on your copy. The tests are grouped as follows:

- *Recording Joint Mobility of the Foot and Ankle - page 119.*
- *Recording Test Results for the Upper Legs and Hips - page 120.*
- *Recording Functional Test Results for the Core - page 121.*

Optional Tests for Pronation and Nerve Entrapment:

- *Recording Results of Optional Tests - page 122.*

Be Honest With Yourself

Please be honest with yourself; each of these functional tests are extremely important and provide valuable information that can help resolve your condition. Some of these tests require a partner to observe you, or perhaps, to videotape you as you perform each test. Record your results as follows:

- **FAIL:** You have difficulties performing the test, or a problem was found.
- **PASS:** You are able to complete the test easily, or NO problem was found.

Note: BEFORE performing the tests, we strongly recommend that you watch the videos we have produced for each test. They are available on our YouTube site (*http://www.youtube.com/kinetichealthonline*). You will need to search for the *Plantar Fasciitis - Functional Testing Play List.* In addition, to ensure *objective analysis* of your results, we recommend that you have someone videotape you as you perform each test. Your cell phone camera works well for recording your test results.

Once you have recorded your test results, you can progress to *Phase 2: Addressing Problems in the PF Kinetic Chain - page 149* where you will build your own, *customized exercise routine* to help complete the resolution of your Plantar Fasciitis.

Recording Joint Mobility of the Foot and Ankle

Carry out the *Functional Tests for Joint Mobility - page 123* to see if joint mobility is a factor in the development of your Plantar Fasciitis. *Print the following test assessment sheet and record your results on the hard-copy.*

Table 6. 1: Record Joint Mobility of the Foot and Ankle

Click for Video	Functional Test	Problem Found (FAIL)	No Problems (PASS)
(video icon)	*1. Testing Dorsiflexion of the Ankle - page 125* YouTube Address: http://youtu.be/ aGPIThv0IQM (2.08 min)	☐ Left Side: _____ cm ☐ Right Side: _____ cm ☐ Other problems noted in the Ankle. _____	☐ Normal Left Side ☐ Normal Right Side
(video icon)	*2. Testing the Mobility of the Big Toe - page 126* YouTube Address: http://youtu.be/ r0galxQ_beU	**MTP Joint** ☐ Left Foot: _____ ☐ Right Foot: _____ **DTP Joint** ☐ Left Foot: _____ ☐ Right Foot: _____ ☐ Other problems noted in either foot. _____	**MTP Joint** ☐ Normal Left Foot ☐ Normal Right Foot **DTP Joint** ☐ Normal Left Foot ☐ Normal Right Foot

Recording Test Results for the Upper Legs and Hips

Carry out the *Functional Tests for the Legs and Hips - page 129* to evaluate the strength, flexibility, and capabilities of the upper legs and hips, both of which are key components of the foot's kinetic chain. *Print the following test assessment sheet and record your results on the hard-copy.*

Table 6. 2: Functional Tests for the Upper Legs and Hips

Click for Video	Functional Test	Problem Found (FAIL)	No Problem (PASS)
	1. Testing Hip Flexion (Thomas Test) - page 130 YouTube Address: http://youtu.be/8D5_fmIbqYk	☐ Right Hip: Restricted ☐ Left Hip: Restricted ☐ Other problems noted in Hips _____	☐ Right Hip: Normal ☐ Left Hip: Normal
	2. Testing Stability of the Lower Extremity - Deep Squat - page 131 YouTube Address: http://youtu.be/_qhE2wxbSts	☐ Anterior View: Problem found ☐ Lateral View: Problem found ☐ Other problems noted in Hips and Upper Legs _____	☐ Anterior View: Normal ☐ Lateral View: Normal
	3. Testing Hamstring Flexibility - page 135 YouTube Address: http://youtu.be/3ISivoJxmmk	☐ Right Hamstring: Restricted ☐ Left Hamstring: Restricted ☐ Other problems noted in Hips and Upper Legs _____	☐ Right Hamstring: Normal ☐ Left Hamstring: Normal

Recording Functional Test Results for the Core

Carry out the *Testing Core Functionality - page 137* to evaluate the strength, flexibility, and capabilities of the core, which serves as the base of stability for the foot's kinetic chain. *Print the following test assessment sheet and record your results on the hard-copy.*

Table 6. 3: Recording Functional Test Results for the Core

Click for Video	Functional Test	Problem Found (FAIL)	No Problem (PASS)
(video)	*1. Core Stability Test 1: Anterior Plank with Alternating Leg - page 137* YouTube Address: http://youtu.be/wDTJx_9iNqk	☐ Left Side: Fatigue before completing test ☐ Right Side: Fatigue before completing test ☐ Other problems noted during Anterior Plank _____	☐ Left Side: Normal ☐ Right Side: Normal
(video)	*2. Core Stability Test 2: Side Bridge with Leg Lift - page 139* YouTube Address: http://youtu.be/wDTJx_9iNqk, 3.11 minutes	☐ Left Side: Fatigue before completing test ☐ Right Side: Fatigue before completing test ☐ Other problems noted during Side Bridge _____ _____	☐ Left Side: Normal ☐ Right Side: Normal
(video)	*3. Core Stability Test 3: Pelvic Raise - Testing the Posterior Chain - page 140* YouTube Address: (YouTube: http://youtu.be/wDTJx_9iNqk, 6.24 minutes)	☐ Left Side: Weak or unstable ☐ Right Side: Weak or unstable ☐ Other problems noted during Pelvic Raise _____ _____	☐ Left Side: Normal ☐ Right Side: Normal

Recording Results of Optional Tests

Not everyone needs to perform the following optional functional examination tests. If you are not experiencing any of the following symptoms, then you do not need to perform these tests:

- Perform the *Wet Foot Test - page 142.* if you have noted abnormal foot motion, pronation, or supination, or have noticed abnormal wear on your shoes. This test will give you a better idea of what type of shoe support you need for your Plantar Fasciitis problem.
- If you have seen indications of nerve entrapment (numbness, altered sensation, or pain along the nerve paths of the feet) then use the *tibial* or *peroneal nerve (page 147)* tests to determine if this is a factor in the development of your Plantar Fasciitis.
- *Print the following test assessment sheet and record your results on the hard-copy.*

Table 6. 4: Record Results of Optional Tests

Click for Video	Functional Test	Problem Found (FAIL)	No Problems (PASS)
	1. Wet Foot Test - page 142 YouTube Address: message URL http://youtu.be/ EeG5q4zn8N4	Right Foot ☐ Flat Arch ☐ High Arch Left Foot ☐ Flat Arch ☐ High Arch	Right Foot ☐ Normal Arch Left Foot ☐ Normal Arch
	2. Functional Test for Tibial Nerve Impingement - page 146 YouTube Address: http://youtu.be/ qwbDfG71dgU	☐ Left Side: ☐ Right Side: ☐ Other problems noted during Tibial Nerve Entrapment Test _____ _____	☐ Left Side: Normal ☐ Right Side: Normal

Table 6. 4: Record Results of Optional Tests

Click for Video	Functional Test	Problem Found (FAIL)	No Problems (PASS)
	3. Functional Test for Peroneal Nerve Impingement - page 147 YouTube Address: http://youtu.be/ Ntm_WfSCip0	☐ Left Side: ☐ Right Side: ☐ Other problems noted during Peroneal Nerve Entrapment Test _____ _____	☐ Left Side: Normal ☐ Right Side: Normal

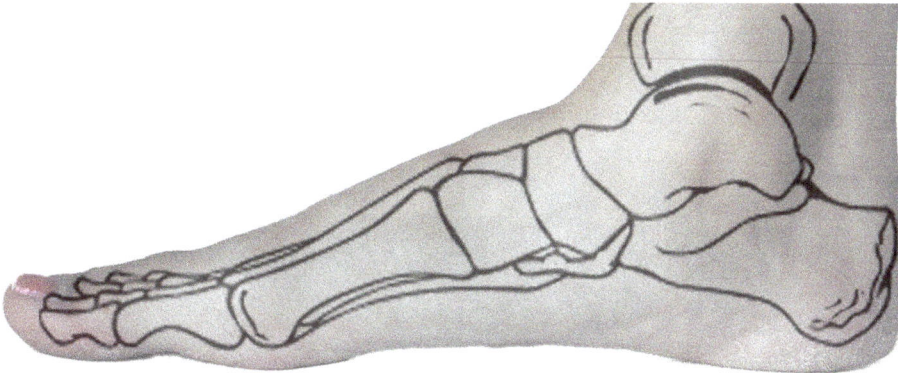

Functional Tests for Joint Mobility

For full resolution of Plantar Fasciitis, it is very important to have good joint mobility in the ankle, foot, and big toe. Ankle dorsiflexion is critical for proper gait, mobility, and the functioning of the foot's kinetic chain. The ankle needs to be mobile and stable, while allowing for both plantar and dorsiflexion of the foot.

In the following example, you can see how poor ankle dorsiflexion can literally affect the entire kinetic chain.

For example, restricted ankle dorsiflexion causes decreased stability in the foot, ankle, knee, hip and back. Even though the action of ankle dorsiflexion involves just one primary action, you can see how almost the entire kinetic chain becomes involved. Hence, multiple problems start to develop, creating a chain of dysfunctions. Unfortunately, each of these new dysfunctions (hip pain, back pain, etc.) can create a cascade of other issues that then perpetuate your Plantar Fasciitis. This is why it is important to address each affected link. otherwise a multitude of other problems can develop along with your Plantar Fasciitis. Similar cascading events can occur due to restrictions in the foot and big toe, once again affecting the entire kinetic web. The following two tests evaluate your joint mobility. Record your results in the table - *Recording Joint Mobility of the Foot and Ankle - page 119.*

Effects of Poor Ankle Dorsiflexion
A Kinetic Chain Example

Copyright 2015: Dr. Brian Abelson and Kamali T. Abelson

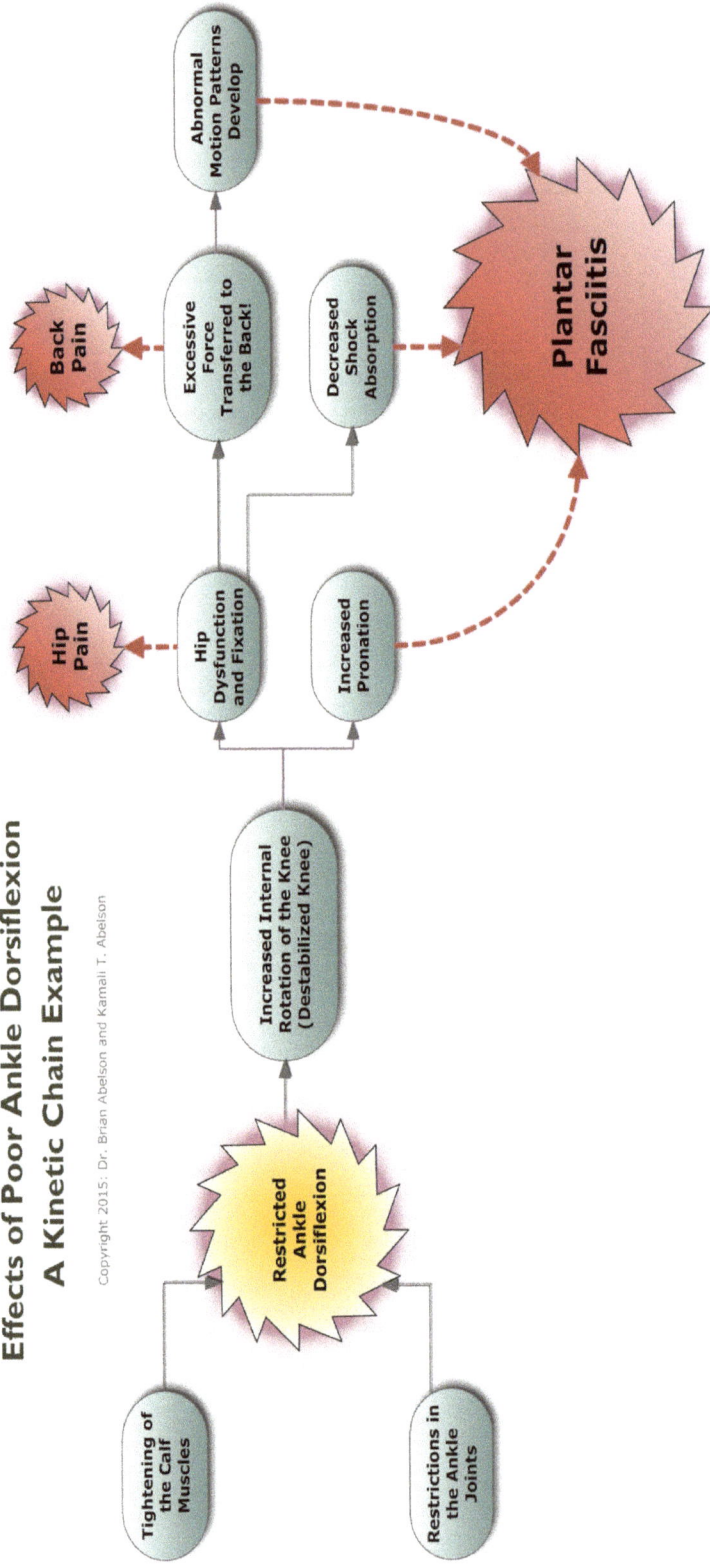

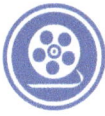

Testing Dorsiflexion of the Ankle

This functional test evaluates the dorsiflexion of your ankle. It is a rather *subtle test*, measured in very small increments, so take your time, and do it carefully. You will need a measuring tape for this test. Be sure to watch the video first!
(YouTube: http://youtu.be/aGPlThv0lQM)

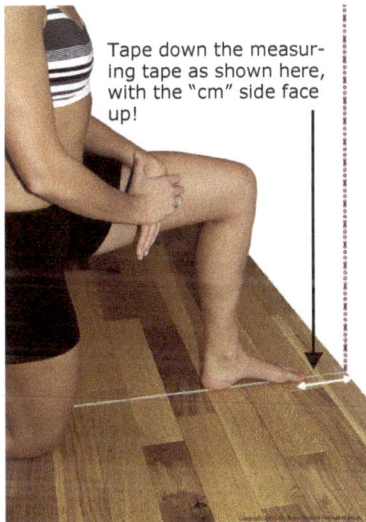

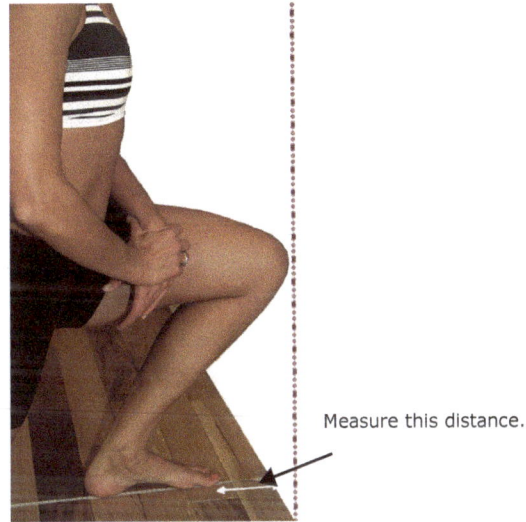

Tape down the measuring tape as shown here, with the "cm" side face up!

Measure this distance.

1. Getting Started:
   - Tape a measuring tape to the floor, making sure the end of it is perpendicular to the wall.

2. Drop down into a kneeling position (as illustrated) with the end of your big toe 10 cm from the wall. Lunge forward and try to touch your knee to the wall. While performing this action, keep your heel down, and drive straight forward over your second toe.
   - If you can touch the wall with your knee, then this will be your starting point of reference.
   - If you cannot reach the wall at 10 cm, move closer until you can reach the wall with your knee. This will then become your starting point of reference.
   - Write down this initial distance.

3. Now, move your foot back in small increments – 0.5 cm at a time – and repeat the forward lunge to the wall. Do this until you find your maximum distance from the wall where you can still touch the wall with your knee.
   - Record this number in *Recording Joint Mobility of the Foot and Ankle on page 119*.
   - This will be a measure of the maximum dorsi flexion for that ankle.

4. Repeat this test for the other ankle, and then compare the two measurements.

Results for Ankle Dorsiflexion Test - If you have a difference of more than two (2) cm between the two legs, it indicates the presence of an imbalance that must be addressed. Mark the test as FAIL if this occurs.

Testing the Mobility of the Big Toe

Having good mobility in the big toe is essential for maintaining normal gait. In this test we will assess two joints – the *metatarsophalangeal joint* (MTP) and the *distal interphalangeal joint* (DIP). (YouTube: http://youtu.be/r0galxQ_beU)

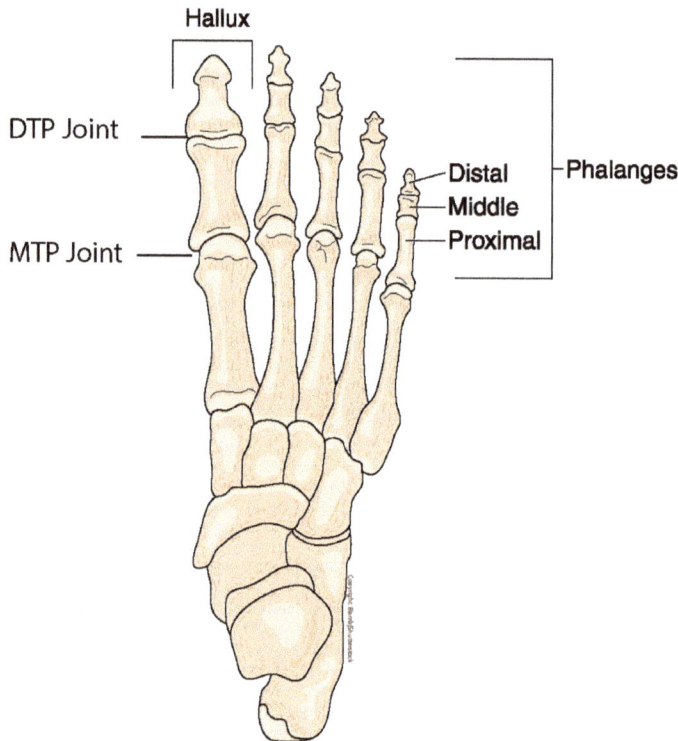

Fig 6.1: DTP and MTP Joints

TIP: We strongly recommend watching the instructional video before attempting this test. This is a very simple test that is well understood after watching the video.

Perform the following two tests to evaluate joint mobility of the DTP and MTP joints in the big toe:

- *Testing the MTP of the Big Toe on page 127.*
- *Testing the DIP of the Big Toe on page 128.*

Testing the MTP of the Big Toe:

1. Getting Started: Take off your shoes and socks.

   ■ Sit down, and cross the leg being tested over the other knee.

2. Test the *metatarsophalangeal joint* (MTP) of the big toe:

   ■ *Lock out the MTP joint* with your hand before performing this test. If you don't do this, you will get invalid test results.

   ■ Test mobility of the MTP in the following six positions: *Flexion, extension, adduction, abduction, clockwise rotation* and *counter-clockwise rotation*.

   ■ Record any restriction that you experience during these tests in *Recording Joint Mobility of the Foot and Ankle on page 119*.

   ■ Continue to Step 3 - Testing the *distal interphalangeal joint (DIP)*.

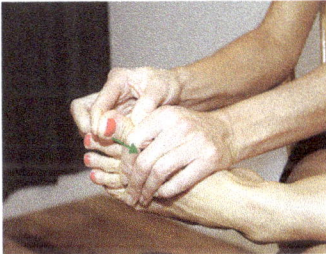
Extension, straighten and extend the big toe.

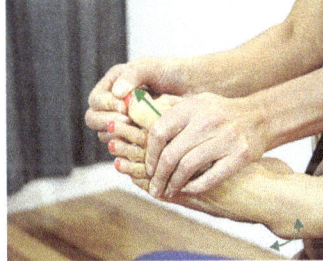
Flexion, curl your big toe downwards.

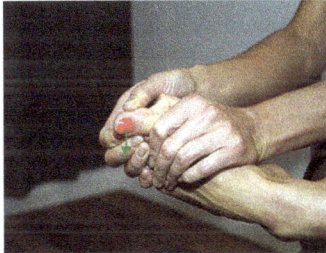
Adduction, bring the big toe towards the others!

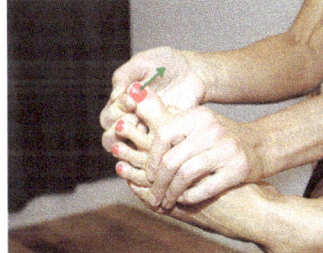
Abduction, move the big toe away from the others!

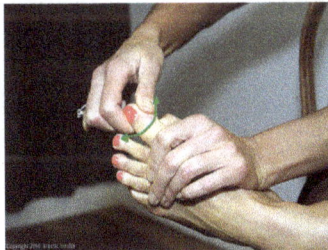
Gently rotate the MTP joint of the big toe.

Testing the DIP of the Big Toe:

1. Now, test the *distal interphalangeal joint* (DIP). Again, test this joint in six positions:

    ■ It is very important to *lock out the DIP joint* with your hand before performing this test.

    ■ Test mobility of the DIP in the following six positions: *Flexion, extension, adduction, abduction, clockwise rotation* and *counter-clockwise rotations.*

    ■ Record any restrictions that you experience during these tests in *Recording Joint Mobility of the Foot and Ankle on page 119.*

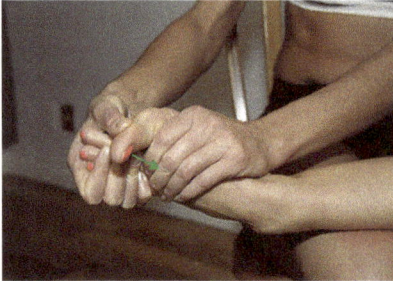

Extension...straighten and extend the big toe.

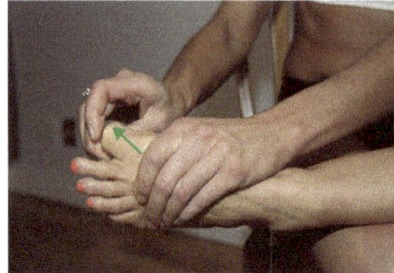

Flexion...curl your big toe downwards.

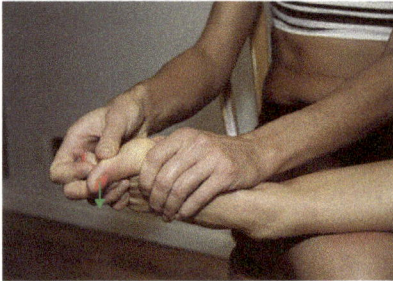

Adduction, bring the big toe towards the others.

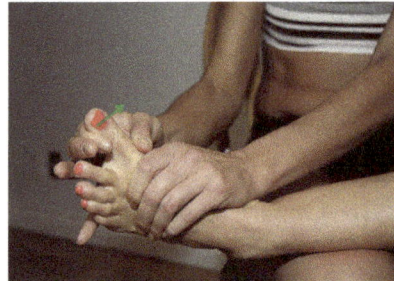

Abduction, move the big toe away from others.

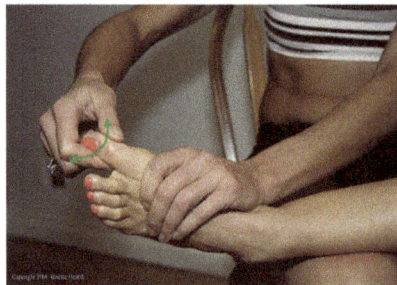

Gently rotate the DIP joint of the big toe.

Functional Tests for the Legs and Hips

You will be performing three (3) functional tests to evaluate structures ranging from your hips to your knees. These three tests will help you to identify if restrictions or muscle imbalances in these structures are a contributing factor to your Plantar Fasciitis. The tests are:

- *Testing Hip Flexion (Thomas Test) - page 130.*
- *Testing Stability of the Lower Extremity - Deep Squat - page 131.*
- *Testing Hamstring Flexibility on page 135.*

Record your results in *Carry out the Functional Tests for Joint Mobility - page 123 to see if joint mobility is a factor in the development of your Plantar Fasciitis. Print the following test assessment sheet and record your results on the hard-copy. - page 119.*

Testing Hip Flexion (Thomas Test)

The Thomas Test is a quick and effective way to assess the flexibility of the muscles that are involved in hip flexion (*psoas, iliacus,* and *rectus femoris*).
(YouTube: http://youtu.be/8D5_fmlbqYk)

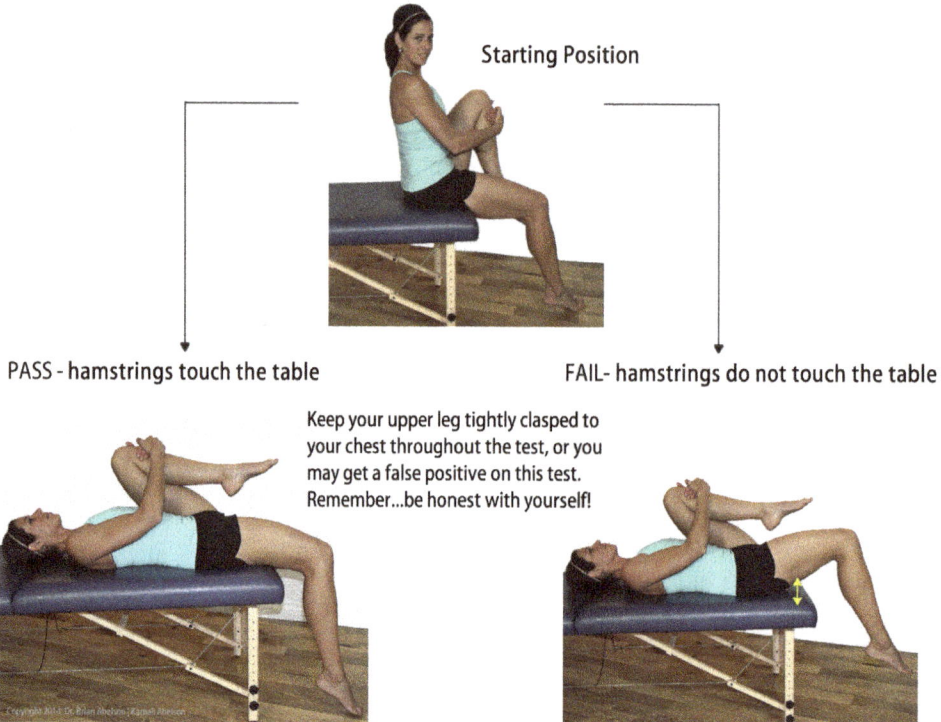

Starting Position

PASS - hamstrings touch the table   FAIL- hamstrings do not touch the table

Keep your upper leg tightly clasped to your chest throughout the test, or you may get a false positive on this test. Remember...be honest with yourself!

TIP: Ask your friend or partner to videotape you as you perform this test. The camera on your cell phone is a convenient tool for recording and viewing your performance. Record both the front and side views of this exercise.

---

1. Starting Position: Sit on the edge of a stable bench or table. Sit right on the bony area of your buttocks (your *ischial tuberosities*)
    - Lift one knee up to your chest, and clasp it with your hands.
    - While *still holding that knee* tight to your chest, lie back (face-up) on the table.
    - Keep both your head and your low back in contact with the table throughout the test. If you allow either your head or your lower back to arch upwards, you will get an invalid test result.
2. Now allow the other leg to drop down, off the edge of the bench.
    - If the back of your leg (*hamstrings*) touches the table, then you have good flexibility in your hip flexors. You can then mark this test as a PASS for that side of your body.
    - If the back of your leg is even slightly off the table, then you have tight hip flexors. Mark this test as a FAIL.

3. Repeat this entire sequence for the other leg and record those results in the table *Carry out the Functional Tests for Joint Mobility - page 123 to see if joint mobility is a factor in the development of your Plantar Fasciitis. Print the following test assessment sheet and record your results on the hard-copy. on page 119*.

Caution: If you do not keep your leg tightly clasped to your chest, you may falsely believe that you have passed this test. When you watch your video, make sure that you have done this test with good form, or you will get invalid results.

Results for Hip Flexion Test - Look at your video (front and side views) to evaluate how *close to horizontal* your lower leg is?

- Does your leg remain tightly clasped to your chest throughout the test. If not, you have to redo the test.
- If your leg is horizontal with the table, or even below the table, then you have good hip flexion. You can then mark this test as a *PASS* result.
- If your leg remains above the table, and you are unable to drop your leg parallel to the table surface *without arching your back*, then you have tight hip flexors. You can then mark this test as FAIL.

Testing Stability of the Lower Extremity - Deep Squat

The Deep Squat is an excellent functional test for assessing motion, synchronization, and stability in the hip, knee, and ankle as they move through a controlled sequence of actions. Difficulties in performing this test can indicate that you have (or will develop) abnormal motion patterns that can cause instabilities in the lower extremities, and eventually lead to Plantar Fasciitis. (YouTube: http://youtu.be/_qhE2wxbSts)

In this test, you will need to observe your motions from both the front (anterior) and side (lateral) positions. Therefore, you will need the assistance of a friend to videotape your actions as you perform the test. Fortunately, just about every phone now has video capablities...so it is easy to do this.

Abnormal, motion patterns during this test can be an indication of poor joint mobility, lack of muscle activation (are the muscles of the hip firing in the proper sequence), or lack of neuromuscular control.

TIP: In order to easily observe the motion of your body as you perform this test, you should wear shorts with no shoes or socks. You should also videotape this test from *both the front view, and the side or lateral view* since it is easy to overlook problems without careful analysis.

Deep Squat - Front View

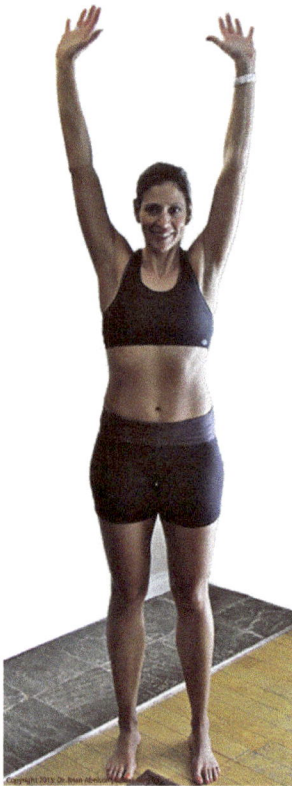

Notice how our model's hip
is dropping down
on her right side.

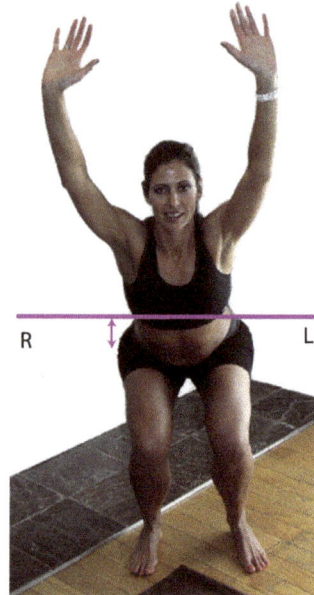

R   L

TIP: Ask your friend or partner to videotape you as you perform this test. The camera on your cell phone is a convenient tool for recording and viewing your performance. Record both the front and side views of this exercise.

1. Stand with feet shoulder-width apart, your arms raised over your head, and the elbows fully extended.

   ■ If you look from the side, your arms should bisect the middle of your body.

2. Slowly squat down (as illustrated) to approximately the height of a chair, then return to the starting position. Repeat this action five times.

   ■ As you perform your squat, sit back into the squat position by bending at your hips first. Try NOT to bend forward at the waist during the squat.
   ■ Try to drop your hips *below* the knees.
   ■ Do not look down when performing the squat.
   ■ Do not allow your heels to come off the ground.

3. Rise back up to your starting position, maintaining good form by raising both your hips and shoulders up at the same rate.

4. Repeat this process five (5) times, while being videotaped from the front.

5. Analyze the anterior view of your deep squat as shown in:

   ■ *Results of your Anterior View of the Deep Squat Test - page 134.*

Deep Squat - Lateral View

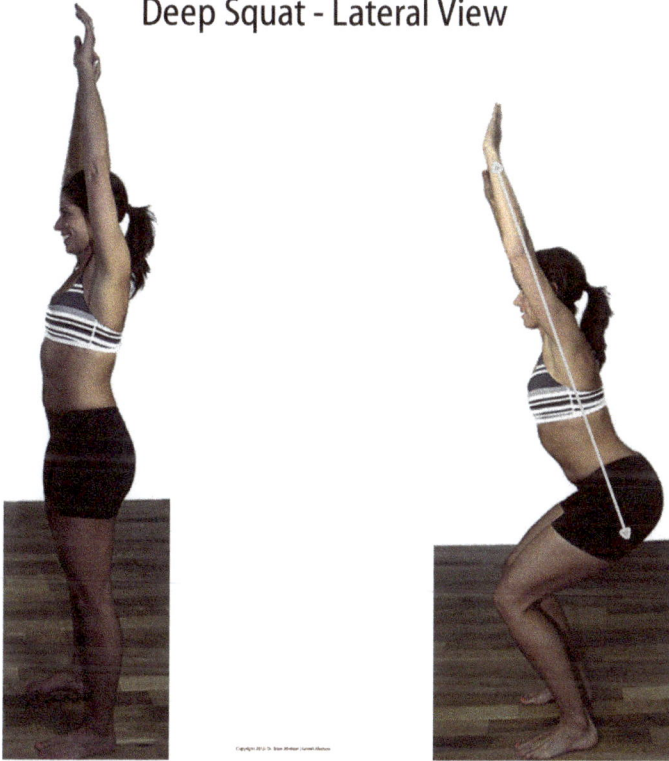

6. Repeat the entire sequence, but this time videotape your actions from the lateral or side view.

7. Analyze the lateral view of your deep squat as shown in:

   ■ *Results of your Lateral View of the Deep Squat Test - page 135.*

Results of your Anterior View of the Deep Squat Test - Your body should move as a single functional unit, with smooth coordination between the motions of your feet, ankles, knees, hips, and core.

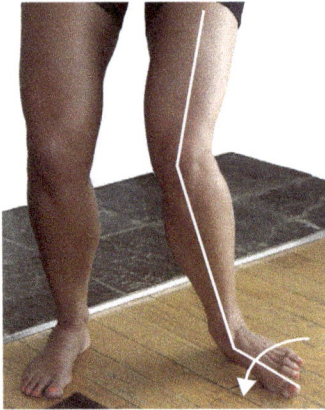

Mark your test as a FAIL if the arches of your feet collapse inwards or your knees point in a different direction than your toes.

This is an indication that your gluteals are deactivated.

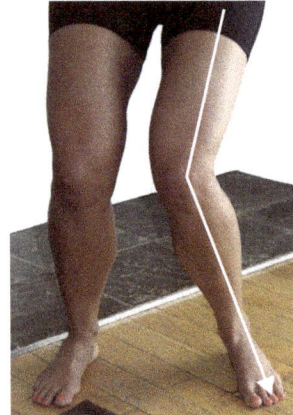

Observe the video of yourself performing the squat and evaluate for the following:

- Are you able to maintain your arms above your head (PASS) or do your arms fall forward as you squat (FAIL)?
- Does one hip drop lower than the other hip (FAIL)? See the picture on *page 131*
- Are the arches of your feet collapsing inwards (FAIL)?
- Are your knees pointing forward in the same direction as your toes (PASS) or are your knees deviating inwards or outwards (FAIL)?
- Are you able to keep your heels on the ground throughout the squat (PASS) or are your heels lifting off the ground (FAIL)?
- Does your back arch or are you leaning forward (FAIL)?

When you observe the results of this test, look for the following:

Table 6. 5: Results of Anterior View of Deep Squat Test

Anterior View: PASS Finding	Anterior View: FAIL Finding
Enter 'PASS' if, for all repetitions, you are able to: - Maintain steady form throughout the test. - Your feet remain aligned straight. - Your knees remain aligned with your feet, and do not extend past your toes.	Enter 'FAIL' if you find that: - Either foot is deviating outwards. - Either hip drops lower than the other. - The arches of either foot are collapsing inwards. - Either knee deviates inwards, or rotates internally. - Either heel lifts off the ground.

Results of your Lateral View of the Deep Squat Test - Once again, as you review the lateral view of your deep squat test, you are looking for the following.

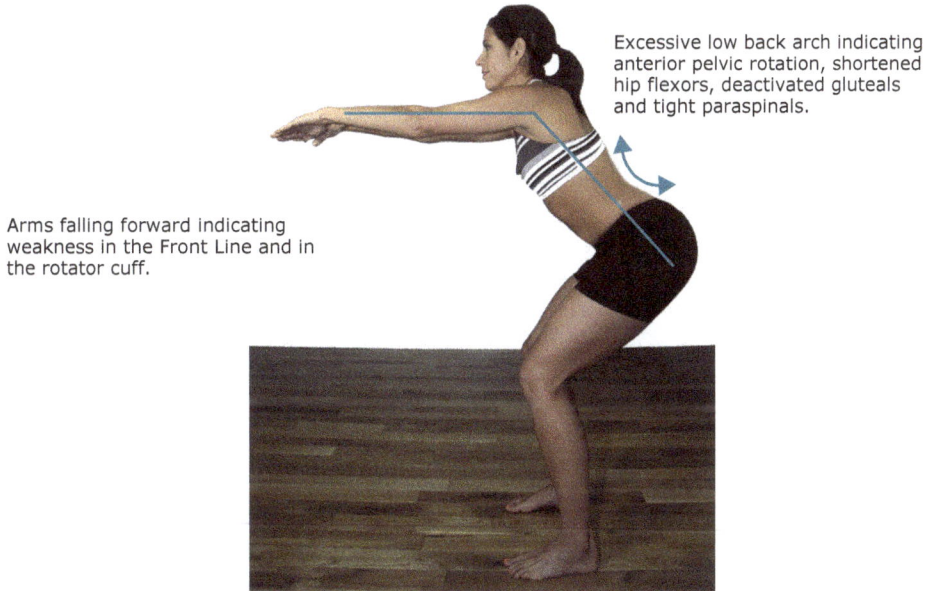

Excessive low back arch indicating anterior pelvic rotation, shortened hip flexors, deactivated gluteals and tight paraspinals.

Arms falling forward indicating weakness in the Front Line and in the rotator cuff.

Table 6. 6: Results of Lateral View of Deep Squat Test

Lateral View: PASS Finding	Lateral View: FAIL Finding
Enter 'PASS' if, for all repetitions, you are able to: ■ If you are *able* to draw a straight line through hip, lumbar spine, shoulder and arm.	Enter 'FAIL' if you find that: ■ You are excessively arching your low back. ■ You are unable to draw a straight line through hip, lumbar spine, shoulder and arm. ■ Your arms drop from the raised position.

Testing Hamstring Flexibility

It is very important to test hamstring flexibility since tight hamstrings have a direct influence on the plantar fascia. See *The Role of the Hamstrings and Quadriceps in PF on page 73* for a more detailed description about how tight hamstrings affect your kinetic chain, gait, and plantar fascia.

To test hamstring flexibility - It is important to perform this test correctly. For example, simply bending over and touching your toes is NOT a good indication that your hamstrings are flexible. This is because you can easily compensate with the muscles of your lower back (lumbar spine) to make it look as if you are flexible, when in actuality, you are not.
(YouTube: http://youtu.be/3ISivoJxmmk. 1.51 min)

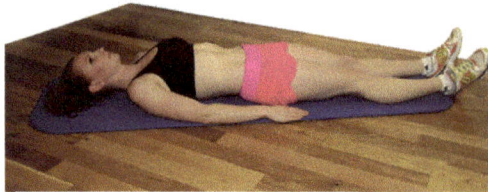

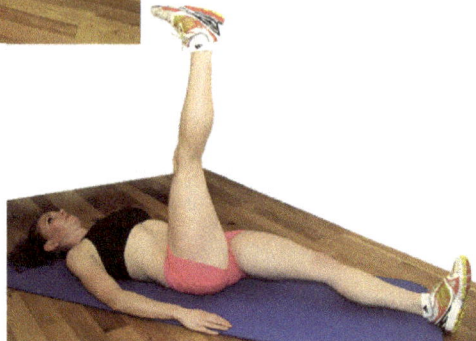

TIP: This test should be observed and videotaped to make it easier to evaluate your results. For convenience, use your cell phone camera! Record both your front and side view.

1. Starting Position: Lie flat on the ground, legs extended and parallel to each other, head resting on the ground, and arms outstretched.
   - Press your low back into the ground, while keeping your head on the ground.
2. Flex your foot (dorsi-flex), lock your knee into it's straight position, and raise that leg up as high as you can (80-to-90° degrees is normal).
   - Do NOT allow either your low back or head to come off the floor.
   - Hold this position for a few seconds. Note how high you are able to raise your leg.
3. Repeat this test for the other leg.
4. Evaluate the video as follows.

Results of Hamstring Flexibility Test - Review the video of yourself doing the hamstring flexibility test. Enter FAIL in the form if you find any of the following in your video:

- Your head or lower back comes off the floor.
- You are unable to raise either of your legs without arching your back, lifting your head, or bending your knee.
- You cannot raise your legs to 80-to-90° degrees off the floor.
- There is a large difference between the flexibility of your two legs.

Testing Core Functionality

You will need to perform three (3) functional core tests. These tests will evaluate your core stability from three directions: *anterior, lateral* and *posterior*. It is very important to perform all three test to get a true picture of your core stability. Remember, being strong in only one direction does not indicate that you have a strong core. A FAIL in any of these three tests indicates that you need to strengthen your core.

Core Stability Test 1: Anterior Plank with Alternating Leg - page 137
(YouTube: http://www.youtube.com/watch?v=wDTJx_9iNqk, 1.24 min)

Core Stability Test 2: Side Bridge with Leg Lift - page 139
(YouTube: http://www.youtube.com/watch?v=wDTJx_9iNqk, 3.00 min)

Core Stability Test 3: Pelvic Raise - Testing the Posterior Chain - page 140
(YouTube: http://www.youtube.com/watch?v=x4HsuvN0T9c)

Core Stability Test 1: Anterior Plank with Alternating Leg

This test is a great way to test your core strength, muscle activation, and neuromuscular control. The Anterior Plank (front bridge) is a common exercise used to strengthen the core. In this case, we will use this exercise to evaluate your core and its relationship to your lower extremities. (
YouTube: http://www.youtube.com/watch?v=wDTJx_9iNqk, 1.24 min)

TIP: Ask your friend or partner to videotape you as you perform this test. The camera on your cell phone is a convenient tool for recording and viewing your performance. Record both the front and side views of this exercise.

1. Lie flat on your stomach with your legs fully extended.
2. Place your elbows shoulder-width apart, hands directly in front of your elbows.
3. Part 1: Lift your body up off the ground, into an anterior plank position, so that only your elbows and toes are supporting the weight of your body.
   - Do not allow your spine to curve down or up.
   - Keep your shoulders relaxed and do not hunch.
4. Your body should form a straight line, from your head to your toes. To test this:
   - Ask a friend to place a broom handle on your back. Ideally the broom handle should touch three points: glutes, mid-back, and head.
   - Hold this position for 15 seconds.

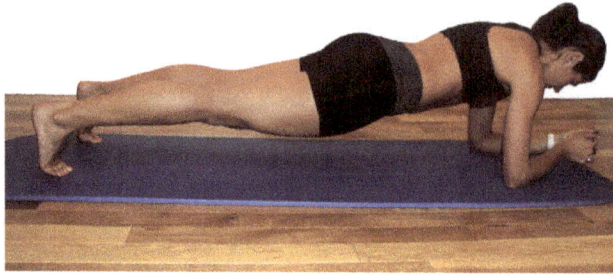

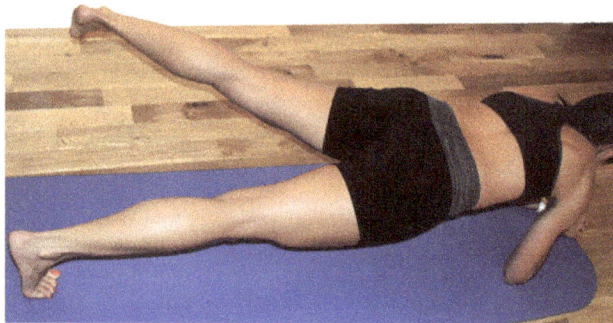

5. Part 2: While still in the plank position, raise your left leg off of the ground and bring it out to the left (as illustrated) and hold for 15 seconds. Be sure to keep that foot off the ground.

6. Return your left leg to the starting position and repeat step 5 for the right leg.

Results for Core Stability Test I: Review the video of yourself doing this test and record your results in *Recording Functional Test Results for the Core on page 121*:

- Enter PASS if you can complete this entire routine with good form (no tilting, collapsing, or shaking).
- Enter FAIL if you cannot hold this position, or if there is a considerable difference between your right or left side, as this indicates that you need to work on your core stability.

Core Stability Test 2: Side Bridge with Leg Lift

The Side Bridge is a great test of your core stability since it activates a large percentage of your core muscles, including both the upper and lower back muscles, *abdominal obliques, rectus abdominus, quadratus lumborum,* and *hip abductor muscles.* (YouTube: http://youtu.be/wDTJx_9iNqk, 3.11 minutes)

1. Lie on your side as shown in the image.

2. Lift your body up off the ground so that your forearm and your feet are supporting the weight of your body as shown in the image.

   ■ Your body should form a straight line, from your head to your feet.
   ■ Do not allow your spine to curve forward or backward.
   ■ Do not allow your body to sag or drop.

3. Hold this position for 15 seconds.

4. Then try to raise your leg, and hold this raised position for 10 seconds and return to the starting position.

5. Repeat this entire procedure for the other side.

Results for Core Stability Test 2: **Review** the video of yourself doing this test and record your results in *Recording Functional Test Results for the Core on page 121*:

■ Enter PASS if you can complete this entire routine with good form (no tilting, collapsing, or shaking).

■ Enter FAIL if you cannot hold this position, or if there is a considerable difference between your right or left side, as this indicates that you need to work on your core stability.

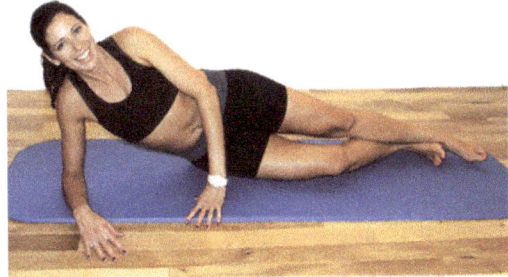

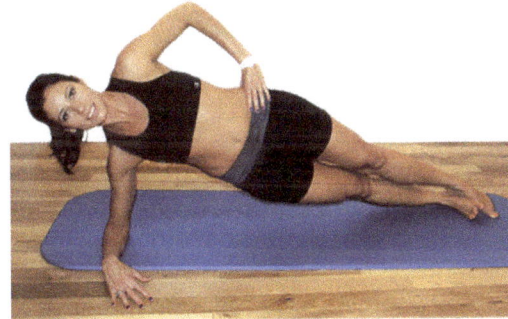

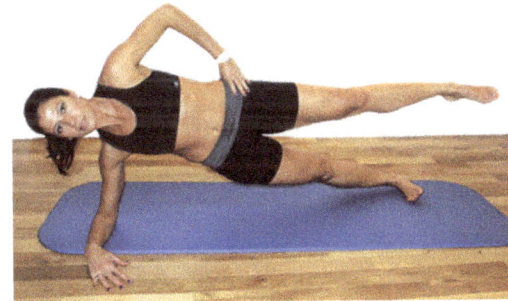

TIP: Ask your friend or partner to videotape you as you perform this test. The camera on your cell phone is a convenient tool for recording and viewing your performance. Record both the front and side views of this exercise.

Core Stability Test 3: Pelvic Raise - Testing the Posterior Chain

The structures of the Posterior Chain - *gluteus maximus* and *hamstrings* (*gracilis, semitendinosus, biceps femoris,* and *semimembranosus*) play an important role in maintaining good muscular balance throughout the core.

A weak posterior chain reduces your strength when performing lunges, squats, jumps, and walking/running. A strong posterior chain, that is well balanced with its anterior chain, protects you from injury, and increases the amount of power you are able to generate through your lower extremities.

To pass this test, you will need to show that you are able to stabilize the posterior chain of muscles in your back, pelvis, and legs. This is a very effective test for evaluating joint stability, muscle activation, and neuromuscular control. Watch the video before performing this test. (YouTube: http://youtu.be/wDTJx_9iNqk, 6.24 minutes)

1. Starting Position: Lay on your back with your knees bent and your arms by your side.
   - Raise your hips up until your abdomen, pelvis, and the tops of your legs form a flat plane.
2. Hold this position, and straighten one leg out, while keeping the top of the thigh parallel with the other thigh.
   - Hold this position for 15 seconds, then return to the starting position.
   - Hold the leg extended and straight without rotating or tipping the pelvis.
   - Hold the leg extended and straight without dropping the leg.
   - Keep your pelvis up.
   - Do not allow your pelvis to rotate or tip as you perform this movement.
3. Now, while maintaining good form, slowly move the straight leg up and down as shown in the video.
   - Repeat this five (5) times, while always keeping the pelvis in neutral position, with no rotation, tipping or dropping.
4. Repeat this test for the other leg.

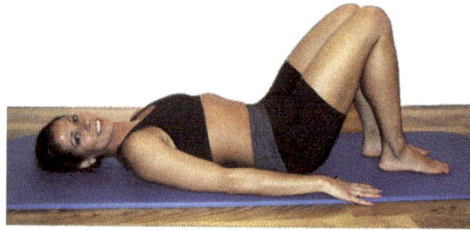

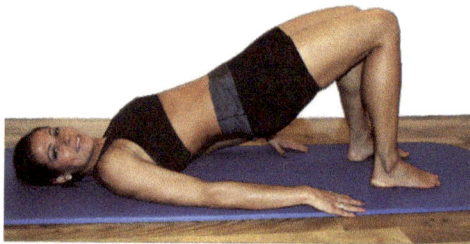

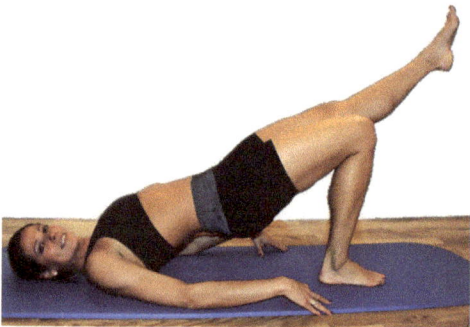

TIP: Ask your friend or partner to videotape you as you perform this test. The camera on your cell phone is a convenient tool for recording and viewing your performance. Record both the front and side views of this exercise.

Results for Core Stability Test 3: Evaluate your performance. Record your results in *Recording Functional Test Results for the Core on page 121*. You should be able to:

- Hold the leg extended and straight without rotating or tipping the pelvis.
- Hold the leg extended and straight without dropping the leg.
- Easily hold your pelvis in a flat-table top position, in both the non-extended and extended leg positions.
- Perform this exercise without experiencing muscle cramping in the *hamstrings*.
- How close to horizontal is your straight leg?
- Are you able to maintain good form with no rotation, tipping, or tilting of the pelvis?

Enter PASS if you are able to easily perform this exercise.

Enter FAIL if you have any trouble performing this test (leg drops, pelvis tips or rotates, or if you experience pain, cramping, or muscle exhaustion during the test). All these are signs of tight hip flexors, and are an indication that you have trouble stabilizing the structures of the lower extremity.

Optional Tests

The following three optional tests provide additional information about your kinetic chain and its associated structures. You may want to perform these tests to identify any additional issues that may be impacting the resolution of your Plantar Fasciitis. These tests will help you to identify if excessive pronation/supination or nerve impingements are impacting your case. See:

- *Wet Foot Test on page 142*.
- *Functional Test for Tibial Nerve Impingement on page 146*.
- *Functional Test for Peroneal Nerve Impingement on page 147*

Record your results in the *Recording Results of Optional Tests on page 122*.

Wet Foot Test

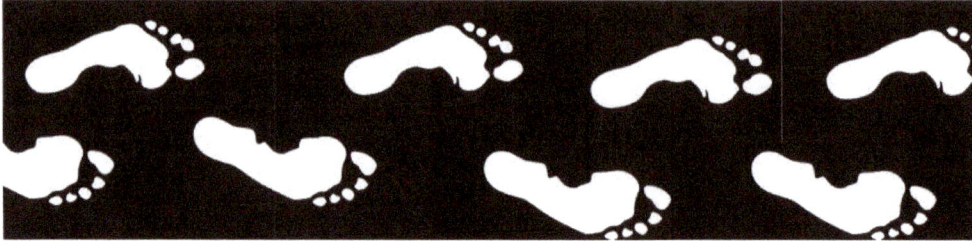

Certain arch types have been associated with an increase in the probability of developing Plantar Fasciitis. Use this simple optional test to identify the *type of arch* in your foot and your *foot type*.

This test can help you to determine the type of shoes that are correct for your body. This test will also help you to determine if you have a normal gait pattern, or excessive pronation or supination patterns. At our *Kinetic Health Clinic*, we often combine this test with motion and gait analysis to obtain an even more accurate diagnosis.

This is an important test to conduct BEFORE you begin your custom exercise program. It is important to wear the right type of shoes before exercising, and during your daily living activities, otherwise, you may exacerbate the problems you are currently having.

To discover your foot type - This test will help to determine what type of shoe support you require. All you need is a shallow basin of water and some heavy-weight, colored paper or a brown paper bag. (YouTube: http://youtu.be/EeG5q4zn8N4)

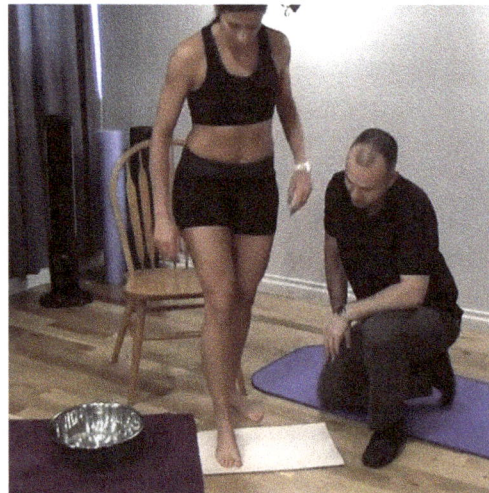

1. Dip the soles of your feet in water.
2. Step briefly onto a tile or on a piece of coloured paper to make an impression of both your feet. It is important to do this in a *weight-bearing* stance (standing up).
3. Look at the type of impression your feet made.

4. Evaluate the results as per the following information and record your results on the form called *Recording Results of Optional Tests on page 122*.
5. Evaluate your results as follows:
   - *Results - Do you have a Normal Arch? on page 143.*
   - *Results - Do you have a Flat Arch? on page 143.*
   - *Results - Do you have a High Arch? on page 144.*

Results - Do you have a Normal Arch? If you have this pattern, then you are a normal pronator.

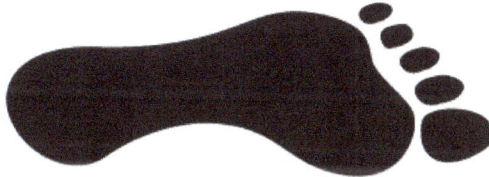

Fig 6.1: Normal Arch

You have a normal arch if your impression looks like this, and your arch is approximately half the width of your foot. This pattern indicates that in all probability:

- You likely strike the floor with your heel when you walk or run. Your foot would then typically roll inwards, and the foot's arch collapses *slightly* inwards (pronates) to absorb the shock of foot impact.
- You probably have normal supination and normal pronation motions in your foot. Remember, some pronation and supination is an important part of the normal shock absorption mechanisms of the foot.
- You either need a **neutral shoe**, or a shoe with **minimal arch support** and some **medial stability** to prevent injuries.

There is usually no need for custom fit orthotics if you have a normal arch. The exceptions are when you are working on concrete floors or are required to spend long hours on your feet.

Results - Do you have a Flat Arch? If your impression shows the entire sole of your foot, then you are most likely flat-footed.

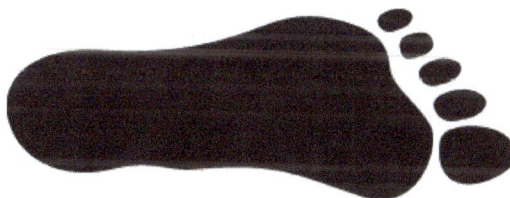

Fig 6.2: Flat-foot Arch

This pattern indicates that in all probability:

- You are prone to abnormal pronation.
- You probably strike the ground on the outside of the heel, and roll excessively inwards.
- Your arch probably collapses inwards too much after foot-strike, resulting in excessive foot motion and an increased risk of injury.
- You probably over-pronate, especially if you have weak hip muscles (external rotators). Strengthening the hip muscles can reduce the over-pronation, and the need for orthotics.
- You may need motion-control shoes for severe pronation, or stability shoes with supportive posts for mild to medium pronation.

You may need orthotics in your shoes. However, I would recommend that you *first* resolve any weakness in the hips, before deciding whether you need orthotics. Remember, some of this over-pronation can often be corrected by strengthening weak gluteal muscles, at which point, the need for orthotics may be eliminated.

Results - Do you have a High Arch? If your impression shows just the ball of your foot, heels, and a narrow line along the arch, then you have a high arch (least common).

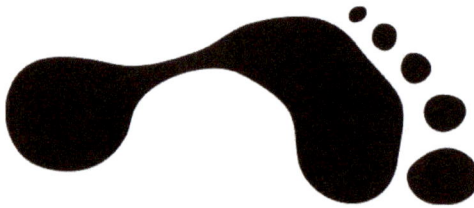

Fig 6.3: High Arch

If this is the case:

- You are prone to abnormal supination.
- Your arch does not collapse enough (under-pronation) to absorb the shock of foot strike, resulting in the force travelling up your leg and injuring structures along that kinetic chain.
- You need shoes with no added stability, softer mid-soles, and normal cushioning to reduce the excessive supination of your foot.
- Do NOT select shoes that reduce or control pronation – that is – do NOT use stability or motion control shoes.
- The best shoe for under-pronators is a neutral shoe, as these shoes have a softer mid-sole to encourage pronation.

Before purchasing orthotics, you need to strengthen any weakness along your foot's kinetic chain before determining if orthotics are necessary.

Effects of Excessive Pronation

Excessive pronation of the foot often results in:

- Calcaneal eversion during pronation.
- Increased tractional forces being placed on the *plantar fascia*.
- Excessive internal *tibial* rotation
- Lowering of the foot's arch.
- Excessive weight being placed on the big toe (*first metatarsal-phalangeal joint*).
- Formation of calluses and bunions.
- Hypermobility of the *metatarsals* can also cause a *Morton's Neuroma* to form. A simple squeeze test of the foot will often show you if this is the case.
- Heel spurs on the *calcaneus* are formed to compensate for these stresses, and are not themselves the cause of Plantar Fasciitis.

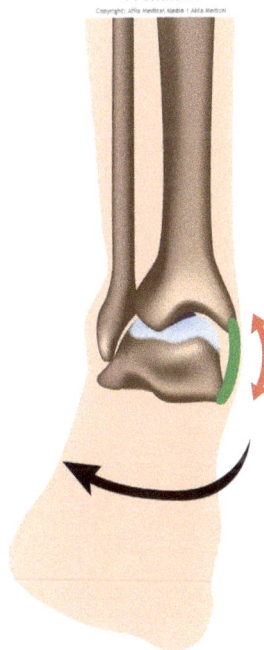

Calcaneus Eversion of the foot caused by excessive **Pronation**

Effects of Excessive Supination

Excessive supination of the foot often results in:

- Calcaneal inversion during pronation.
- External tibial rotation.
- Foot's arch does not collapse enough due to under-pronation, leading to poor shock absorption in the Gait Cycle.
- Weight bearing occurs on the outside edge of the foot, causing increased stress on the 4th and 5th metatarsal-phalangeal joints.
- Formation of calluses on the foot.
- Increased risk of inversion sprains or injury to the cuboid due to foot positioning during gait.

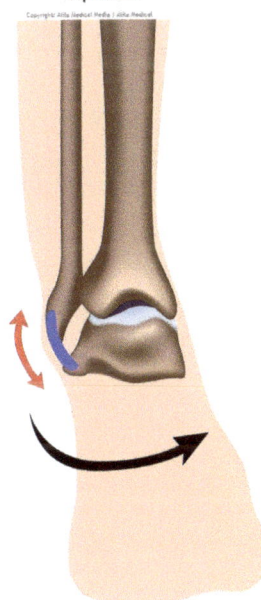

Calcaneus Inversion of the foot caused by excessive **Supination**

Functional Test for Tibial Nerve Impingement

The *tibial nerve* is often involved in sciatica as well as in foot pain. In your foot the *tibial nerve* divides into *medial and lateral plantar nerves*. Altered sensations in the foot could be due to compression of these nerves. Nerve impingements, or compressions of the *tibial nerve,* can negatively impact the long-term resolution of Plantar Fasciitis. The following simple evaluation will help you to determine if *tibial nerve* impingement is a factor in your Plantar Fasciitis. See *Common Nerve Compression Sites for PF on page 87* for more information.

(YouTube: http://youtu.be/qwbDfG71dgU)

TIP: It is best to have a partner assist you in performing this test.

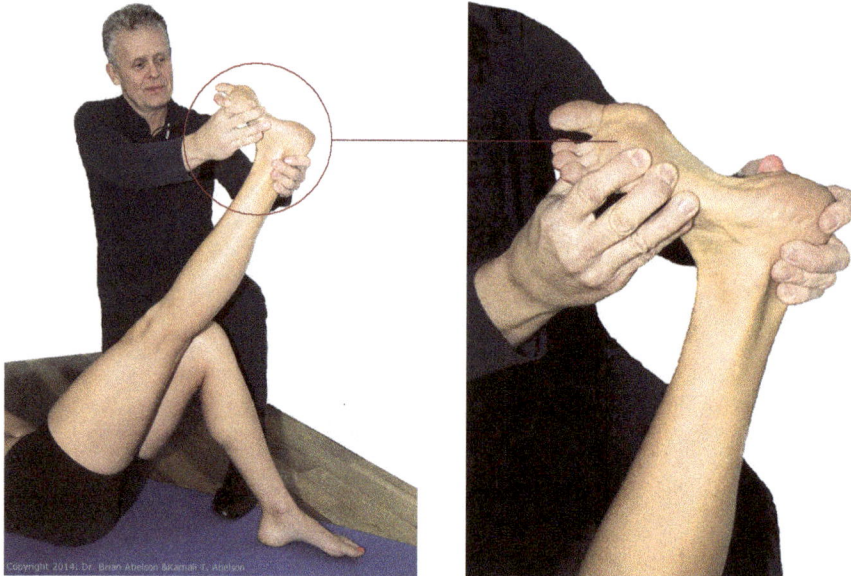

1. Starting Position: This is a **3-part test.** Note your results for each part of the test.
    - Lie face up, with the leg to be tested lying straight and with the knee extended, and its foot in an everted (turned outward), dorsi-flexed position (pulled back towards your body).
    - Ask your friend to grasp your foot, and *evert* (turn outwards) the foot even further, as shown in the above diagram.
2. **FIRST**: Raise your leg to about 35 degrees, keeping your foot in the everted position throughout. This position will help to stretch the *tibial nerve.*
    - Note any changes in symptoms (tingling, burning, sharp pain, or altered sensation) along the foot and lower leg. This is an indication that the *tibial nerve* could be involved in your problem.

3. **SECOND**: Slowly raise the leg higher (keeping the foot everted) and note if any nerve symptoms increase or change. This includes symptoms such as: *tingling, burning, sharp pain, or altered sensations*. This is an indication that the tibial nerve is involved in your problem.

4. **THIRD**: Do this portion if there is NO increase in symptoms during the SECOND part of the test.
   - Flex your neck forward.
   - Move your hip inward (adducted).
   - Note if any nerve symptoms increase or change. This includes symptoms such as: *tingling, burning, sharp pain, or altered sensations*. This is an indication that the *tibial nerve* is involved in your problem.

5. Repeat this entire test for the other leg if you have Plantar Fasciitis on both feet.

Results for Tibial Nerve Entrapment - If you experience any symptomatic changes in steps 2 through 5, then mark this test as a **FAIL** on your form for *Recording Results of Optional Tests on page 122*. This indicates that you will need to add *tibial nerve* flossing exercises to your exercise protocol.

See *Phase 2: Addressing Problems in the PF Kinetic Chain on page 149* for more details about how to release these entrapped or restricted nerves.

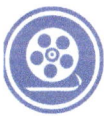

Functional Test for Peroneal Nerve Impingement

The peroneal nerve, which is a branch of the sciatic nerve, innervates muscles along the side of the leg (peroneus longus, peroneus brevis, and the short head of the biceps femoris). This nerve has both sensory and motor functions and, when injured, can lead to decreased ankle and foot stability. Entrapment of this nerve can effect the function of these muscles and may manifest as foot drop and numbness and tingling along the side of the leg. This can lead to abnormal walking and running patterns that can eventually lead to the development of Plantar Fasciitis.

Peroneal Nerve Test - This is a simple test you can perform to see if you have a *Common Peroneal Nerve* entrapment. The *peroneal nerve* is often injured in ankle sprains, but can also be involved in sciatica. You will need someone to assist you to perform this test. (YouTube: http://youtu.be/Ntm_WfSCip0)

TIP: It is best to have a partner assist you in performing this test.

---

1. Starting Position:
   - Lie face up, with your knees bent, and feet flat on the ground.
2. Assistant: Raise one leg until the thigh is perpendicular to the floor.
   - Keep the foot and ankle relaxed
   - Keep that knee slightly bent.

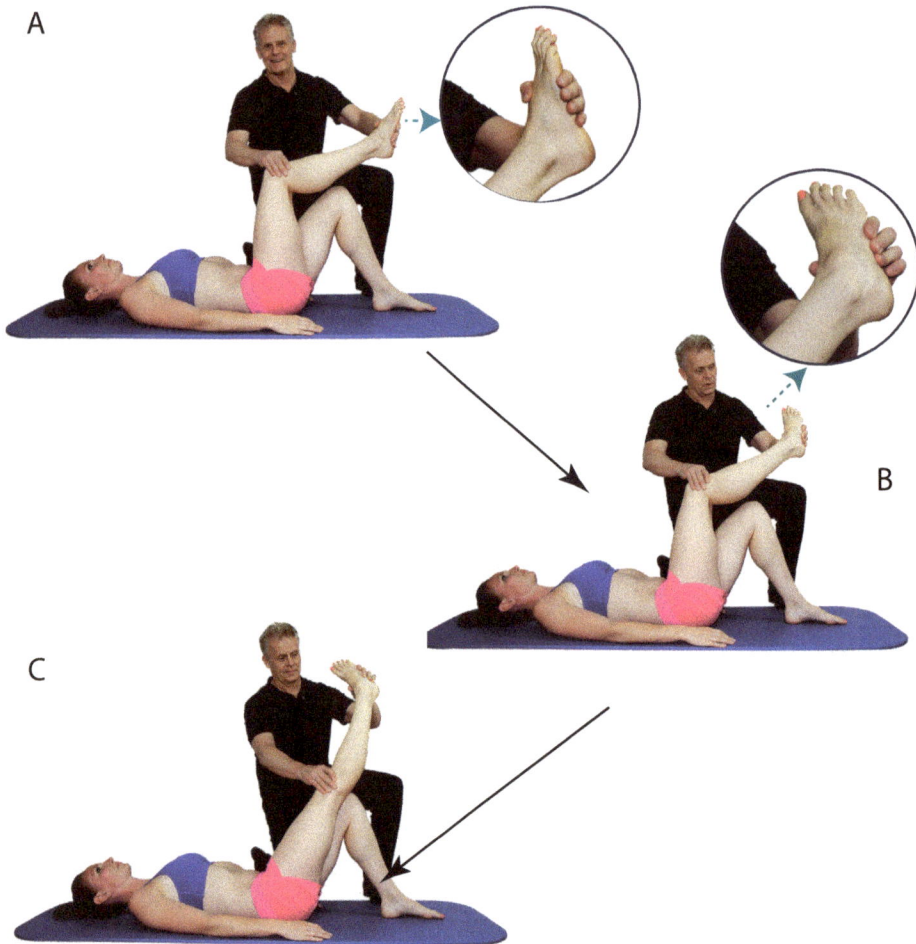

Copyright 2014: Kinetic Health | Dr. Brian Abelson

3. Assistant: Place one hand on the knee, and the other on the bottom of the foot.
   - Invert the foot (turn it towards the center of the body).
   - With the food inverted, straighten the leg.
   - Observe the effects.
4. Assistant: Repeat for the other leg.

Results for Peroneal Nerve Entrapment: If there are problems with **entrapment** of the *peroneal nerve*, you will feel numbness, tingling, and pain along the outside of the lower leg, ankle, or foot.

If this occurs, mark this test as a **FAIL** on your form for *Recording Results of Optional Tests on page 122*. This indicates that you will need to add *peroneal nerve* flossing exercises to your exercise protocol.

See *Phase 2: Addressing Problems in the PF Kinetic Chain - page 149* for more details about how to release these entrapped or restricted nerves.

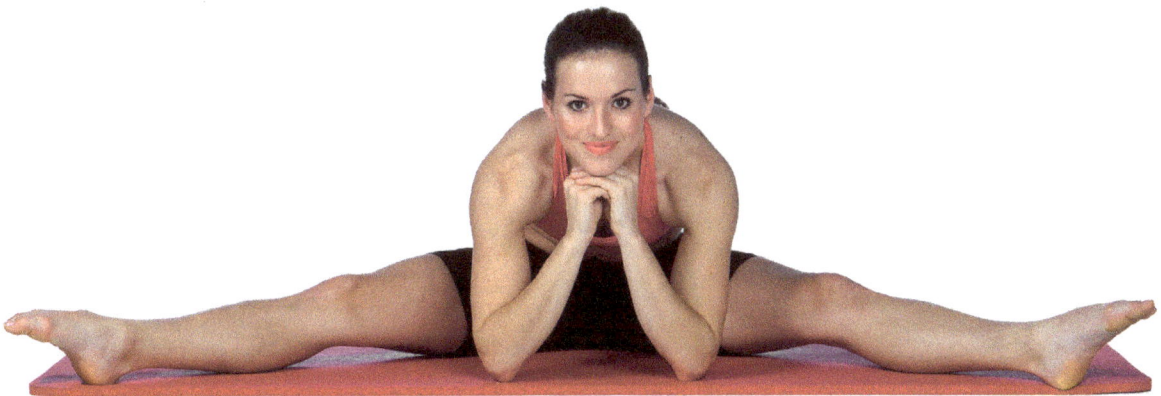

Copyright: Shutterstock|dean bertoncelj

Phase 2: Addressing Problems in the PF Kinetic Chain

In this Chapter

Now that you have completed the first four weeks of exercises (where you addressed problems *local* to the area of your Plantar Fasciitis), you can begin to address your kinetic chain issues (if your Plantar Fasciitis is not already fully resolved).

Every person who suffers from Plantar Fasciitis will have his (or her) own unique combination of factors, injuries, and biomechanical disabilities that affect their kinetic chain, and their healing process. This section of the book helps you to build a *customized exercise routine* that is based on the results of *your own biomechanical analysis*. (See *Recording your Functional Test Results - page 118* for more details.)

How can I fit even more exercises into my life?

Don't worry; I know that you are probably asking yourself how are you possibly going to find the time to add even more exercises to your daily program. As I said, don't be concerned, we have reduced the contents of all the Foundational Routines to give you more time to incorporate these new exercises into your program. These new routines are labelled as 'Condensed Foundational Routine for' and are much shorter than the ones your performed during the first four weeks.

Start with a Condensed Foundational Protocol

We continue your healing process by performing specifically selected exercises that address *the most common* **kinetic chain related** *causes of Plantar Fasciitis.*

Write your results on the tables provided on the subsequent pages. Since most of us live time-limited, busy days, we have *reduced the contents* of the *Foundational Routines* to give you the time you need to include the additional exercises that are needed to fully resolve your Plantar Fasciitis.

Everyone does the following *condensed foundational routines for Phase 2.*

- *Condensed Foundational Stretching Routine for PF on page 151.*
- *Attention: To prevent injuries, be sure to perform 10 - 20 minutes of cardiovascular exercise to warm-up these structures BEFORE stretching. (See "The Importance of Aerobic Warm-ups" - page 163). It is very important to perform this full stretching routine on each of days 1, 2, 3, 4, 5, and 6. on page 151.*
- *Condensed Foundational Strengthening Routine for PF on page 152.*

Based on your test results, you will be adding additional exercises to these condensed foundational routines as described in *Build Your Kinetic Chain Routine for PF on page 154.*

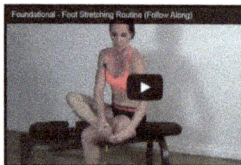

Try the Follow-Along Videos for the Stretching and Myofascial Release protocols - You may want to use these follow-along videos to perform the stretches and myofascial releases of your feet.

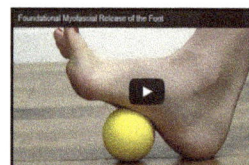

But we do recommend taking the time to first watch and understand each exercise by watching it's associated YouTube video.

- **Follow-Along Stretching Foot Flexors:** http://youtu.be/HEJ_O7EX8C4.
- **Follow-Along Myofascial Release of the Foot:** http://youtu.be/lk8byu8UGoo.

Caution: Attention: To prevent injuries, be sure to perform 10 - 20 minutes of cardiovascular exercise to warm-up these structures BEFORE stretching. (See "The Importance of Aerobic Warm-ups" - page 163). It is very important to perform this full stretching routine on each of days 1, 2, 3, 4, 5, and 6.

Condensed Foundational Myofascial Release Routine for PF

Perform the following *condensed myofascial release exercises* on *days 1, 2, 3, 4, 5, and 6.*

Table 7. 1: Condensed Foundational Myofascial Release for Plantar Fasciitis

	Follow-Along Foundational Myofascial Release of the Foot
	For detailed instructions on how to do each exercise, see *Foundational Myofascial Release of the Foot - page 185*.

Condensed Foundational Stretching Routine for PF

Perform the following *condensed stretching exercises on days 1, 2, 3, 4, 5, and 6.* Add other exercises to this routine based on your test results.

Table 7. 2: Condensed Foundational Stretching Routine for Plantar Fasciitis

	Follow-Along Foundational Foot Stretching Routine
	For detailed instructions on how to do each exercise, see *Foundational Foot Stretching Routine - page 176*.
	Stretching the Calf Muscles - page 196.

Condensed Foundational Strengthening Routine for PF

Perform the following *condensed strengthening routine on days 2, 4, and 6.* Add other exercises to this routine based on your test results.

Table 7. 3: Condensed Foundational Strengthening Routine for Plantar Fasciitis

	Theraband Strengthening of the Foot Routine on page 218.
	Salsa Towel Crunch on page 220.
	Pen and Loonie Exercise on page 221.

Addressing Kinetic Chain Issues for PF

Please review the findings of your tests now in order to determine which *additional exercises* are needed to solve your Plantar Fasciitis. Remember a FAIL (or positive finding) in a test indicates that you have a problem in this area that needs to be addressed.

Use the following flowchart as a visual guide to find the exercises that will help to resolve the kinetic chain issues identified in your test results and then add the appropriate exercises to your Condensed Foundational Routines. Alternatively, you can see the more detailed charts in the following sections to identify and jump to your exercises.

- *Attention: To prevent injuries, be sure to perform 10 - 20 minutes of cardiovascular exercise to warm-up these structures BEFORE stretching. (See "The Importance of Aerobic Warm-ups" - page 163). It is very important to perform this full stretching routine on each of days 1, 2, 3, 4, 5, and 6. on page 151.*
- *Condensed Foundational Stretching Routine for PF on page 151.*
- *Condensed Foundational Strengthening Routine for PF on page 152.*

Addressing Problems in the Plantar Fasciitis Kinetic Chain

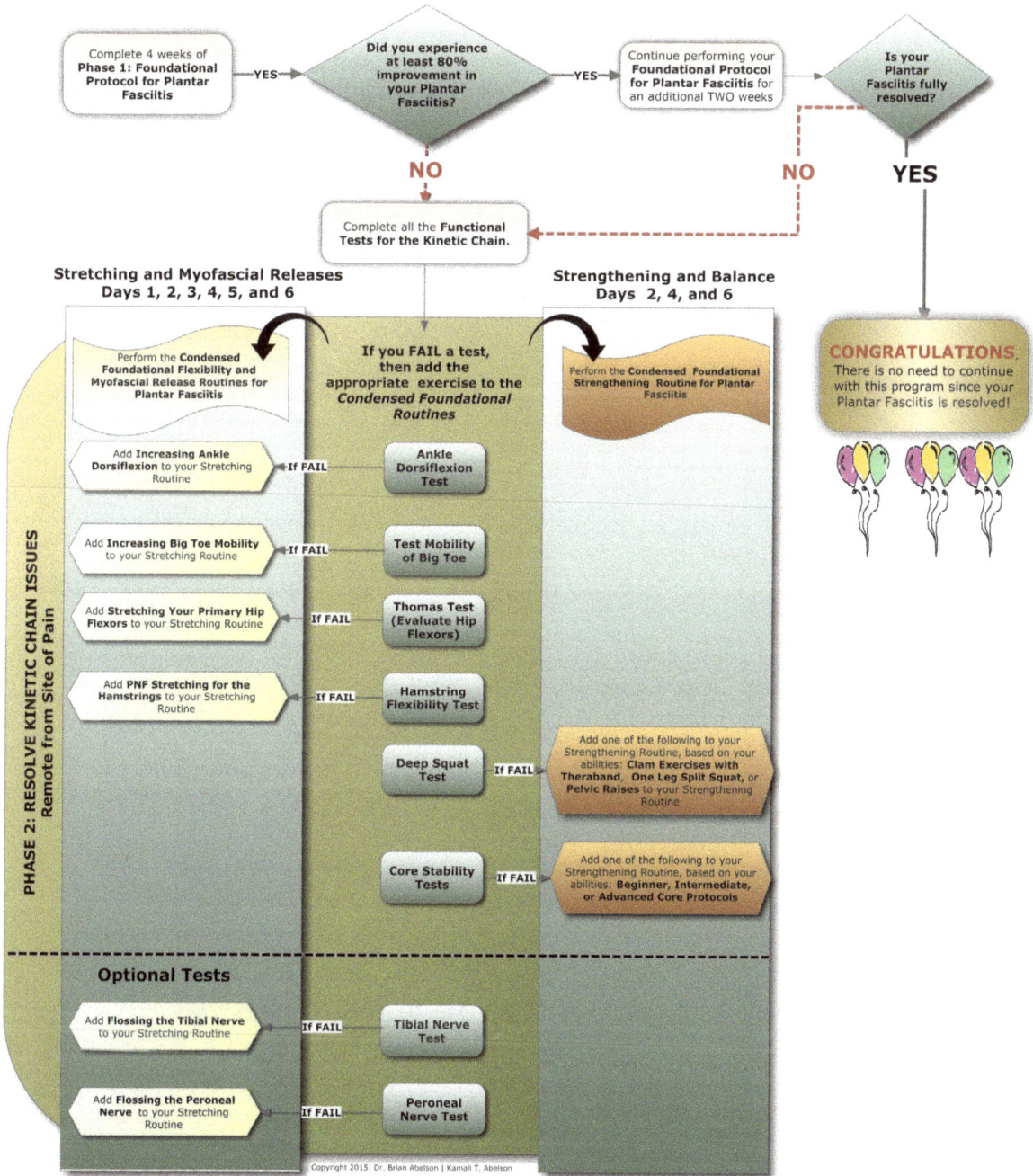

Complete 4 weeks of **Phase 1: Foundational Protocol for Plantar Fasciitis** —YES→ Did you experience at least 80% improvement in your Plantar Fasciitis? —YES→ Continue performing your **Foundational Protocol for Plantar Fasciitis** for an additional TWO weeks → Is your Plantar Fasciitis fully resolved?

NO ↓

NO (from Foundational Protocol)

YES ↓

Complete all the **Functional Tests** for the Kinetic Chain.

Stretching and Myofascial Releases
Days 1, 2, 3, 4, 5, and 6

Strengthening and Balance
Days 2, 4, and 6

PHASE 2: RESOLVE KINETIC CHAIN ISSUES Remote from Site of Pain

Perform the **Condensed Foundational Flexibility and Myofascial Release Routines for Plantar Fasciitis**

If you FAIL a test, then add the appropriate exercise to the **Condensed Foundational Routines**

Perform the **Condensed Foundational Strengthening Routine for Plantar Fasciitis**

CONGRATULATIONS. There is no need to continue with this program since your Plantar Fasciitis is resolved!

| Add Increasing Ankle Dorsiflexion to your Stretching Routine | ←If FAIL | Ankle Dorsiflexion Test |

| Add Increasing Big Toe Mobility to your Stretching Routine | ←If FAIL | Test Mobility of Big Toe |

| Add Stretching Your Primary Hip Flexors to your Stretching Routine | ←If FAIL | Thomas Test (Evaluate Hip Flexors) |

| Add PNF Stretching for the Hamstrings to your Stretching Routine | ←If FAIL | Hamstring Flexibility Test |

Deep Squat Test —If FAIL→ Add one of the following to your Strengthening Routine, based on your abilities: Clam Exercises with Theraband, One Leg Split Squat, or Pelvic Raises to your Strengthening Routine

Core Stability Tests —If FAIL→ Add one of the following to your Strengthening Routine, based on your abilities: Beginner, Intermediate, or Advanced Core Protocols

Optional Tests

| Add Flossing the Tibial Nerve to your Stretching Routine | If FAIL | Tibial Nerve Test |

| Add Flossing the Peroneal Nerve to your Stretching Routine | If FAIL | Peroneal Nerve Test |

Copyright 2015. Dr. Brian Abelson | Kamali T. Abelson

Build Your Kinetic Chain Routine for PF

Evaluate your test results, and for each FAIL in a test, add the following recommended exercises to the appropriate **Condensed Foundational Routines** (*page 150*). You will need to perform this new sequence of exercises for a minimum of four weeks in order to effectively resolve your identified kinetic chain issues.

- *Attention: To prevent injuries, be sure to perform 10 - 20 minutes of cardiovascular exercise to warm-up these structures BEFORE stretching. (See "The Importance of Aerobic Warm-ups" - page 163). It is very important to perform this full stretching routine on each of days 1, 2, 3, 4, 5, and 6. on page 151.*
- *Condensed Foundational Stretching Routine for PF on page 151.*
- *Condensed Foundational Strengthening Routine for PF on page 152.*

TIP: Photocopy the next few pages and mark your results on those pages. Use those pages to track your exercises.

Phase 2: Stretching & Myofascial Release Routine for PF

Use the following tables to build your customized stretching and myofascial release routine, one which addresses your specific kinetic chain issues.

| Everyone must do these condensed foundational routines on days 1-to-6.

Time: 8–10 minutes per foot. | Condensed Foundational Stretching Routine for PF ------ page 151.

and

Condensed Foundational Myofascial Release Routine for PF ----- page 151. | ■ Stretching the Foot's Flexors ------ page 176.
■ Stretching the Extensors of the Foot ------ page 181.
■ Foundational Myofascial Release of the Foot ------ page 185. |

Table 8: Build your Stretching/Myofascial Routine for the Kinetic Chain

For this Functional Test...	Pass	Fail	If Fail...Add This!	Exercises in this Routine
Testing Hip Flexion (Thomas Test) ------ page 130	☐	☐	*Stretching the Hip Flexors on page 201.*	■ Stretching your Primary Hip Flexors ------ page 202. ■ Stretching the Quadriceps - Secondary Hip Flexors ------ page 203.

Table 8: Build your Stretching/Myofascial Routine for the Kinetic Chain

For this Functional Test...	Pass	Fail	If Fail...Add This!	Exercises in this Routine
Testing Hamstring Flexibility ------ page 135	☐	☐	*Single Leg PNF - Hamstring Stretch on page 204.*	■ Single Leg PNF - Hamstring Stretch ------ page 204.
Functional Test for Tibial Nerve Impingement ------ page 146 - Optional Test	☐	☐	*Tibial Nerve Flossing Exercises - page 208*	■ Mobilizing the Tibial Nerve - Seated ------ page 210. ■ Tensioning the Tibial Nerve - Supine: ------ page 209.
Functional Test for Peroneal Nerve Impingement ------ page 147 - Optional Test	☐	☐	*Flossing the Peroneal Nerve - Supine Mobilization on page 212.*	■ Flossing the Peroneal Nerve - Supine Mobilization ------ page 212. ■ Mobilizing the Peroneal Nerve - Seated Position ------ page 213.

Phase 2: Strengthening Routine for PF

Use the following table to build your customized Strengthening Routine to address your specific kinetic chain issues. In some cases, we have provided multiple options; choose the exercise that you can perform with good form.

TIP: Just like in Phase 1, you can perform the Stretching and Myofascial Release exercises in the morning, and the Strengthening Exercises in the evening.

Everyone must do this **Condensed Strengthening Routine.** Time: 8–10 minutes per foot.	Condensed Foundational Strengthening Routine for PF ----- page 152	■ Theraband Strengthening of the Foot Routine ------ page 218. ■ Salsa Towel Crunch ------ page 220. ■ Pen and Loonie Exercise ------ page 221.

Table 9: Build your Strengthening Routine for the Kinetic Chain

For this Functional Test...	Pass	Fail	If Fail...Add This!	Exercises in this Routine
Testing Dorsiflexion of the Ankle ------ page 125	☐	☐	*Increasing Dorsiflexion of the Foot with a Theraband on page 205.*	Increasing Dorsiflexion of the Foot with a Theraband ------ page 205.
Testing the Mobility of the Big Toe ------ page 126	☐	☐	*Increasing Mobility of the Big Toe on page 206.*	Increasing Mobility of the Big Toe ------ page 206.
Testing Stability of the Lower Extremity - Deep Squat ------ page 131	☐	☐	Choose **ONE** of these exercises - based on your physical ability.	■ One Leg Split Squat - (Bulgarian Split Squat) ----- page 225 – OR ■ Pelvic Raise: Beginner to Intermediate ------ page 227 – OR ■ Strengthening Hip Abductors with the Suspended Clam Exercise - ----- page 226.
Testing Core Functionality ------ page 137 Add *ONE* of the *Beginner, Intermediate*, or *Advanced* Core Stabilization Routines if you failed any of the Core Tests.	☐	☐	Choose **ONE** of the following Core Stabilization Routines - based on your physical ability. Time: 15-20 minutes for both legs.	■ Basic Core Stabilization Routine for PF ------ page 216 – OR ■ Intermediate Core Stabilization Routine for PF ------ page 216 – OR ■ Advanced Core Stabilization Routine for PF ------ page 216.

Plantar Fasciitis

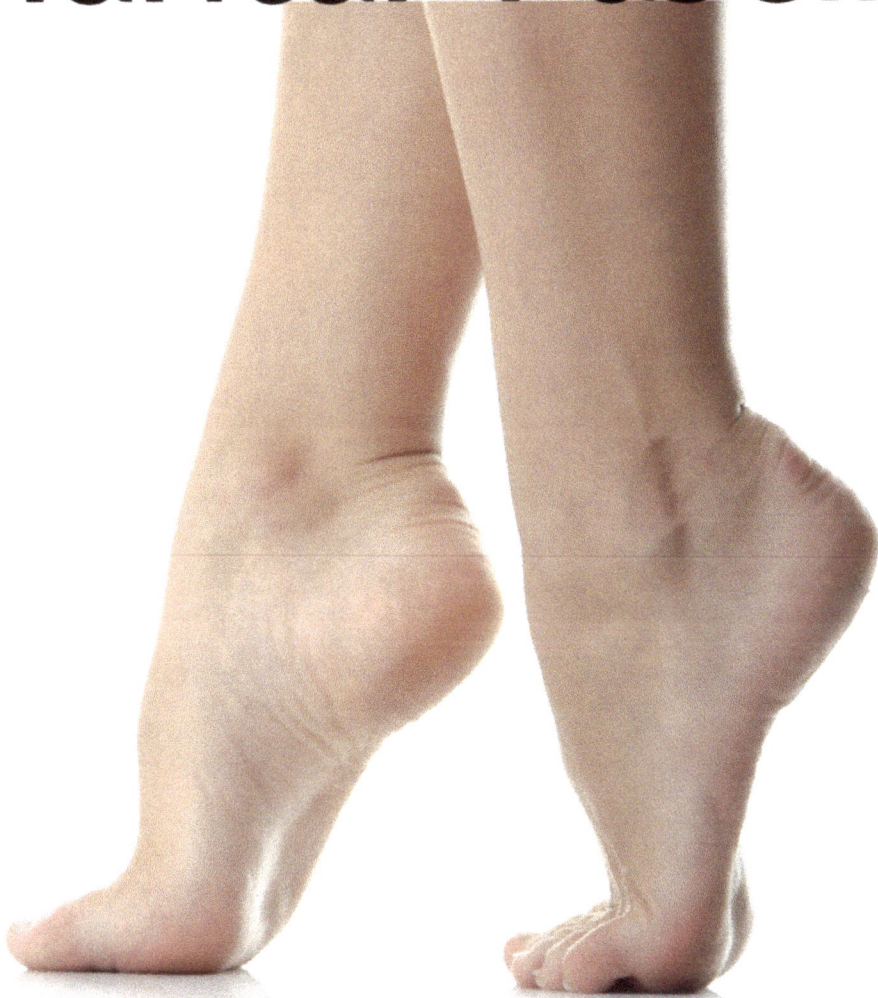

Exercise Routines

for Plantar Fasciitis

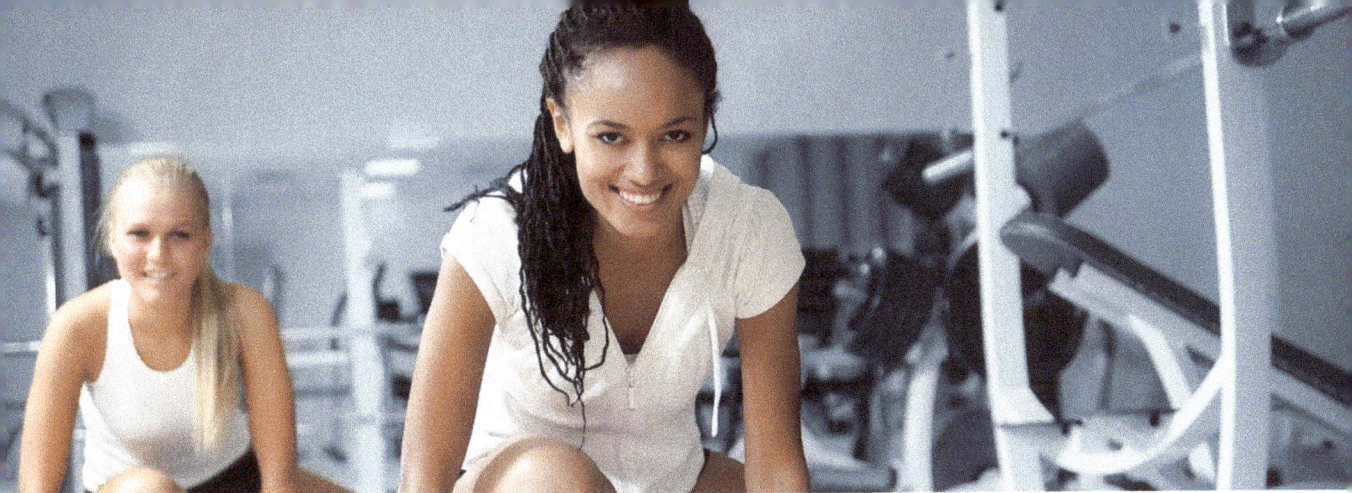

Why Exercise is Essential

In this Chapter

Note: This chapter is all about WHY exercise plays such an important role in helping you achieve a full resolution of any musculoskeletal condition. If this interests you, then please read on. Or, if you would prefer to get started on the exercises, you can jump straight to *Stretching & Myofascial Release Exercises for PF on page 171* and *Strengthening Exercises for Plantar Fasciitis on page 215*.

In many cases, exercise alone may be sufficient to resolve your case of Plantar Fasciitis. But in other cases, you may require a combination of both therapy and exercise in order to achieve a full resolution. For both instances, to achieve a complete long-standing resolution, you will need to practice a specific combination of exercises that focus on flexibility, strength, myofascial release, and joint mobility.

In addition, several other key factors (such as aerobic warm-ups and sufficient sleep and rest) can play significant roles in resolving this condition.

- *The Importance of Stretching and Myofascial Release Exercises - page 160.*
- *The Importance of Strengthening Exercises - page 162.*
- *The Importance of Nerve Flossing Exercises - page 163.*
- *Involving Your Core - page 167.*

The Importance of Stretching and Myofascial Release Exercises

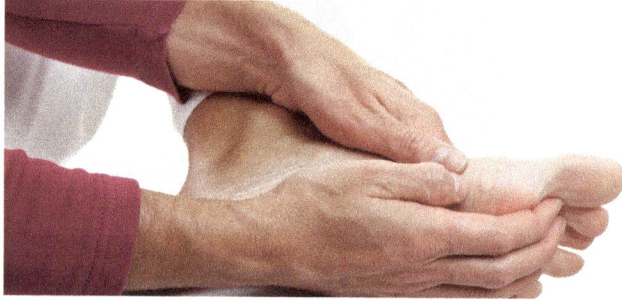

If you really want to resolve your Plantar Fasciitis, there are some key physiological factors that you just cannot get around. One very important factor is the process of *tissue remodelling*. The tissues of the body remodel according to the forces placed upon them. Without the right combination of stretching, strengthening, and proprioceptive exercises, you cannot expect to obtain full resolution of Plantar Fasciitis.

Remodelling Tissues with Stretches

During the *Regenerative Phase* of an injury, the body creates and lays down collagen to repair the injured area. Without exercise, this collagen is laid down in random directions, resulting in the formation of weak scar tissue that inhibits motion. By performing the correct stretching exercises, you can cause the majority of new tissue to be laid down with the same fiber orientation as the tissue that is being repaired – allowing this new tissue to properly perform its function (once the healing phase is complete), and even increasing the strength and functionality of these structures.

See the following topics for more information about the stretches you need to perform to resolve Plantar Fasciitis:

- *Shin Flexibility and Myofascial Release Routine - page 189*
- *Calf Flexibility and Myofascial Release Routine - page 195*
- *Stretching the Hip Flexors - page 201*.

Stretching Tips

Keep the following stretching tips in mind as you perform the stretches in your routine.

Customize the stretches for maximum benefit - As you work through the stretches in our book, feel free to customize the stretches to work better for you. For example:

- Try to stretch until you feel a slight pulling sensation (but not pain).
- Change the *angle* of your stretch in order to obtain the maximum benefit from an exercise.
- Hold the '*stretched*' position until the stretched muscle relaxes.
- Increase the degree of stretch each time.

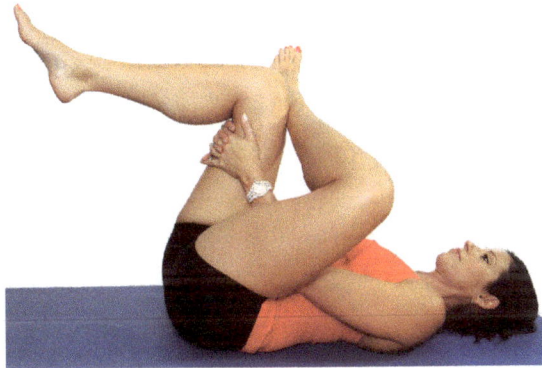

Use your breath to power your stretches - Use your breath to help you stretch and lengthen your tissues. The slow, rhythmic motion of your lungs (your respiratory pump) as it depresses your diaphragm causes a downward force on your internal organs. This classic Yoga and Tai Chi principle has a very positive effect on your circulatory function, and increases the rate of healing.

- Always *exhale* as you lengthen the tissue, or as you move into the stretch.
- Slow deep breathing helps to relax your body by increasing the parasympathetic activity of your nervous system.

Avoid bouncing during the stretch - Bouncing (or ballistic motions) can cause your muscles to suddenly contract when stretched again, resulting in increased risk of injury. There are some stretches that require small bounces, but these are usually used for dynamic warm-ups during athletic or performance training. Some exercises in this book do require short pulsations, but these are controlled movements and are not ballistic motions. In general, do **NOT** bounce when performing the stretching exercises in this book.

The Importance of Strengthening Exercises

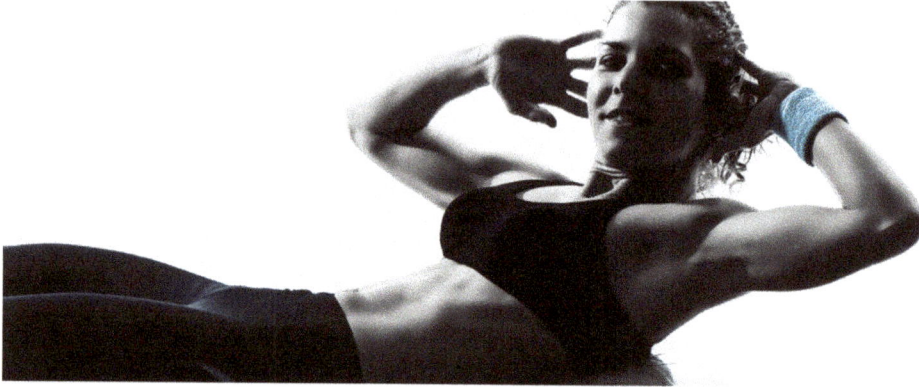

Biochemically, strength training is one of the key factors that works to naturally increase the levels of *Human Growth Hormone (HGH)*. This increase is known as the *EIGR Response* or *Exercise Induced Growth Hormone Response.*

As we age, the levels of HGH naturally decrease. This is unfortunate since decreased secretion of growth hormone is (in part) responsible for decreases in lean body mass, increases of adipose-tissue mass (fat), and the thinning of the skin that occurs with old age. Obviously, it would be a great thing if we can stop these negative effects from occurring in our body by naturally increasing levels of HGH.

Remodelling Tissues with Strengthening Exercises

Strength training plays a key role in *tissue remodelling* during both the *regenerative* and *remodelling* phases. Every time you injure yourself, your body lays down new tissue to repair itself.

This new tissue is initially very fragile, thin, and easily torn or re-injured. Strength or weight training places stress upon these new tissues, causing them to go through a process of *remodelling*. During this process, the new tissue literally converts from one type of collagen into a different type which is up to 10x thicker and 10x stronger. But, this collagen conversion only occurs when you apply continued stress upon the tissue...as you would with weight and strength training exercises.

The amazing thing is that this remodelling of the tissues can, with the right stimulus, happen at any age, even for those in their 80's or 90's.[35] So, no matter what your age or physical condition, you need to incorporate strength training into your exercise routines. See the following topics for more information about using strengthening exercises for resolving Plantar Fasciitis:

■   *Strengthening Exercises for Plantar Fasciitis - page 215*.

The Importance of Nerve Flossing Exercises

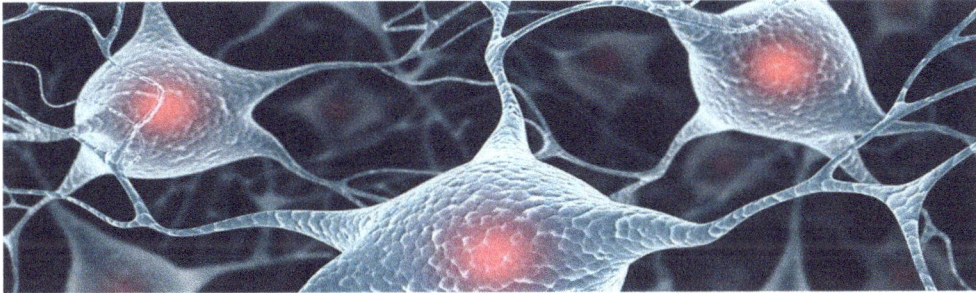

We sometimes find that patients who are suffering from Plantar Fasciitis will also present with symptoms of numbness, tingling, or altered sensations along their foot and lower legs. These symptoms often present in a very specific pattern, and are often related to very specific nerves that have been restricted by inflammation or tight muscles. To address this issue, we typically use a combination of nerve flossing and pin-and-stretch exercises that release the trapped or restricted nerve.

The Importance of Aerobic Warm-ups

It may sound a little strange when we tell you to "warm up" your entire body, especially when you feel that your pain is localized in one area, such as your foot, jaw, neck, or shoulder, and you just want to get started on resolving that particular issue.

But this initial aerobic workout (lasting for 10 to15 minutes) is one of the *first* things you should do before you ever begin working on your injured or restricted areas, and definitely before you begin any exercise routine.

---

35.   *Effects of Human Growth Hormone in Men over 60 Years Old.* Daniel Rudman, M.D., Axel G. Feller, M.D., Hoskote S. Nagraj, M.D., Gregory A. Gergans, M.D., Pardee Y. Lalitha, M.D., Allen F. Goldberg, D.D.S., Robert A. Schlenker, Ph.D., Lester Cohn, M.D., Inge W. Rudman, B.S., and Dale E. Mattson, Ph.D. N Engl J Med 1990; 323:1-6July 5, 1990DOI: 10.1056/NEJM199007053230101.

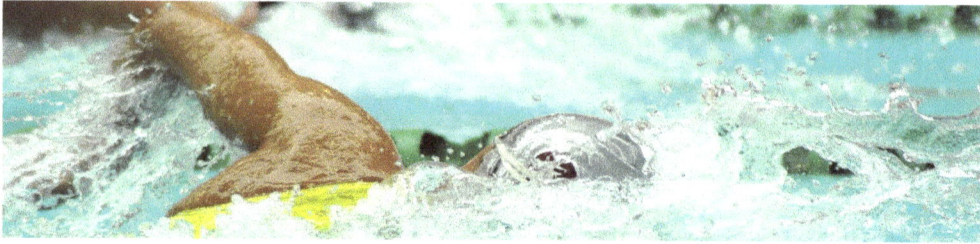

What Happens During Aerobic Warm-ups

The aerobic warm-up helps to prepare your body, both physically and mentally, for the upcoming exercises by:

- Increasing circulation to your tissues.
- Preparing your heart for the upcoming exertions.
- Warming your tissues and thereby reducing your chances of injury.
- Making your muscles more flexible and ready for action.
- Priming and preparing your nervous system for new instructions.
- Improving your reaction times.
- Speeding healing of existing injuries.
- Increasing the mitochondrial function of your cells.

Improving Cellular Function with Aerobic Exercises

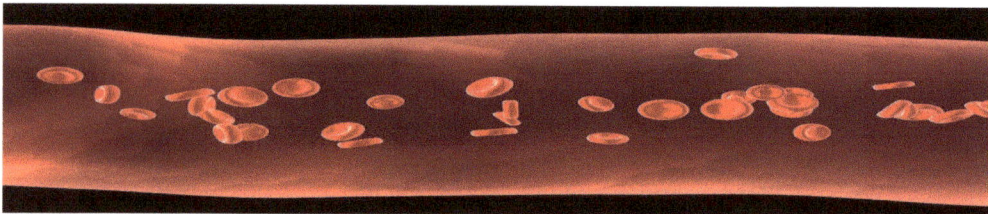

Aerobic exercise is the fastest way to increase the strength and function of your cardiovascular system. By increasing the density of capillaries, you are able to get more nutrients into your muscular tissue, thereby helping them to heal and perform better.

The increased density of capillaries means that you are better able to eliminate the waste by-products of healing and metabolism from your cells, again allowing them to perform more efficiently.

Aerobic exercise also increases the function of mitochondria in your cells. This increased mitochondrial function immediately boosts your body's ability to generate power and energy since your mitochondria are the principal energy generators for your cells.

Mitochondria convert existing nutrients into ATP (adenosine triphosphate), a form of energy that is readily usable by all the cells in your body. Your body uses this energy to perform all of its functions – from healing existing injuries, to eliminating waste, to powering your muscles when you walk, talk, or perform any action.

As we age, or when we injure ourselves, our ability to produce ATP decreases. Exercise is one of the few factors that will naturally increase ATP production to give you increased energy.

Aerobic Warm-Ups...How they helped resolve my injury!

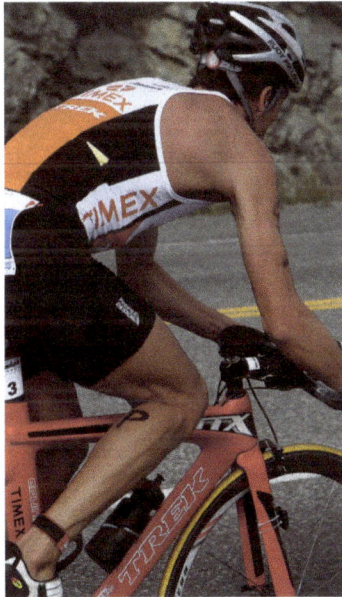

I have had a personal experience that showed me the importance of cardiovascular warm-ups as they relate to recovering from an injury.

I am speaking about an injury for which most people would never perform an aerobic workout. A few years ago I suffered from a severe case of *Bell's Palsy* (weakness of the nerve that innervates and controls the muscles for facial expression) on one-half of the face.

Bell's Palsy left me with the muscles of one-half of my face paralyzed and expressionless. I was told it would take 3 to 6 months before normal nerve function would be restored!

I was unwilling to live with this condition for that long and immediately researched means for reducing this time frame. One of the first things I did after getting Bell's Palsy was to get on my road bike/wind trainer for at least 20 to 30 minutes each day. I followed this up with TMJ massage and a variety of jaw, neck, and shoulder exercises.

To everyone's amazement, I recovered fully, with complete neuromuscular control of the muscles in my face, within about a month. I am convinced that my daily aerobic exercise is one of the major reasons I got over this condition in about a third of the normal time. The aerobic exercises I did every day resulted in increased circulatory function and improved mitochondrial activity (energy production)!

So take the time to do your aerobic warm-up before doing these exercise programs...you will be amazed at the difference it makes in your healing, recovery, power, and strength development!

So What is a Good Warm-up?

A good warm-up should include all the large muscles of your body and include movements that increase your heart rate and breathing. With Plantar Fasciitis, a good warm-up in an exercise that does not further aggravate your condition. Most of our Plantar Fasciitis patients are still able to use a stationary bike, swim, or use an elliptical machine.

■ **Swim for 20 minutes**. If you are doing the front crawl, make sure you breathe from both sides. You don't want your warm-up to create neuromuscular imbalances because you breathe from just one side of your body.

■ **Use an elliptical or ski machine for 10–to–20 minutes**. Both are good for reinforcing a cross-crawling pattern, which helps establish good neuromuscular control, as well as for warming up all the big muscles of your body.

■ **Ride a stationary bike for 10–to–20 minutes**. This option is not my first choice due to the lack of motion in the upper extremity. In terms of bike types, I prefer the use of upright bikes much more since you can maintain better posture, especially if you have a history of back pain.

■ **Go for a brisk 10–to–20 minute walk**. Make sure you move your shoulders and swing your arms. Good upper extremity motion takes the stress off your back and helps you to store and release energy from your core. Don't walk at a slow pace, this will not achieve the desired results and is actually quite hard on your back compared to brisk walking.

■ **Jog, or run for 10–to–20 minutes**. If you are not a runner, start with a brisk walk interspersed with a few short jogs. If you are a runner, make sure you maintain a good upright posture with good shoulder movement, and make sure you land on the middle of your feet. No toe or heel running as this deactivates your gluteals and causes a lot of other problems. Treadmills are fine but do not increase your elevation too much.

This is a good opportunity to *listen* to your body, and recognize any injury, tight spots, or restrictions that you may have to accommodate during your exercise routine. The following are some common warm-ups that we recommend to our patients.

Working within your Aerobic and Anaerobic Zones

Your warm-up, like all initial aerobic activity, needs to be performed within your aerobic zone. This is the range within which you want your heart to operate while you are performing your aerobic exercise. Think of your aerobic zone as the base which you must first establish for rehabilitation, and also for moving into the higher levels of performance in your chosen activity.

Calculating your aerobic zone - Use the following formula to calculate your *aerobic zone*:

1. Subtract your age from the number **220**.
    - For example, if I am **40** years old, then **220 - 40 = 180**.
2. Obtain the low end of your aerobic range by multiplying the result of step 1 by **0.6**.
    - In our example: **180 * 0.6 = 108**
3. Obtain the high end of your aerobic range by multiplying the result of step 1 by **0.7**.
    - In our example: **180 * 0.7 = 126**

This is your *aerobic heart rate zone* within which you need to work to develop your aerobic capacity. It is the zone which will best speed your recovery from an injury. If you work above this zone you run the risk of injury. If you work below this zone, you will not achieve the maximum benefits provided by your aerobic warm-up.

TIP: I strongly recommend purchasing and using a heart-rate monitor. These are relatively inexpensive, and are a great tool for ensuring you stay within your aerobic zone.

Involving Your Core

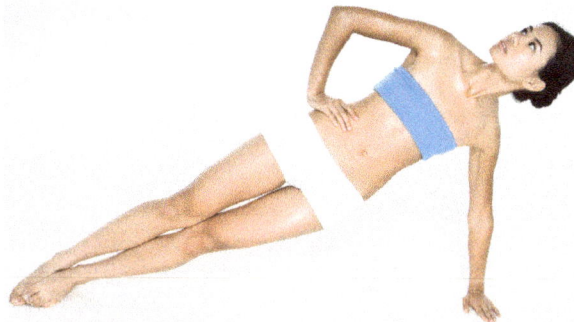

It doesn't matter what type of exercise you are performing; all exercises require good posture and solid support from your core. Your core is the foundation and source of all your movements, providing a stable base for all arm, leg, and neck motions. Your ability to maintain good posture is greatly dependent upon your core stability!

If you have a stable, balanced, elastic core, then you can easily transfer energy from the center of your body to all your extremities! This process of first storing energy, and then releasing it, is very similar to how a spring mechanism works. A compressed spring contains stored energy. When the spring releases, the stored energy is released to allow the spring to expand. The muscles of your core act like a spring, compressing or tightening to store energy, and expanding to release the stored energy for use in movement!

Having the ability to store and release energy from your core is a fundamental aspect of injury resolution and athletic performance. It does not matter how fit you currently are, what your age is, or what your current health status is...you can always improve the quality of your core.

If you do not have a strong core, you rob yourself of much needed power and energy, and make yourself more susceptible to injuries.

Bracing Your Core

Many of our exercises require you to activate, brace, and otherwise involve your core! One of the key ways that all exercises can be converted into *core* exercises is through the process of **bracing**. I first learned about this process from Dr. Stuart McGill, Department Chair of the Spine Biomechanics Laboratory at the University of Waterloo.

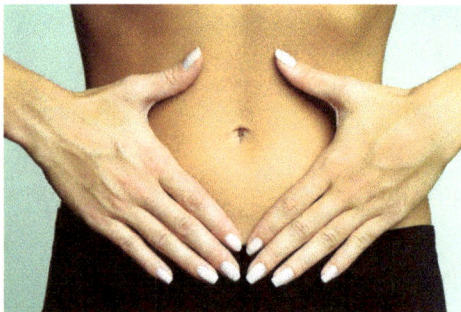

Bracing refers to the process of "*contracting all the muscles in the abdominal wall without drawing or pushing in*"[36]. This is very different from the common advice given by some trainers to suck in (or hollow-out) your abdominals or to contract (pull in) your Transversus Abdominis muscle (TVA). In fact, Dr. McGill's research has shown that the action of *pulling in* your TVA actually **de-activates your paraspinal muscles** causing increased instability by creating or reinforcing abnormal neuromuscular patterns.

---

36.   Ultimate Back Fitness and Performance, 3rd Edition, Stuart McGill PhD. 2004, Wabuno Publishers, BackFitPro Publishers.

Basically, bracing is the process of gently pushing out while contracting all of your abdominal muscles. This process also forces your paraspinal muscles to tighten at the same time.

The process of bracing creates a belt or corset around the core of your body, giving you a base of stabilization. This base of stability allows you to direct energy from your core to your extremities.

TIP: For a better understanding of your core, I recommend reading Dr. Stuart McGill's book, "**Ultimate Back Fitness and Performance**".

How to Brace your Core

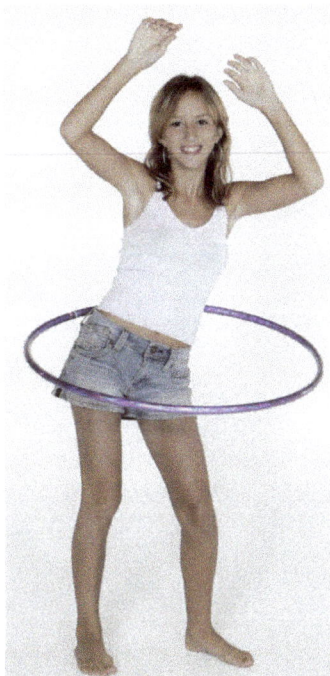

Bracing is accomplished by gently pushing *out* your abdominal wall while tightening your back at the same time. This is actually quite a simple procedure once you get used to it. When bracing is done correctly, you will almost immediately feel like you have a stronger core.

Another way to quickly learn how to brace is by using a hula-hoop. That's right...your childhood toy can help you brace properly, especially when you use a weighted hula-hoop. Hula-hooping forces you to brace all your abdominal and back muscles at the same time.

Many adults are surprised to discover just how difficult hooping can be initially, especially when their children find it to be so easy. This is because children generally have better core strength than their parents.

Just five minutes of hula-hooping a day can substantially increase your core stability.

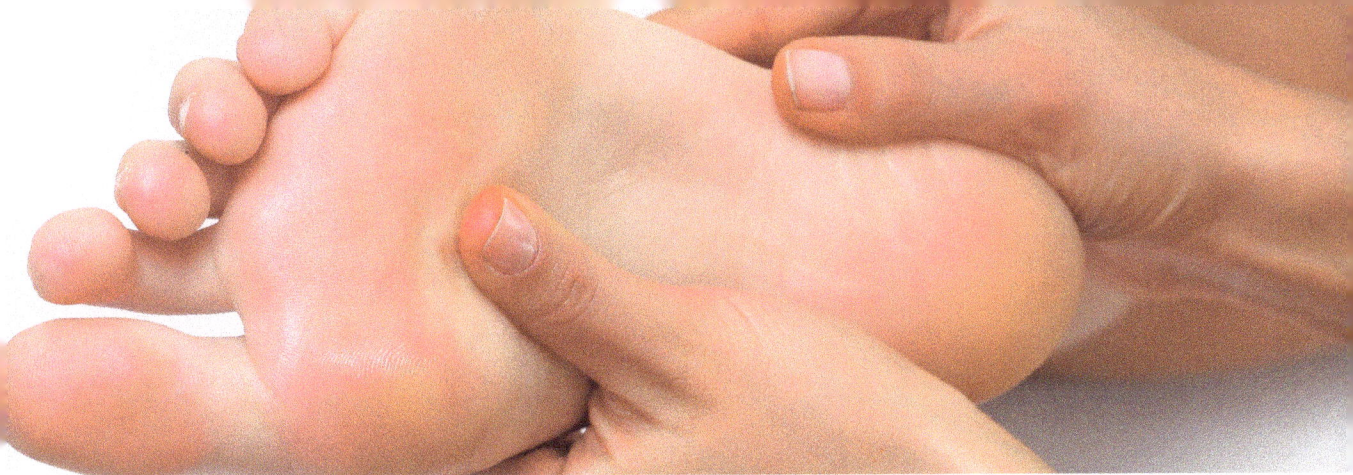

Stretching & Myofascial Release Exercises for PF

In this chapter

TIP: For all stretches, it is important to FIRST perform 10-to-20 minutes of cardiovascular warm-ups. This can be any one of cycling, swimming, or elliptical machine.

This chapter shows the stretching and myofascial release exercises that we recommend for treating Plantar Fasciitis. We will be using a combination of myofascial release, passive and dynamic stretches, along with PNF (*proprioceptive neuromuscular facilitation*) stretching.

For more information about the anatomical structures and kinetic chain relationships of the structures in these exercises, you can explore the contents of *The Anatomy Behind Plantar Fasciitis on page 49*.

About Scheduling Your Workout

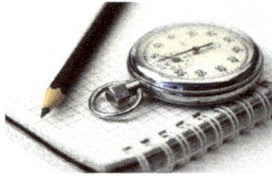

As much as possible, try to complete your customized stretching and myofascial release routine *all at once*, as one complete sequence of exercises. This option gives you the most powerful and effective healing and recovery.

On the other hand, if you find that your time is extremely limited, it is okay to divide the stretching and myofascial release sections into two different times of the same day. Just be sure to perform all of the exercises listed under *The Foundational Foot Flexibility and Myofascial Release Protocols - page 175* at once, within one session.

How Much Time Will It Take?

You **must** to do the full routine for *each foot that has Plantar Fasciitis.* (However, if you have Plantar Fasciitis in just one foot, then you do NOT have to do this routine for the unaffected foot.)

Once you are familiar with the exercise routine, stretching of the flexors and extensors of *both* feet will only take about five (5) minutes per foot. The *Foundational Myofascial Release of the Foot on page 185* will take an additional 3 to 5 minutes per foot. Total time required for both stretching and myofascial release:

- One foot involved: 8 to 10 minutes.
- Both feet are involved: 16 to 20 minutes.

Learning these Routines

You will be able to learn these stretching and myosfascial release protocols in a short period of time. Initially, I would recommend that you perform the stretching protocol after watching our YouTube video presentations. After that you should be able to simply refer to the photos in this book if you need a quick reminder.

TIP: Each exercise in these protocols has an associated YouTube video. For our online readers, simply click the video icon beside the exercise, and if you have internet access, you will be able to immediately watch the video. If you are reading a hard-copy of this book, simply type the YouTube address into your internet browser and learn how to perform each exercise.

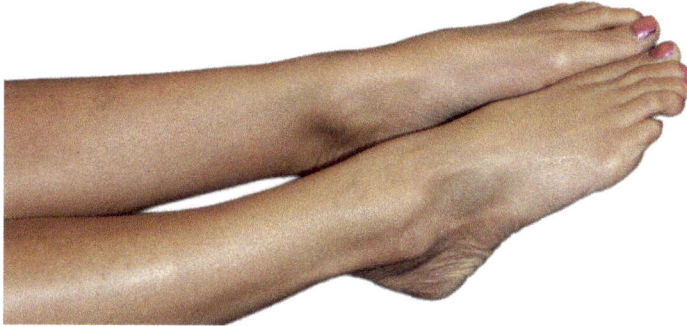

How Are These Exercises Organized

Remember, the goal is to *stretch over-active and tight muscle groups*, while *strengthening weak or over-stretched* muscles. Refer to the chapters *Phase 1: Foundational Protocol for Plantar Fasciitis - page 107* and *Phase 2: Addressing Problems in the PF Kinetic Chain - page 149* to identify exactly **which** exercises YOU need to do.

For your convenience, we have divided the exercises into the following sections:

Foundational Flexibility and Myofascial Release Routine:

- *Stretching the Foot's Flexors on page 176.*
- *Stretching the Extensors of the Foot on page 181.*
- *Myofascial Release of the Foot on page 187.*

TIP: Each of these foundational routines has an accompanying 'follow-along' video that you can access from our YouTube site. Use these videos to get you started.

Shin Flexibility and Myofascial Release Routine:

- *Stretching the Tibialis Anterior on page 190.*
- *Myofascial Release of the Shins on page 191.*
- *Tiger Tail - Myofascial Release of the Shins on page 192.*
- *Stretching and Releasing the Peroneals on page 193.*

Calf Flexibility and Myofascial Release Routine:

■ *Stretching the Calf Muscles on page 196.*
    ■ *Part 1: Stretch the Gastrocnemius: on page 196.*
    ■ *Part 2: Stretch the Soleus: on page 197.*
■ *Myofascial Release of the Calf on page 198.*
    ■ *First Exercise – Myofascial Release of the Calf with a Foam Roller: on page 198.*
    ■ *Second Exercise – Myofascial Release of the Calf with a Soft-Ball: on page 199*

Hip Flexor Stretching and Myofascial Release Routine:

■ *Stretching your Primary Hip Flexors on page 202.*
■ *Stretching the Quadriceps - Secondary Hip Flexors on page 203.*

Hamstring Stretching Exercises:

■ *Single Leg PNF - Hamstring Stretch on page 204.*

Joint Mobility Exercises:

■ *Increasing Dorsiflexion of the Foot with a Theraband on page 205*
■ *Increasing Mobility of the Big Toe on page 206.*

Nerve Flossing Exercises:

■ *Tensioning the Tibial Nerve - Supine: on page 209.*
■ *Mobilizing the Tibial Nerve - Seated on page 210.*
■ *Flossing the Peroneal Nerve - Supine Mobilization on page 212.*
■ *Mobilizing the Peroneal Nerve - Seated Position on page 213.*

TIP: The icon on the left indicates that we have produced a video demonstrating this exercise, test, or procedure. These videos are hosted on YouTube. If your e-reader supports appropriate internet, you can simply click on the icon to start the video OR click on the accompanying link to view this video from your e-reader's browser.

The Foundational Foot Flexibility and Myofascial Release Protocols

The *Foundational Foot Flexibility and Myofascial Release Protocol* must be performed by everyone who suffers from Plantar Fasciitis, no matter what their test results indicate. These protocols should be performed on days **Day 1, 2, 3, 4, 5,** and **6**.

- The *Foundational Flexibility Routine* will stretch key structures that perform the essential actions of dorsi and plantar flexion, as well as inversion and eversion of the foot. Some of these structure are very superficial while other run deep, such as the three muscles that run under your calf muscles.
- The *Foundational Myofascial Release Routine* will help to break up restrictions and adhesions that have formed under your feet. These protocols should be performed from days 1-through-6.

Just remember, the muscles of the foot are like the tires on your car. When just one of your tires is out of alignment, it can affect the motion of the entire vehicle. In the same way, a problem in just one muscle of your foot can result in the development of a cascade of *abnormal motion patterns* throughout your entire body. The exercises in the *Foundational Flexibility and Myofascial Release Routine* will help you to balance the structures of your foot so that they work in a proper and synchronized manner.

For those of you (anatomists, practitioners, and engineers) who like to know exactly which structures are being stretched in your foot, here is the list:

Your Foot's Flexors:

- Flexor digitorum longus.
- Quadratus plantae.
- Flexor hallicus longus.
- Flexor digitorum brevis.
- Flexor hallicus brevis.
- Flexor digiti minimi brevis.

Your Foot's Extensors:

- Extensor hallicus longus.
- Extensor digitorum longus.

For more details about these structures and their function, read *The Anatomy Behind Plantar Fasciitis on page 49.*

Foundational Foot Stretching Routine

Our entire **Foundational Foot Stretching Routine** incorporates a carefully selected set of foot stretches that work the critical flexors and extensors of the foot and toes. This routine (to be performed by everyone) includes the following three sets of exercises. Don't worry, although this list looks long, once you learn these, it will only take about **8 minutes** to complete the entire set.

The Foundational Foot Flexibility and Myofascial Release Protocols on page 175 consists of the following three sets of exercises. Do the full routine for each foot that is experiencing Plantar Fasciitis:

- Stretching the Foot's Flexors ------ page 176.
  - Stretching the Foot's Long Flexors ------ page 177.
  - Stretching the Big Toe's Long Flexors ------ page 178.
  - Stretching the Short Flexors of the Foot ------ page 179.
  - Stretching the Short Flexors of the Big Toe ------ page 180.
- Stretching the Extensors of the Foot ------ page 181.
  - Stretching the Foot's Long Extensors ------ page 181.
  - Stretch the Big Toe's Long Extensors ------ page 182.
  - Stretch the Foot's Short Extensors ------ page 183.
  - Stretch the Big Toe's Short Extensors ------ page 184.
- Foundational Myofascial Release of the Foot ------ page 185.

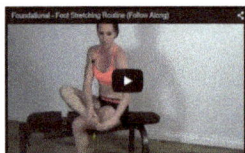

Want to know more? - Use our *"Follow Along Foundational Foot Stretching Routine Videos"* to stretch the foot's flexors. But we do recommend taking the time to first watch and understand each exercises by watching it's accompanying detailed YouTube video. **Watch this follow-along video:** http://youtu.be/HEJ_O7EX8C4

Stretching the Foot's Flexors: Your foot's flexors lie under the calves, and are the muscles that help you to point the foot, and point the toes. The longer foot flexors originate under your calf muscles, while the shorter flexors lie along the bottom of the foot. You must stretch both the flexors and extensors in order to obtain a full resolution of your condition.

This is a four-part stretch that should only take a few minutes to complete the entire sequence. *Do the full combination for each leg.*

- Stretching the Foot's Long Flexors ------ page 177.
- Stretching the Big Toe's Long Flexors ------ page 178.
- Stretching the Short Flexors of the Foot ------ page 179.
- Stretching the Short Flexors of the Big Toe ------ page 180.

TIP: Perform all four parts of this exercise on one leg before performing the same series on the other leg. If you only have Plantar Fasciitis on one foot, then only perform this exercise on the affected side of the body.

Stretching the Foot's Long Flexors: This combination of dynamic and static actions primarily stretches the *flexor digitorum longus* muscle, increases flexion of toes 2-thru-5, and aids in inversion and plantar flexion of the foot. Holding the stretch in the flexed (dorsi-flexed) position also stretches the *plantar fascia*.

Watch this video: (http://www.youtube.com/watch?v=kEBnqg5nnyM, @ 0.47 minutes)

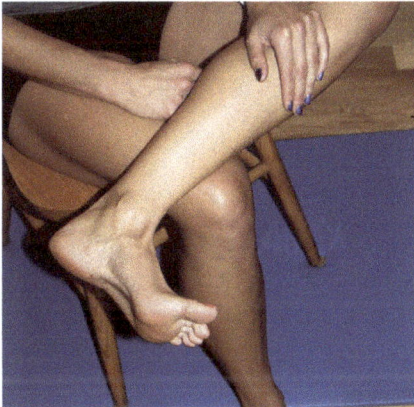

Keep your foot dorsi-flexed, and gently pulse your toes, holding each pulse for 3 seconds. End by holding the full flexed position for 15 seconds.

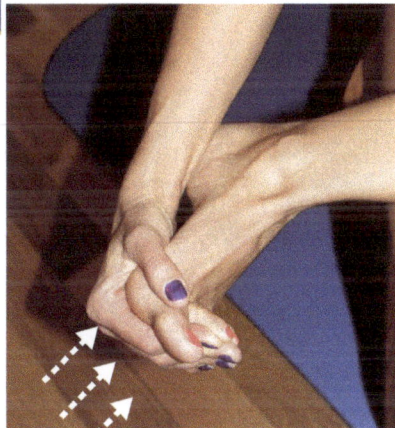

1. Starting position: Sit on a chair, with one leg crossed over the other knee, foot relaxed.
   - Rest your hand along the bottom of the foot, so that your fingertips lie over your toes. You will be using your fingers to push the toes back.
   - Keep your toes relaxed, and your foot dorsi-flexed as shown in this image.
2. Gently push your toes UP, for a 3-count pulse, and then bring your toes back to the starting position.
   - Immediately push your toes UP again for another 3-count pulse. This is the dynamic phase of the exercise.
   - Repeat this action five (5) times.
3. After the 5th pulse, hold the stretch in the fully flexed (dorsiflexion) position for a count of 15 (a static stretch).
4. Stay in the same seated position and proceed onto stretching the *Stretching the Big Toe's Long Flexors on page 178* (next set of instructions).

Stretching the Big Toe's Long Flexors: This combination of dynamic and static actions primarily stretches the *flexor hallucis longus* muscle. This muscle flexes the big toe, and assists in inversion and plantar flexion of the foot.

Watch this video: (http://www.youtube.com/watch?v=kEBnqg5nnyM, @ 1.35 minutes)

Keep your foot dorsi-flexed, and gently pulse your big toe, holding each pulse for a 3-count pulse.

End by holding the fully flexed position of the big toe for 15 seconds.

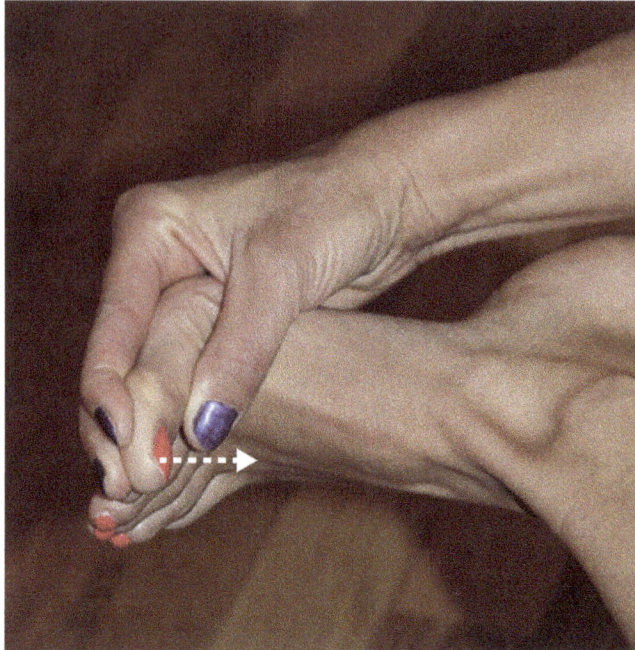

1. Starting position: Stay in the same-seated position as in the previous exercise (*Stretching the Foot's Long Flexors on page 177*), sitting on a chair, with one leg crossed over the other knee, foot in dorsi-flexed position.

2. Perform a similar motion to the first exercise, except this time focus on the big toe.
   - Use your fingers to push *just your big toe upwards*, while keeping your foot in a stable position.
   - Start by pushing your big toe UP for a 3-count pulse, then bring your big toe back to the starting position.
   - Immediately push your big toe UP again for another 3-count pulse. This is the dynamic phase of the exercise.
   - Repeat this action five (5) times.

3. After the 5th pulse, hold the big toe stretch in the fully flexed (dorsiflexion) position (for a static stretch).
   - Hold the stretch for a count of 15.
   - It is important to maintain enough pressure to feel the stretch, but not so much pressure as to cause any type of sharp pain.

4. Stay in the same-seated position and proceed to *Stretching the Short Flexors of the Foot on page 179*.

Stretching the Short Flexors of the Foot: This combination of dynamic and static actions stretches two very important short flexors of the foot, including the *flexor digitorum brevis* (which flexes the *proximal interphalangeal joints* of toes 2-thru-5) and the *quadratus plantae* (which assists in flexing toes 2-thru-5 and modifies line-of-pull for the *flexor digitorum longus*). **Watch this video:** (http://www.youtube.com/watch?v=kEBnqg5nnyM, @ 2.25 minutes)

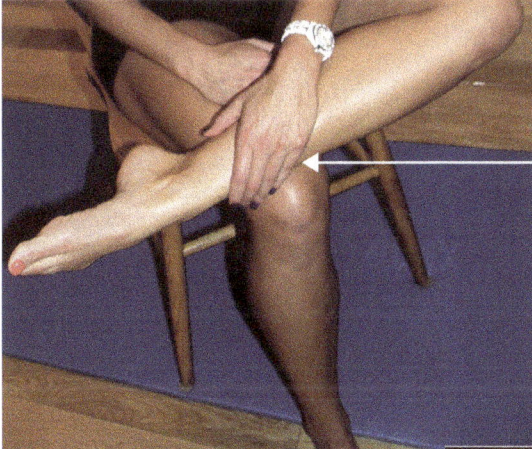

Keep your foot plantar flexed, isolating the long muscles from action by grasping the ankles.

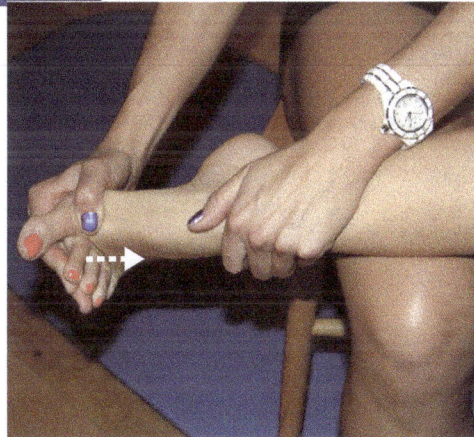

Each pulse should last for 3 counts. End by holding the toes in the fully flexed position for 15 seconds.

1. Starting position: Sit on a chair, with one leg crossed over the other knee, foot relaxed.
    - Point your foot (plantar flexed).
    - With one hand, isolate the long muscles by clasping your ankle. Now all the actions you perform will be completed by the short muscles of the foot.
    - Keep your toes relaxed, and your foot plantar-flexed as shown in this image.
2. Use your hands to push and pulse your toes for a 3-count pulse, then bring the toes back to the starting position (this is the dynamic stretch).
    - You should feel the stretch from the heel to the toe.
    - Make sure you keep your foot pointed throughout the exercise.
    - Pulse your toes about five (5) times.
3. After the 5th pulse, hold the stretch for the toes in the fully flexed (dorsiflexion) position (for a static stretch). Hold the stretch for a count of 15.
4. Continue with the next stretch *Stretching the Short Flexors of the Big Toe on page 180*.

Stretching the Short Flexors of the Big Toe: This combination of dynamic and static actions primarily stretches the *flexor hallicus brevis* muscle. This muscle flexes the big toe joint (*proximal phalanx*).

Watch this video: (http://www.youtube.com/watch?v=kEBnqg5nnyM, @ 3.30 minutes)

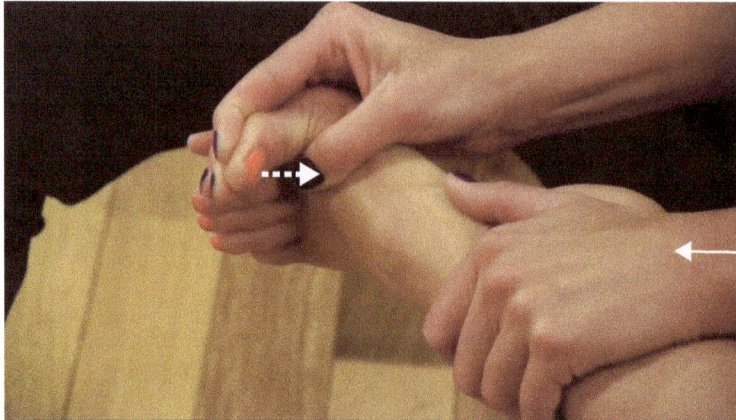

Keep your foot plantar flexed, isolating the long muscles from action by grasping the ankles.

Hold each pulse for 3 seconds. End by holding the big toe in the fully flexed position for 15 seconds.

1. Starting position: Sit on a chair, with one leg crossed over the other knee, foot relaxed.
    - Point your foot (plantar flexed).
    - With one hand, isolate the long muscles by clasping your ankle. Now all the actions you perform will be completed by the *short muscles* of the foot.
    - Keep your toes relaxed, and your foot plantar-flexed as shown in this image.

2. Use your hands to push and pulse your big toe for a 3-count pulse, then bring your big toe back to the starting position (dynamic stretch).
    - Pulse your big toe about five (5) times.
    - You should feel the stretch from the heel to the toe.

3. After the 5th pulse, hold the stretch for the big toe in the fully flexed (dorsiflexion) position (for a static stretch). Hold the static stretch for a count of 15.

4. Now that you have completed this series for one leg, you can repeat the entire sequence (*Stretching the Foot's Flexors on page 176*) for the other leg (if you are suffering from Plantar Fasciitis on both feet).

Note: If you only have Plantar Fasciitis on one foot, you can move onto the next section to stretch the extensors of the affected foot. See *Stretching the Extensors of the Foot on page 181* for the next phase.

Stretching the Extensors of the Foot: Your extensors help you to bring your toes up, and your foot closer to your shins (dorsiflexion). The longer foot extensors lie along the front of the leg (the shins), while the shorter extensors lie along the top of the foot. These extensors form the oppositional muscles of the flexors. It is important to stretch both flexors and extensors in order to obtain full resolution of your plantar fasciitis. This a four-part stretch. *Do the full routine for each leg.*

- Stretching the Foot's Long Extensors ------ page 181.
- Stretch the Big Toe's Long Extensors ------ page 182.
- Stretch the Foot's Short Extensors ------ page 183.
- Stretch the Big Toe's Short Extensors ------ page 184.

Stretching the Foot's Long Extensors: This combination of dynamic and static stretches works the *extensor digitorum longus*. This muscle extends toes two (2) through five(5), and assists in eversion and dorsi-flexion of the foot.
(**Watch this video:** http://www.youtube.com/watch?v=kEBnqg5nnyM, @ 4.07 minutes)

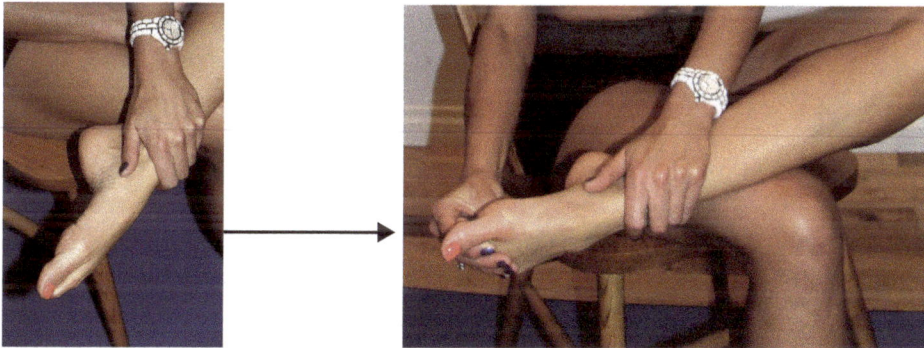

1. Starting position: Sit on a chair, with one leg crossed over the other knee, foot relaxed.
   - Keep your toes relaxed, and your foot *pointed* and plantar-flexed as shown in this image. Grasp your ankle to stabilize the foot.
   - Wrap the fingers of your other hand around the *front of your toes*, so that your fingers can pull the toes towards your body. If necessary, brace your thumb against the bottom of your foot so you can better control the pulses.
2. Gently pull, and pulse your toes, with each pulse lasting for three (3) counts (this is the dynamic stretch).
   - Pulse your toes about five (5) times, taking three counts for each pulse.
3. After the 5th pulse, hold the stretch in the fully flexed (plantar-flexion) position (for a static stretch). Hold the stretch for a count of 15.
4. Now move onto the next phase of this exercise – *Stretch the Big Toe's Long Extensors on page 182.*

Stretch the Big Toe's Long Extensors: This combination of dynamic and static stretches works the *extensor hallicus longus*. This muscle extends the big toe and assists in dorsiflexion of the foot.

Watch this video: (http://www.youtube.com/watch?v=kEBnqg5nnyM, @5.30 minutes)

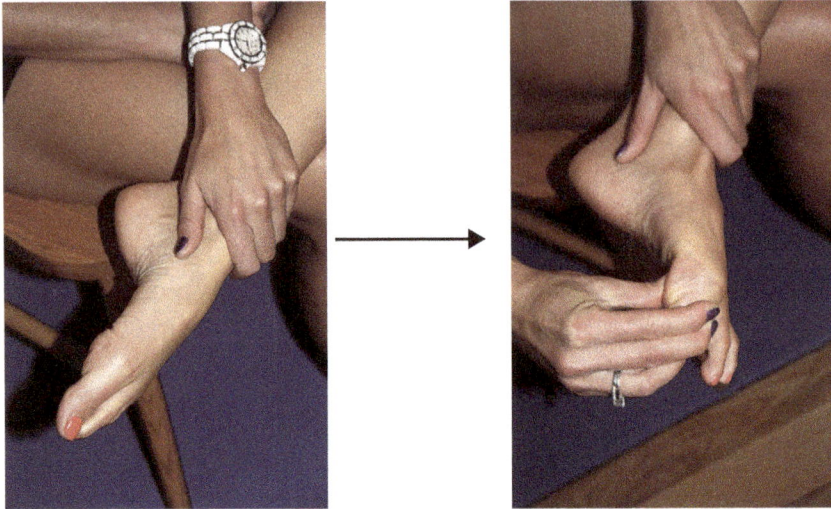

1. Starting position: Sit on a chair, with one leg crossed over the other knee, foot relaxed.
    - Keep your toes relaxed, and your foot pointed and plantar-flexed as shown in this image. Grasp your ankle to stabilize the foot.
    - Wrap the fingers of your other hand around the *front of your big toe*, so that your fingers can pull the big toe towards your body. Use your fingers and thumb to stabilize the joint of the big toe.
2. Gently pull, and pulse your big toe, using three (3)counts to complete each pulse (dynamic stretch).
    - Pulse the big toe about five (5) times, taking three counts for each pulse.
3. After the 5th pulse, hold the stretch for the big toe, in the fully flexed (plantar-flexion) position (for a static stretch).
    - Hold this static stretch for a count of 15.
4. Now, continue to the next exercise in this combination, *Stretch the Foot's Short Extensors on page 183.*

Stretch the Foot's Short Extensors: This combination of dynamic and static exercises uses a combination of pressure and motion to stretch the *extensor digitorum brevis*. This muscle extends all the joints of your toes two (2) through four (4).

Watch this video: (http://www.youtube.com/watch?v=kEBnqg5nnyM, @ 6.13 minutes)

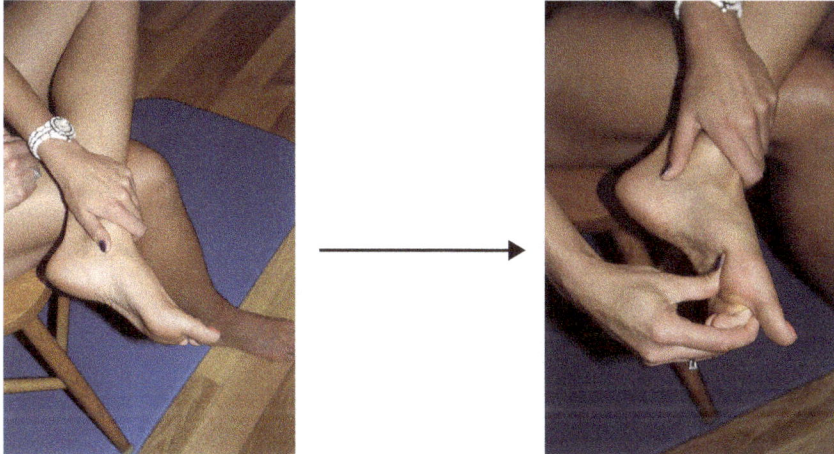

1. Starting position: Sit on a chair, with one leg crossed over the other knee, foot relaxed.
    - Keep your toes relaxed, and your foot in a neutral, relaxed position as shown in this image. Grasp your ankle to stabilize the foot.
    - Wrap the fingers of your other hand around the *front of your toes*, so that your fingers can pull the toes towards your body. If necessary, brace your thumb against the bottom of your foot so you can better control the pulses.
2. Gently pull, and pulse your toes, using three (3) counts to complete each pulse (this is the dynamic stretch).
    - Pulse the toes about five (5) times, taking three counts for each pulse.
3. After the 5th pulse, hold the toes in the fully flexed (plantar-flexion) position (a static stretch) for a count of 15.
4. Continue on to the next part of this exercise – *Stretch the Big Toe's Short Extensors on page 184.*

Stretch the Big Toe's Short Extensors: This combination of dynamic and static motions stretches the *extensor hallicus brevis*. This muscle extends the big toe (*proximal phalanx*).
Watch this video: (http://www.youtube.com/watch?v=kEBnqg5nnyM, @ 5.30 minutes)

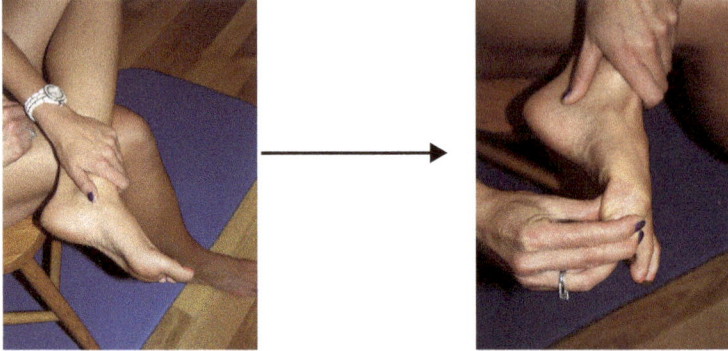

1. Starting position: Sit on a chair, with one leg crossed over the other knee, feet relaxed.
   - Keep your toes relaxed, and your foot in a neutral position as shown in this image. Grasp your ankle to stabilize the foot.
   - Wrap the fingers of your other hand around the *front of your big toe*, so that your fingers can pull the big toe towards your body. Use your fingers and thumb to stabilize the joint of the big toe.
2. Gently pull, and pulse your big toe, holding each pulse for three (3) seconds (this is the dynamic stretch).
   - Pulse the big toe about five (5) times, taking three counts for each pulse.
3. After the 5th pulse, hold the stretch for the big toe in the fully flexed (plantar-flexion) position (for a static stretch). Hold this static stretch for a count of 15.
4. Repeat this entire sequence (*Stretching the Extensors of the Foot on page 181*) for the other leg (if you have Plantar Fasciitis on both feet).

Note: If you only have Plantar Fasciitis on just one foot, then you do NOT need to repeat this exercise sequence for the unaffected leg. Otherwise, repeat this entire sequence on the other foot.

Foundational Myofascial Release of the Foot

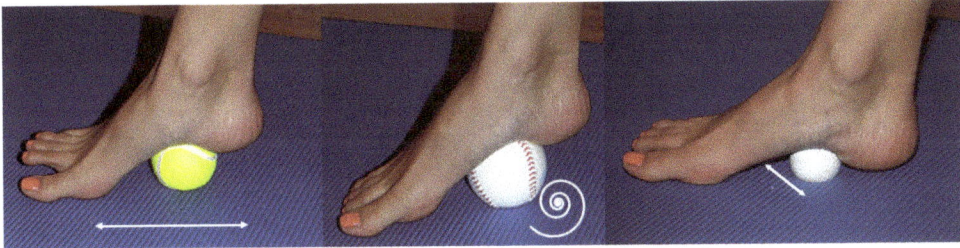

This series of exercises combines self-myofascial and pin-and-stretch techniques to help you effectively release the soft-tissue structures on the bottom of your foot. To perform these exercises you will need a dense ball, such as a lacrosse ball. You will first 'warm up' the tissues of the foot, and then perform myofascial release and pin-and stretch. Take a few minutes to watch and follow-along with the video for this exercise. Watch this Video: http://youtu.be/lk8byu8UGoo

- *Warm-Up of the Foot - page 185.*
- *Myofascial Release of the Foot - page 187.*

TIP: Use the *Follow-Along Foundational Myofascial Release of the Foot YouTube Video* to perform these exercises. In addition to the follow-along video, the video icon beside each of the myofascial exercises links to a separate YouTube video with detailed step-by-step instructions.

Warm-Up of the Foot:
Make sure to perform both part A and B of the warm-up exercise in order to prime the soft-tissues under your foot prior to releasing them. Use a tennis ball for the warm-up. Watch this Video: (http://youtu.be/lk8byu8UGoo, @ 7 min)

Part A: Priming the Tissues of your Foot: Prepare the foot for the next step.

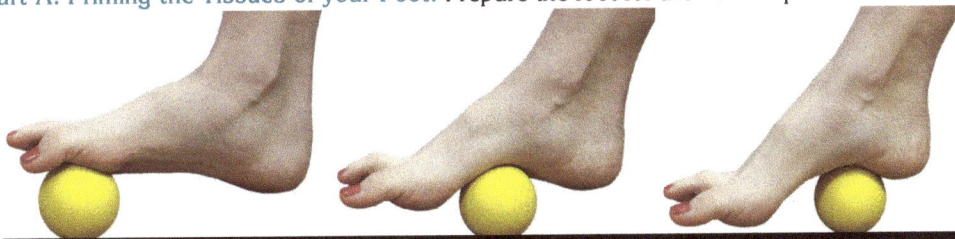

Copyright 2015: Dr. Brian Abelson | Kamali Abelson

1. Starting Position: Stand with one foot resting comfortably on a tennis ball.
2. Roll the ball back and forth **across** the entire length of the bottom of your foot.
   - Roll lengthwise as well as in circles.
   - Make sure to roll the inside, middle and outside part of the bottom of your foot.
   - Roll in a rhythmic and smooth motion.
3. Perform this action for 30 to 60 seconds.
4. Repeat for the other foot if you have Plantar Fasciitis in both feet.

Part B: Engage your Parasympathetic Nervous System: By combining slow deep breathing with compression you will train your body to become *"parasympathetic dominant"*. This process engages the parasympathetic part of your autonomic nervous system - the part the helps to slow your heartbeat, dilate blood vessels and relax muscles. The end result is that you will be able to release the structures at the bottom of the foot in a much more effective way. Watch this Video: (http://youtu.be/lk8byu8UGoo, @ 7.45 min)

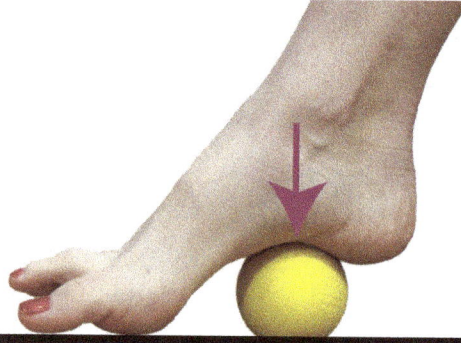

1. Now that you have performed the warm-up exercise, roll the tennis ball over to a tender point on the bottom of your foot and stop there.

2. Hold this position and push your foot into the ball so that you compress the tissue.
    - Use enough force so that you feel the compression, but do not push too hard.
    - You should experience moderate tenderness, but not excruciating pain.

3. Now take in a deep breath, expanding your diaphragm to fill your lungs fully, and hold your breath for one second and then exhale in a relaxed manner.
    - Breathe with your abdomen.
    - Breathing should be slow and relaxed.

4. Perform this exercise for 60 seconds (this will help engage your parasympathetic nervous system).

5. Work your way around the bottom of your foot and combine compression and breathing to help release all the tender areas you find.

Myofascial Release of the Foot: This self-myofascial release exercise uses a lacrosse ball to create a shear force that releases the soft-tissue structures on the bottom of your foot. A shear force acts on a structure in a direction that is perpendicular to the line of fibers within that structure. If you look at the soft-tissue fiber orientation of the bottom foot, you will see that the fibres run predominantly length-wise (from heel to toe) and are parallel to each other. Rolling the ball side-to-side (perpendicularly) across these fibers will create a shear stress between the soft-tissue layers resulting in a more effective release of adhesions and increasing circulation within that area.

Watch this Video: (http://youtu.be/lk8byu8UGoo, @ 8.40 min)

Shear Force Release of the Foot: Be sure to perform both part A and B of the warm-up exercise (*Warm-Up of the Foot - page 185*) before you start.

Watch this Video: (http://youtu.be/lk8byu8UGoo, @ 8.40 min)

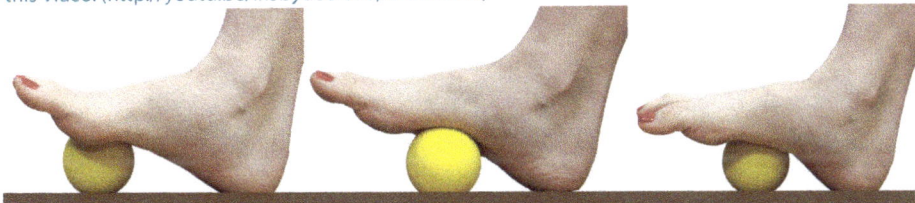

Copyright 2015: Dr. Brian Abelson | Kamali Abelson

1. First Foot Position: Stand and raise your foot up while keeping your heel on the ground. Position the ball under your foot just behind your toes so that the pads of your forefoot rest on the ball.

    ■   Keep your heel on the ground during this entire exercise.

2. Roll the ball side-to-side across the bottom of your foot.

    ■   Roll the ball in short rhythmic motions from side-to-side to create shear stress.
    ■   Use compression while rolling the ball. Stay within your pain limits.
    ■   Spend enough time in each area to feel a release.
    ■   If you come across a tender area, roll it out for an extra 15-20 seconds in order to release it.

3. Repeat this entire exercise in three sections: front, middle, and the back of the bottom of the foot. For each section, release three areas: inside, middle and outside of the bottom of foot.

4. Second Foot Position: Once you've completed this exercise for the three sections and corresponding areas of the foot, change your foot position:

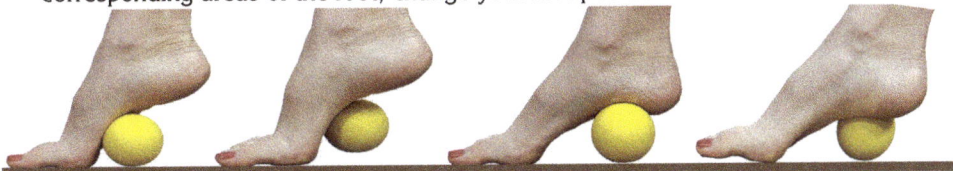

Copyright 2015: Dr. Brian Abelson | Kamali Abelson

Perform side-to-side and rotational movement along the entire length of the foot, while keeping the toes firmly planted on the ground.

    ■   Raise your heel and go up onto your toes.
    ■   Position the ball under your foot.
    ■   Keep your toes on the ground for the rest of this exercise.

5. Repeat step 2 above.

6. Repeat for the other foot if you are experiencing Plantar Fasciitis in both feet.

Pin and Stretch for the Foot: Pin and Stretch exercises were developed and taught by Ida Rolf as early as the 1930's. These exercises are both highly effective and yet simple to perform. They will help you to release adhesions and restrictions that form between soft-tissue layers. Watch this Video: (http://youtu.be/lk8byu8UGoo, @ 12.30 min)

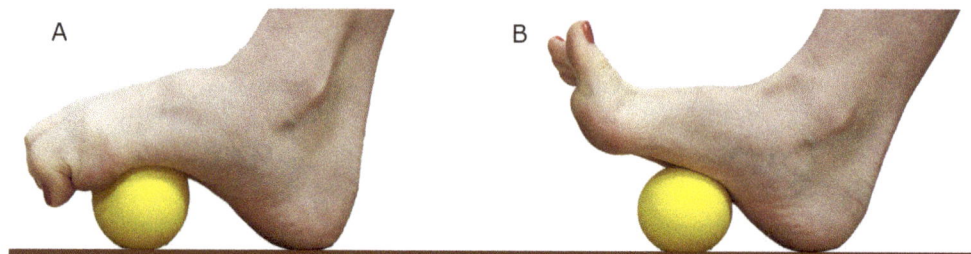

A   B

Copyright 2015: Dr. Brian Abelson | Kamali Abelson

Be sure to perform both part A and B of the warm-up exercise (*Warm-Up of the Foot - page 185*) before you start.

1. Starting Position: Stand and place the ball under your foot just behind your toes so that the pads of your forefoot rest on the ball.

    - Keep your heel on the ground during this entire exercise.

2. Point your toes down so that your foot curls over the ball and hold this position.

    - Compress the ball with your foot to "*pin*" the tissues down.
    - Use enough force to release the soft-tissues, but stay within your pain limits.

3. Pull your toes back towards you to *stretch* the tissue, and then point them down again.

    - Maintain compression.
    - "Perform this dynamic stretch 3 to 5 times.

4. Hold the last stretch in a static position.

    - Pull your toes towards you.
    - Hold for 10 seconds.

5. Repeat this entire exercise in three sections: front, middle, and back of the bottom of the foot. For each section, release three areas: inside, middle and outside of the bottom of foot.

TIP: This process may feel uncomfortable, but it should not cause any sharp, or acute pain. If you find that you are overly sensitive, then ice-massage your feet before doing this exercise. You may also want to consider using a night splint (on a short-term basis) to break the cycle of re-injury, and help your feet adapt and heal more quickly. See *Using a Night Splint for Plantar Fasciitis on page 248* for more information.

Shin Flexibility and Myofascial Release Routine

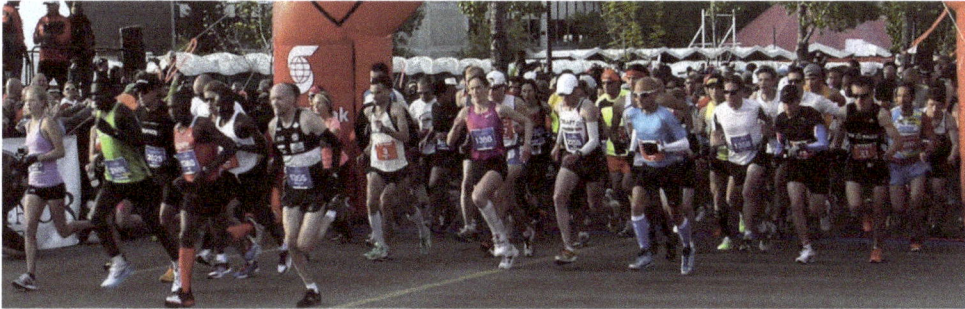

The muscles of your shins play an incredibly important role in the resolution of Plantar Fasciitis. Firstly, your shins act as shock absorbers, dissipating force as you walk or run. Secondly, these muscles control foot impact (during eccentric contraction).

Your shin muscles act as the antagonists to your calf muscles. Tight, restricted shins will neurologically inhibit your calf muscles, forcing them to work unnecessarily harder. Restrictions in the shin muscles also leads to the formation of restrictions in the calf muscles, which in turn is directly related to an increase in the occurrence of Plantar Fasciitis.

The lack of strong, flexible, and unrestricted shins causes a lack in the motion control that is needed to resolve Plantar Fasciitis.

Perform the following stretches if you have identified restrictions in your shins.

- *Stretching the Tibialis Anterior on page 190.*
- *Myofascial Release of the Shins on page 191.*
- *Tiger Tail - Myofascial Release of the Shins on page 192.*

TIP: If you find any tender or restricted areas while performing these stretches, massage them with your fingertips, while working your way up-and-down the entire length of the *tibialis anterior* muscles (shins).

Stretching the Tibialis Anterior: This specific stretch for the *tibialis anterior* muscle combines both dynamic (with movement) and static (no movement) stretching techniques, and can be used for both prevention and treatment of injuries such as bunions, shin splints, and plantar fasciitis. The *tibialis anterior* (TA) muscle allows you to lift (dorsiflex) your foot and toes so that you can clear the ground when walking and running. It also helps you to control the lowering of your foot and toes at the beginning of the stance phase of running or walking.

Restrictions that form in the TA muscle can adversely affect your ability to control these actions. If the TA becomes very tight and restricted, a compression syndrome can also develop in the anterior compartment within which the muscle is located, preventing the runner from properly controlling the lowering of the foot to the ground (*eccentric contraction*), resulting in a slapping action of the foot on the ground.

Watch this video: (YouTube -http://youtu.be/6Z6XM63x2TM)

Stretching the Tibialis Anterior (TA) Muscle

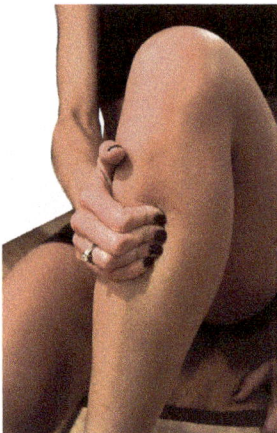

| Locate your shin bone and squeeze your fingers into the TA | Plantar-flex your foot and pull upwards with your fingers | Dorsiflex your foot while maintaining the upwards pull with your fingers |

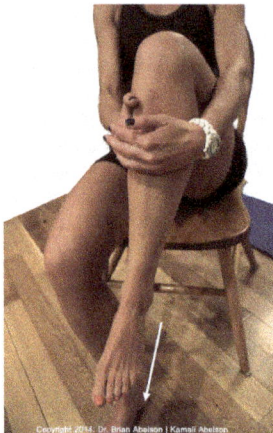

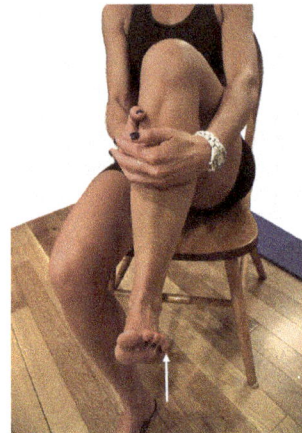

1. Starting Position: Perform this exercise for each leg.
   - Sit in a chair, raise one knee, and with your fingertips, locate your shin bone.
   - Point your foot downwards (plantar-flexed), and keep it in this position until step 3.
   - Move your fingertips towards the outside edge of the shin bone until you drop off the bone, into the muscle belly of the *Tibialis Anterior*.

2. Reinforce your fingers with your other hand, and squeeze them into the *Tibialis Anterior* muscle, *pulling upwards* at the same time.

3. Now, keeping your hands in this position, point your foot down (*plantar flexion - toes away from the shins*) and then pull your foot back up (*dorsiflexion - toes towards your shins*).
   - Repeat this action five (5) to six (6) times, in short pulses, at this location.
   - Follow this with a 5-second hold in the *dorsiflexed position*.

4. Then move your fingers down your shin, and repeat step 3 for this next location. Keep doing this until you have covered the full length of your shins (about 5-to-8 times).

5. Repeat this exercise on the other leg. It should take you a total of three (minutes) to complete this exercise for both legs.

Myofascial Release of the Shins: Myofascial release of the shins is commonly missed in the treatment protocols for Plantar Fasciitis. The following two exercises help to release the structures of the shins, especially the *tibialis anterior* (TA) muscle. The TA has a direct fascial connection into the IT band, as well as into the arch of the foot (*medial cuneiform* and *first metatarsal*).[37] **Watch this video:** (YouTube - http://youtu.be/jQLeVPXjlTQ, @ 1.27 minutes)

Releasing these structures can initially feel quite painful, but this pain will quickly pass after just a few sessions. Use one of the following exercises to release your shins:

- *Foam Roller - Myofascial Release of the Shins on page 191*
- *Tiger Tail - Myofascial Release of the Shins on page 192*

Foam Roller - Myofascial Release of the Shins: Foam rollers come in a variety of densities and hardness. Select a foam roller that you are able to use without excessive force or pain.

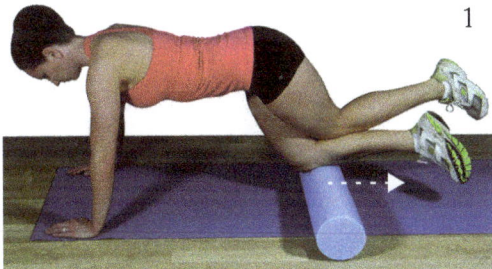

1

If you notice an area that is particularly tight, roll over that specific area for an additional 15-20 seconds on just that tender or restricted area in order to release those soft-tissues.

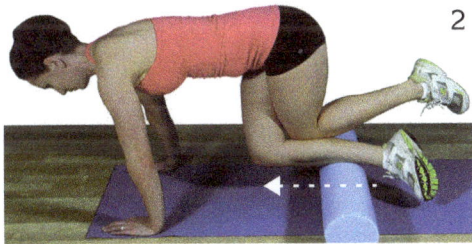

2

You should be able to complete this myofascial release, for both legs, in about three (3) minutes.

1. Starting position: Place the foam roller horizontally on the mat.
   - Kneel down and place your knee on the roller, as shown in Image 1.
   - Place the palms of your hands on the mat to stabilize your upper body.
   - Slightly rotate your leg so the outside fleshy part is against the roller to avoid rolling on your tibia bone.
   - Lift the opposite leg and place its knee behind the leg on the roller.
2. Use your weight to roll the foam roller from the top of your shins, all the way down towards the ankle. Include small side-to-side motions to create shear forces that break adhesions and increase circulation between tissue layers.
3. Once the roller reaches the ankle, reverse directions, and return to just below the knee.
4. Repeat for 15-20 times.
5. Now reverse your legs and repeat for the opposite side of your body.

---

37. Anatomy Trains, 2nd Edition, Myofascial Meridians for Manual and Movement Therapist, Thomas W. Meyers, Churchill Livingstone, Copyright: 2009

Tiger Tail - Myofascial Release of the Shins: The *Tiger Tail* is a specialized rolling pin (where the rolling pin is covered in thin foam) that is designed to release soft-tissue restrictions. It is an ideal tool for deep tissue massage along the length of the shins and calves. There are several other similar devices, but we have found the Tiger Tail to be the most effective and versatile. **Watch this video:** (YouTube - http://youtu.be/jQLeVPXjlTQ, @ 2.55 minutes)

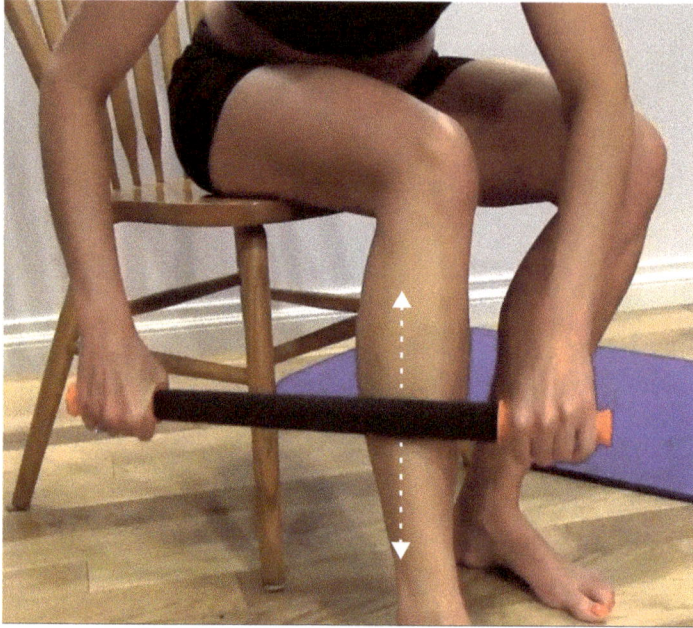

1.   Starting Position: Sit on a chair with a *Tiger Tail* or *other similar device* in your hands.

2.   Start by rolling the *Tiger Tail* back-and-forth across the muscles at the front and outside part of the shin (*tibialis anterior, extensor digitorum longus, extensor hallicus longus, peroneus longus, peroneus brevis, and peroneus tertius muscles*).

   ■   Apply enough pressure to release the areas of restriction, but not enough pressure to cause you acute pain. In most cases, this exercise will feel good as the restrictions are released.

3.   Repeat this action 15-20 times.

   ■   If you notice an area that is particularly tight or restricted, then work over that tender or restricted area for an additional 15-20 seconds to release those soft-tissues.

   ■   Try to move the Tiger Tail at different angles, or try rotating your foot back and forth slowly as you perform this release. This will add shear stress to this exercise, helping to release restrictions and increase circulation between the tissue layers.

4.   Repeat this process on the other leg.

   ■   The entire exercise, for both legs, should take a total of three to four minutes.

Stretching and Releasing the Peroneals: Injuries to the *peroneal* muscles often occur during an ankle sprain (inversion sprain). Chronic injuries of the *peroneal* muscles are often associated with ankle instability, and can involve numerous structures along the kinetic chain. The *peroneals* run along the outside of leg, below the knee (*fibula*), down the side of the leg, around the ankle (*lateral malleolus*), and insert under the foot (at the first *metatarsal*)[38]. The *peroneus longus* (on the lateral side) and the *tibialis posterior* (on the medial side) support the arch of the foot.

This exercise releases restrictions in the *peroneus longus* and *peroneus brevis* (also known as the *fibularis longus* and *fibularis brevis*). These muscles lie along the outside of your lower leg. They help you to push off through the ankle (*plantar flexion*) and stabilize the lower extremity (by maintaining the *transverse arch* of your foot). Perform the following two stretches on the involved leg(s).

- *Peroneal Stretch on page 193.*
- *Myofascial Release of the Peroneals on page 194.*

Peroneal Stretch: The peroneals are often difficult to stretch and are often neglected in most stretching routines. This peroneal stretch stretches both the *peroneus longus* and *peroneus brevis*. Many people find this supported stretch (using a strap or towel) to be highly effective.
Watch this video: (YouTube - http://www.youtube.com/watch?v=g38uNfDGVwI, @ min=2.03)

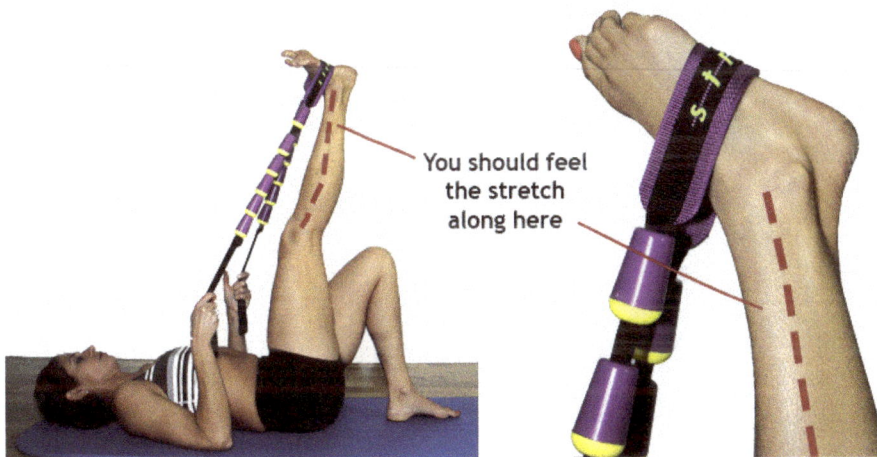

You should feel the stretch along here

1. Starting position: Sit on the floor, with one leg straight.
   - Wrap either a strap or towel around your foot as illustrated.
   - Keep your foot turned in (inverted).
   - Holding the strap in your hands, lie back on the floor.
2. Raise your leg straight up, while keeping your foot in the turned-in position (inverted).
   - Increase the tension on the strap or towel until you feel a stretch along the *peroneal* muscles.
   - Hold this position for 10-15 seconds.
3. Repeat the exercise three or four times on each affected leg.

38. Dananberg, H, Understanding the impact of muscle weakness. Podiatry Today. Vol 15. Issue #4 April 1 2002. pp 60-62. http://www.podiatrytoday.com/article/290

Myofascial Release of the Peroneals: One of the most effective ways of releasing the peroneal muscle is to use the foam roller in the sitting position. A travel roller works very well since it is smaller than standard rollers.

Watch this video: (YouTube - http://www.youtube.com/watch?v=g38uNfDGVwI, @ min=2.56).

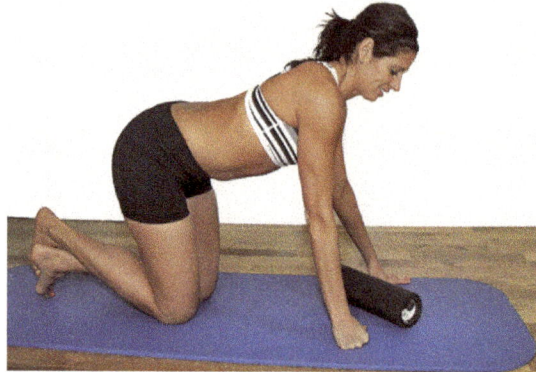

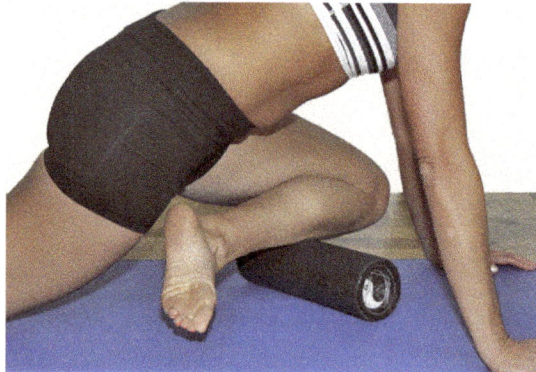

1. Starting position: Sit with one leg stretched back, and the other leg folded forward as shown.

    - ◼ Place the front leg on the foam roller as illustrated.
    - ◼ The roller should be against your peroneal muscles.

2. Start by rolling back and forth in short sections, applying as much pressure as you need to release the peroneal restrictions. This can be an intense experience, but should *not* be a painful procedure.

    - ◼ Roll back and forth 5-to-10 times along each section of the peroneal muscles.
    - ◼ Add side-to-side and circular motions at each stage to increase the shear force that releases restrictions and increases circulation in that area.
    - ◼ Once you finish one area, move the foam roller down your leg to the next section, and repeat.

3. Repeat this procedure until you reach the ankle.

4. Repeat this exercise on the other leg.

Calf Flexibility and Myofascial Release Routine

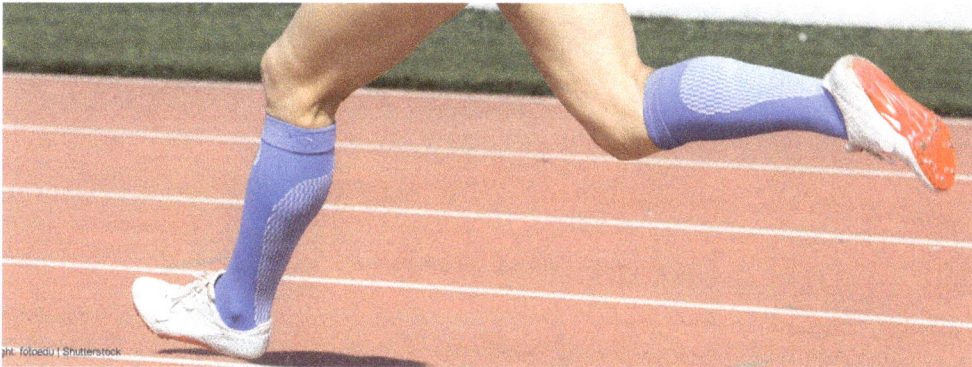

Several studies have found a correlation between tight calf muscles (*gastrocnemius* and *soleus*) and Plantar Fasciitis. The calf muscle complex is often referred to as the *triceps surae*, its most important function is plantar flexion (lifting of the heel off the ground, or rising up on your toes). Tight restricted calf muscles are almost always accompanied by tight hamstrings, and numerous compensations in the core of your body.[39]

Restrictions and adhesions in your calf muscles must be released in order to fully resolve any cases of Plantar Fasciitis. Upon contraction, your calf muscles not only pull your heel up (causing forward motion), but they also act as the antagonist muscles to the actions of your shins (which control how your feet strike the ground with every step). Any restrictions or tension in the calf will result in decreased shin strength, causing biomechanical imbalances along the kinetic chain. See *The Role of the Shins & Calves in Plantar Fasciitis - page 64* for more information about the importance of these structures in resolving Plantar Fasciitis.

Caution: For all stretches, it is important to FIRST perform 10 to 20 minutes of cardiovascular warm-ups. This can be cycling, swimming, or an elliptical machine.

---

39. Labovitz, J. M.; Yu, J., The Role of Hamstring Tightness in Plantar Fasciitis. Foot & Ankle Specialist 2011, 4 (3), 141-144.

Stretching the Calf Muscles: This two-part exercise stretches both the *gastrocnemius* and *soleus* muscles with a combination of dynamic (with movement) and static (no movement) stretching techniques. The variations in heel position can help you to determine and isolate the affected areas, and help to increase calf flexibility.
Watch this video: (YouTube - http://youtu.be/JSzCfi0wbcA)

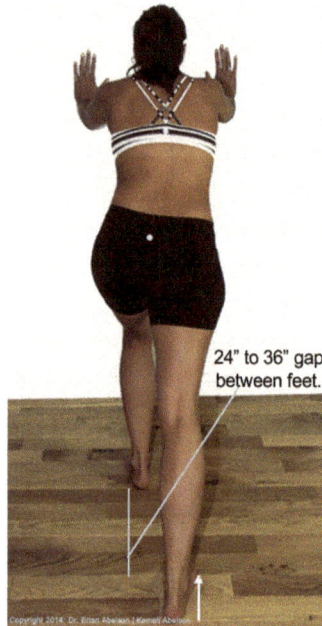

Stretching the Calf (Gastrocnemius) Muscles

You should be able to complete this exercise, for both legs, in about 3 minutes.

Rotate your ankle to the inside and outside, paying attention to when you feel tension in the ankle. Stretch in that position until you feel a release.

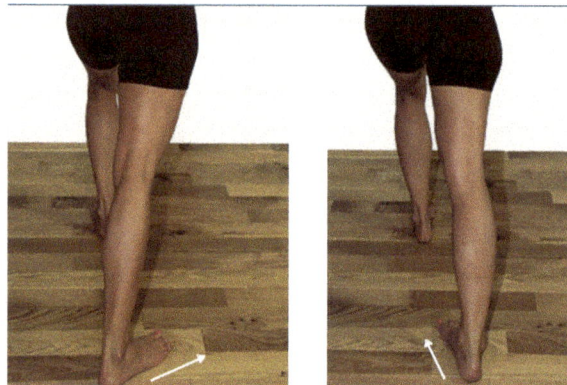

24" to 36" gap between feet.

1. Face the wall and place the palms of your hands against the wall.
   - Support your upper body by bracing your arms against the wall.
   - Move one leg back about 2 to 3 feet, making sure that both feet are facing directly forward, and the heel of your back foot remains firmly planted on the ground.
   - Lean forward towards the wall.

Part 1: Stretch the Gastrocnemius: (YouTube - http://youtu.be/JSzCfi0wbcA, 0.15 minutes)

2. Now bend the front leg slightly, while keeping the back leg extended and straight. You should feel tension closer to the knee than to the ankle.

3. Rotate or angle your heel to the inside and to the outside, paying attention to where you feel the tension in your calf.

4. Once you find the point of tension, hold this position and perform 3-4 *dynamic pulses* followed by a *static stretch* for 15-to-20 seconds, or until you feel a release of the tension.

5. Repeat this *gastrocnemius* stretch two to three times (2-to-3 times), and then repeat with the other leg. It should take about 3 minutes to perform this stretch on both legs.

Part 2: Stretch the Soleus: **Watch this video:** (YouTube - http://youtu.be/JSzCfi0wbcA, @ 1.50 minutes)

Stretching the Calf (Soleus) Muscles

You should be able to complete this
exercise, for both legs, in about 3 minutes.

Rotate your ankle to the inside and outside, paying
attention to when you feel tension in the ankle.
Stretch in that position until you feel a release.

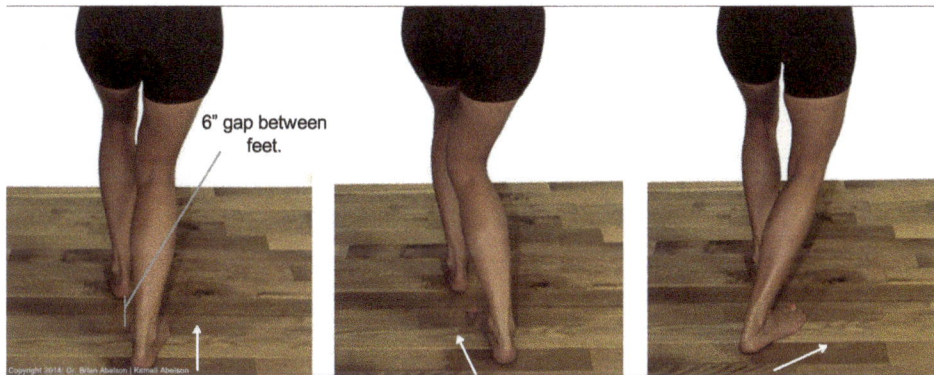

6" gap between feet.

1. Now, bring the back leg forward until there is a 6-inch gap between the two feet. Keep both feet pointing straight forward, with heels firmly planted on the ground throughout the stretch.

2. Bend *both legs* to create a stretch along the *soleus* muscle of the back leg. You should feel tension closer to the ankle than to the knee for this stretch.

3. Next, rotate or angle your heel to the *inside* and to the *outside*, paying attention to where you feel the tension.

4. Once you find the **point of tension**, perform 3-4 *dynamic pulses* followed by a *static stretch* for 15-20 seconds, or until you feel a release of the tension.

5. Repeat this *soleus* stretch two to three times (2 to 3 times), and then repeat with the other leg. It should take about 3 minutes to perform this stretch on both legs.

Myofascial Release of the Calf : In addition to stretching, it is very important to actually *release the restrictions* within the calf muscles. To do this, we are providing **three** types of myofascial release exercises for the calf - the first is with a *foam roller*, the second is with a *soft ball,* and the third is with a *tiger tail* roller. Perform these myofascial releases on the same day as the stretching exercises (but you can choose to do it at a different time of that same day). Perform one of these exercises to release your calf muscles.
Watch this video: (YouTube - http://youtu.be/Q4rCu53K_gw)

First Exercise – Myofascial Release of the Calf with a Foam Roller: This method covers a large area of the calf and is less forceful.
Watch this video: (YouTube - http://youtu.be/Q4rCu53K_gw, @ 0.14 minutes)

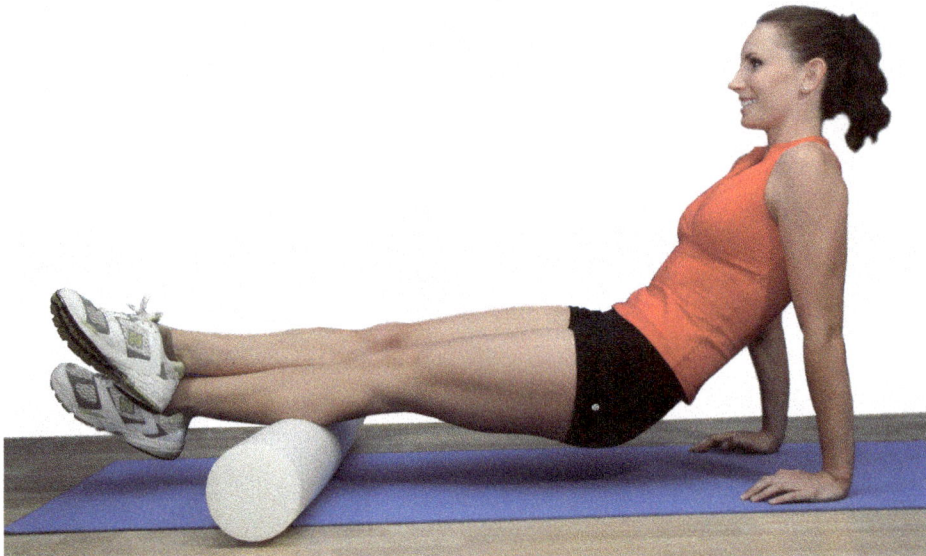

1. Starting Position: Sit on the mat with the foam roller placed horizontally under the fleshy part of the calf muscles.
   - Use the palms of your hands to stabilize your upper body as shown in this image.
   - Cross the right ankle over the left ankle.
   - Lift your body up so that your hips clear the floor.
2. Slowly roll the foam roller from the top of the calves to the heels.
   Stop and reverse directions. Repeat for 45-60 seconds.
   - If you notice an area that is particularly tight, stop and rest over that tender point for an additional 20-30 seconds.
   - Include some side-to-side motions at each stage to increase the shear stress on the tissues, making it easier to release adhesions, and to improve circulation in those tissues.
3. Now reverse your legs and repeat for the opposite side of your body.

TIP: Variation - If you find that there is too much stress on your arms, you can use one leg to stabilize your body. Just place the foot of the other leg flat on the ground to reduce shoulder stress and achieve better control while using the roller.

Second Exercise – Myofascial Release of the Calf with a Soft-Ball: This method is very effective at addressing restrictions in your calf muscles that require deeper, more intensive attention. The softball allows for a broader range of motion, since you can use both linear and circular motions along the fleshy areas of the calf. Though this is more intense than a foam roller, it remains my first choice for myofascial release of the calf muscles.

Watch this video: (YouTube - http://youtu.be/Q4rCu53K_gw, @ 1.30 minutes)

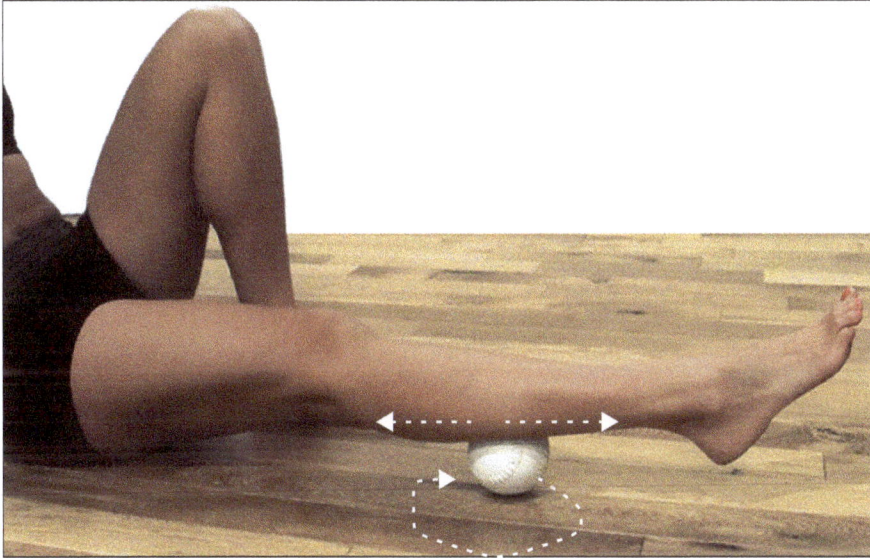

1. Starting Position: Sit on the mat with a soft-ball (baseball) under your calf muscle.
    - Use the palms of your hands to stabilize your upper body
    - Keep the other leg bent to stabilize your body.
    - Lift your hips off the ground by using your arms and the bent leg.

2. Roll the ball up and down the length of your calf. Cover the middle, inside, and outside of your calf muscles.
    - Alternate the up-and-down motion with circular motions. Do this for 30 to 60 seconds.
    - Include some side-to-side motions at each stage to increase the shear stress on the tissues, making it easier to release adhesions, and to improve circulation in those tissues.
    - If you notice an area that is particularly tight, stop and rest over that tender point for an additional 20-30 seconds.

3. Now reverse your legs and repeat for the opposite side of your body.

TIP: Depending on your tolerance, you can use balls of different densities to increase or decrease the amount of pressure exerted on your tissues.

Third Exercise – Myofascial Release of the Calves with a Tiger Tail: The *Tiger Tail* is a specialized rolling pin (the rolling pin is covered in thin foam) which is designed to release myofascial restrictions. There are numerous brands available on the open market that achieve similar results, but personally, have found the Tiger Tail to be one of the most effective. **Watch this video:** (YouTube - http://youtu.be/Q4rCu53K_gw, @ 2.15 minutes)

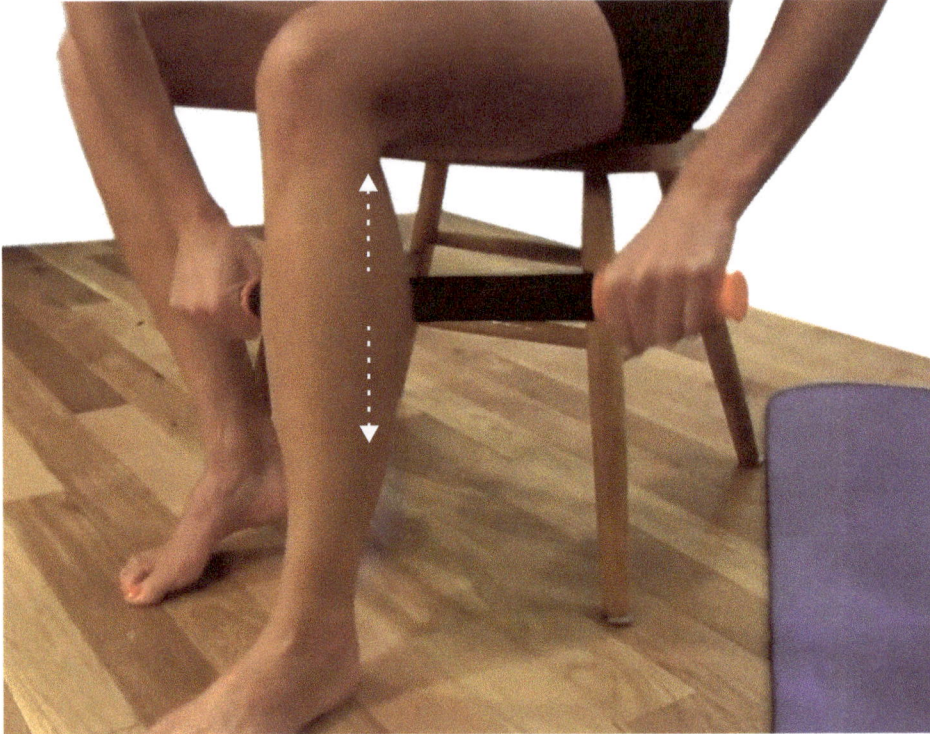

1. Starting Position: Sit on a chair with a *Tiger Tail* or *other similar device* in your hands.

2. Start by rolling the *Tiger Tail* up-and-down the full length of your calf muscles. Apply enough pressure to feel it in the deeper tissues, without causing intense pain. Make sure you cover the inner and outer sides of the calf muscle.

3. Repeat this action 15-20 times.
    - If you notice an area that is particularly tight or restricted, then be sure to work over that tender or restricted area for an additional 15-20 seconds to release those soft-tissues.

4. Change the vector as you move up and down the calf muscles. By moving the roller at a slight diagonal, you will increase the level of shear stress and make it easier to release adhesions between the tissues, and increase circulation in this area.

5. Repeat for the other leg.

Stretching the Hip Flexors

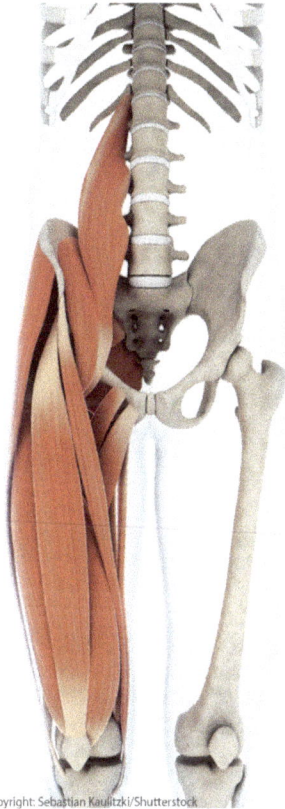

Hip flexors are the muscles that lift your leg when you walk, or help you to move your thigh towards the abdomen. The *iliacus, psoas major*, and *psoas minor* are the primary movers for hip flexion. Together, these three structures are known as the *iliopsoas* muscle.

Hip flexors play an important role in maintaining the stability and function of your lower extremities. In addition to acting as the primary hip flexor, the *iliacus* and *psoas* muscles act as the antagonist to your *glutes* (your primary shock absorbers). Through the process of reciprocal inhibition, tension in these structures will inhibit gluteal function, and increase the amount of shock experienced by the other muscles of your body when you walk or run.

If you lead a lifestyle in which you are always sitting, these muscles will be pulled into a shortened contracted position, leaving them very tight. Tight hip flexors can leave you with limited power when walking or running, and can have a direct impact on your Plantar Fasciitis.

Copyright: Sebastian Kaulitzki/Shutterstock

Perform the exercises in the following section if your tests showed restrictions in the hip flexors.

- *Stretching your Primary Hip Flexors on page 202.*
- *Stretching the Quadriceps - Secondary Hip Flexors on page 203*

Caution: For all stretches, it is important to FIRST perform 10 to 20 minutes of cardiovascular warm-ups. This can be cycling, swimming, or elliptical machines.

Stretching your Primary Hip Flexors: This is both a dynamic and static stretch of your primary hip flexors – the *psoas* and *iliacus* muscles. It is important to stretch both these muscles, as they are the antagonist, or oppositional muscles for the gluteals. If these are tight, you will decrease the stability of the entire lower extremity.

Watch this video: (YouTube - http://youtu.be/NMvFE--4jXw)

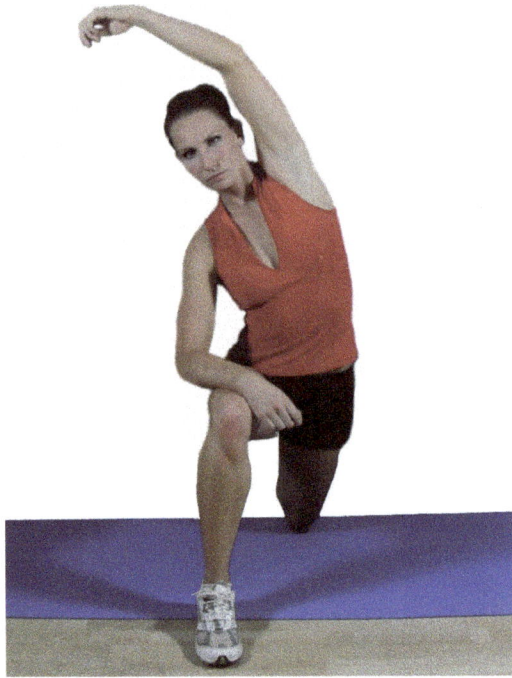

1. Starting position:
    - Get into a front-lunge position, and rest the back knee on the ground.
    - Rest your forearm on the bent leg.
    - Raise the other arm over your head.
    - Push your pelvis forward.
2. Exhale, push forward with your pelvis, and reach over to the opposite side as shown here. You want to stretch both the *iliacus* and *psoas*. Make sure your arm reaches over your head – otherwise only the *iliacus* is stretched.
3. Bring your arm back to your side and relax your pelvis. Repeat from step 2, and with each repetition, bring your arm over and push your pelvis forward.
4. Start by performing 5 dynamic stretches, and then hold the static stretch for 20-30 seconds.
5. Repeat from step 1 for the opposite side.

Stretching the Quadriceps - Secondary Hip Flexors: Your quadriceps are your weaker hip flexors (*secondary hip flexors*). All four quadriceps are powerful extensors of the knee, and have the additional task of stabilizing the knee cap (*patella*) during walking or running. These structures often become restricted when your primary hip flexors become tight. When your primary hip flexors are unable to perform their normal tasks (due to restrictions) then that force is transferred into your secondary hip flexors. These restrictions must be released in order for your primary hip flexors to function properly.

Watch this video: (YouTube - http://youtu.be/NMvFE--4jXw, @ 1:35 minutes)

Basic Quadricep Stretch

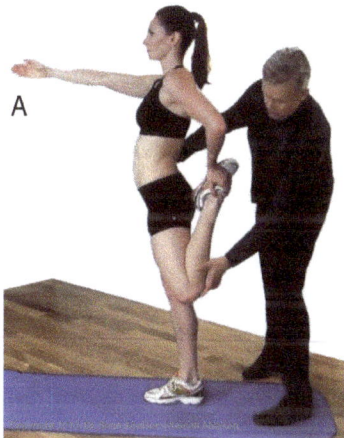

A

Advanced Quadricep Stretch

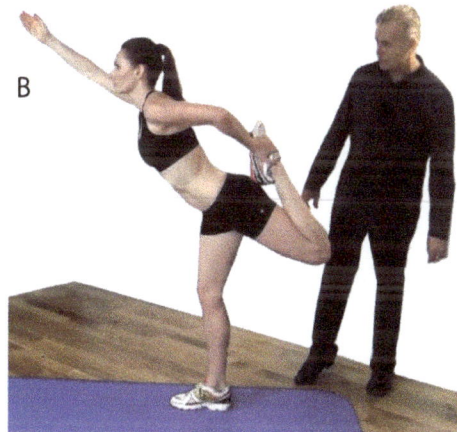

B

1. Starting Position: See Image A.
   - Stand straight, with both feet on the ground.
   - Bring one leg back, bending at the knee.
   - Grip the top of that foot with your hand to hold it in position.
   - Keep your hips tucked in and forward facing, chest up.
2. Stretch your other arm out in front of you to help maintain your balance.
3. Now push outwards with your foot (away from the buttocks), while at the same time resisting this motion with your hand. At the same time, push your pelvis forward.
   - Ensure your bent knee does not move outward, and stays tucked close to the standing leg throughout this stretch. *See Image A: Basic Quadricep Stretch*.
4. Hold this stretch for 15-to-20 seconds.

TIP: You can increase the stretch by bending your upper body forward, reaching forward with your extended arm, while maintaining your hold on your foot. Again, hold for 15 seconds, and repeat 3 to 5 times on each side. *See Image B: Advanced Quadricep Stretch.*

---

5. Repeat this exercise 3 to five (5) times for each leg.

Single Leg PNF - Hamstring Stretch: Having good hamstring flexibility is a key component of resolving Plantar Fasciitis. There are direct fascial connections between your hamstrings, calf muscles (*gastrocnemius*), *Achilles tendon*, and *plantar fascia*. Essentially, tight hamstrings force you to walk or run on the toes (metatarsals). This reduces shock absorption by your foot (through the windlass mechanism), transmits force back up your body, and causes a multitude of problems.

Watch this video: (YouTube - http://youtu.be/BJI5uPhWM6U)

TIP: If you find that you do not have the flexibility to straighten your leg, use a stretching strap to assist in straightening the leg.

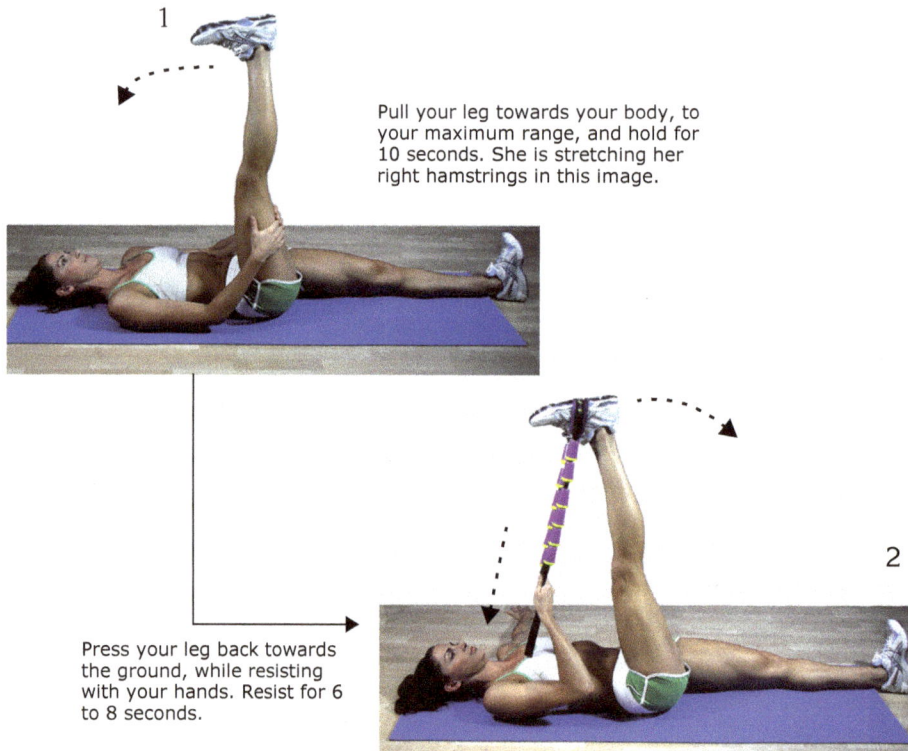

1

Pull your leg towards your body, to your maximum range, and hold for 10 seconds. She is stretching her right hamstrings in this image.

2

Press your leg back towards the ground, while resisting with your hands. Resist for 6 to 8 seconds.

1. Starting position: Lay on your back on a mat.
   - Bend your leg as if you were bringing your knee to your chest.
   - Once your knee is perpendicular to the floor, straighten your leg as far as you can. To increase the stretch, use a stretching device as shown.
2. Grasp your thigh with your hand and hold this position for 10 seconds. See image 1.
3. Now press your leg *back down* against your hand (while using your hands to resist that action) for 6 to 8 seconds.
4. Next, release, and pull your leg even further towards your body and hold for 10 counts.
5. Repeat this process 4-to-5 times, each time increasing the degree of stretch.
6. Repeat for the other leg.

Increasing Joint Mobility

The following exercises increase the joint mobility of your foot, knees, and ankle.

Increasing Dorsiflexion of the Foot with a Theraband: This is a great exercise for increasing ankle mobility. In this exercise you will be moving the ankle joint posterior, while the *tibia* (shin bone) moves forward. Over time, you will find that your ankle mobility will increase considerably. For this exercise, you will need a mat or towel, a dowel or a broom handle, and a length of Theraband (since the theraband is broad, it can be comfortably wrapped around the ankle). This exercise is quite simple, but we do recommend watching the video to learn how to easily setup and prepare for this exercise.
Watch this video: (YouTube - http://youtu.be/UVcS6kP5aPc)

1.

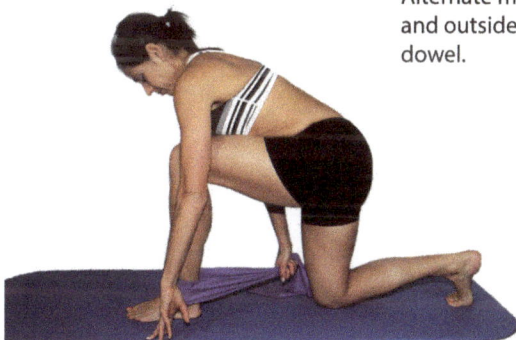

2.

Lunge forward so that your knee moves past the dowel. Alternate moving inside and outside of the dowel.

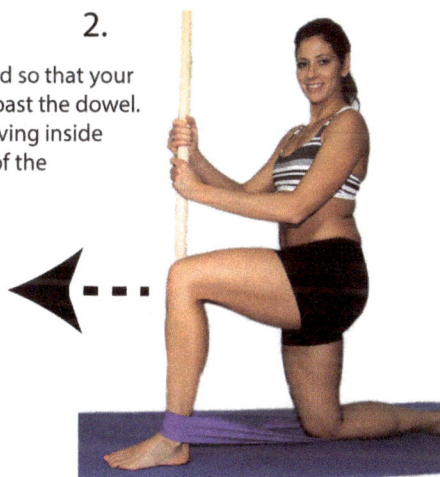

1. Starting position:
   - ■ Kneel on the mat (or towel) and wrap the Theraband or rubber tubing around your ankle.
   - ■ Bring tension into the Theraband and place the band under the other knee to hold it in place. See image 1.
   - ■ Adjust the position of the front foot until you have a fair amount of tension.
   - ■ Take the dowel and place it just in front of the ankle, along the inside of your leg.
2. While maintaining the tension on the Theraband, lunge forward so that your knee moves past the dowel.
3. Now draw your knee back. On the next pass, take your knee past the inside of the dowel. With each pass, alternate moving your knee past the inside, then the outside of the dowel.
4. Perform 10 to 15 repetitions, 2 to 3 sets on each leg.

Increasing Mobility of the Big Toe: Having good mobility in the joints of the big toe is essential for maintaining a normal gait. Unfortunately, the two main joints of the big toe (*metatarsophalangeal joint (MTP)* and the *distal interphalangeal joint (DIP)*) are common sites of restriction. In addition, the most common site of arthritis in the foot is at the base of the big toe. The following exercise is a simple and effective way to release restrictions in these key joints. **Watch this video:** (YouTube - http://youtu.be/rS7tZQTFEV0)

TIP: Watch this video before performing this exercise. It is a very effective and simple exercise that is well understood after watching the video.

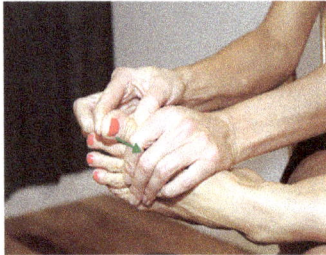
Extension, straighten and extend the big toe.

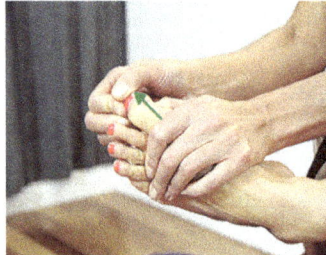
Flexion, curl your big toe downwards.

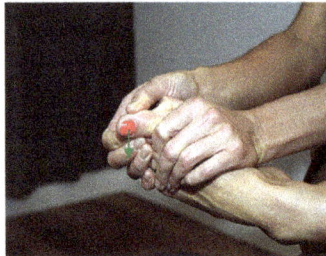
Adduction, bring the big toe towards the others!

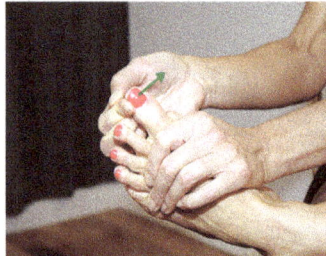
Abduction, move the big toe away from the others!

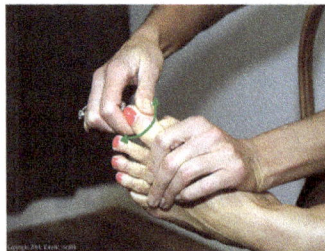
Gently rotate the MTP joint of the big toe.

1. Starting position: Sit on a chair, with one leg crossed over the knee, feet relaxed.
    - Relax your toes, foot and ankle.
2. Lock-out the *metatarsophalangeal joint* (MTP):
    - Lock-out the MTP joint by grasping it with your hand. Use the hand that is on the same side as the leg that is crossed over to lock out the joint.
    - Make sure that the MTP joint remains locked for this entire exercise.
    - Grasp your big toe with the other hand.

3. Now mobilize this joint five times, in each of the following six positions: *flexion, extension, abduction, adduction, clockwise rotation* and *counter-clockwise rotation*.

    ■ Perform 5 mobilizations in one position before moving on to the next position.

    ■ Follow the sequence in the order that it is listed above. Start with five *flexions*, then five *extensions*, and so forth until you have mobilized the big toe in all six positions.

    ■ Movement should be slow and rhythmic.

    ■ Make sure to move the joint through its full range of motion.

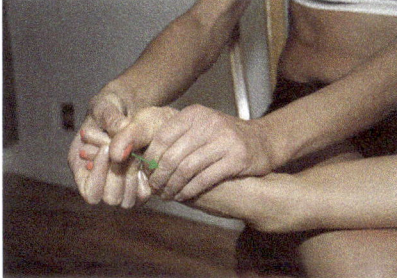

Extension...straighten and extend the big toe.

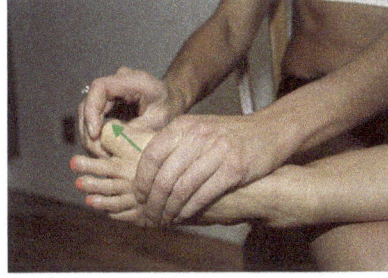

Flexion...curl your big toe downwards.

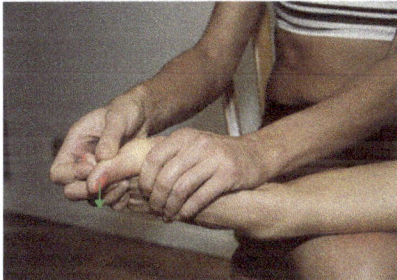

Adduction, bring the big toe towards the others.

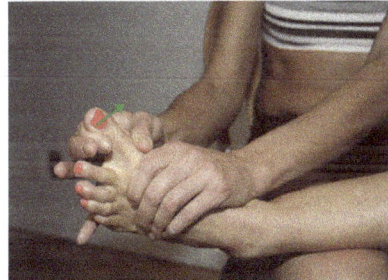

Abduction, move the big toe away from others.

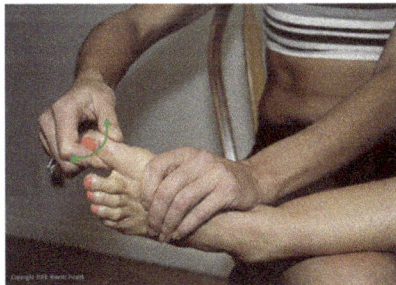

Gently rotate the DIP joint of the big toe.

4. Now, lock-out the *distal interphalangeal joint* (DIP):

    ■ Lock out the DIP joint by grasping it with your hand. Use that same hand positions as in step 2 above.

    ■ It is very important that the DIP joint remains locked during this entire exercise.

    ■ Grasp the end of your big toe with the other hand.

5. Repeat step 3, for the DIP joint.

Nerve Flossing for Plantar Fasciitis

Use the following nerve flossing exercises if you identified issues in the *tibial* and *peroneal* nerves in the *Functional Test for Tibial Nerve Impingement - page 146* and *Functional Test for Peroneal Nerve Impingement - page 147*.

- *Tensioning the Tibial Nerve - Supine: - page 209.*
- *Mobilizing the Tibial Nerve - Seated - page 210.*
- *Flossing the Peroneal Nerve - Supine Mobilization - page 212.*
- *Mobilizing the Peroneal Nerve - Seated Position - page 213.*

See *Common Nerve Compression Sites for PF - page 87* for more information about these issues.

Tibial Nerve Flossing Exercises

Watch this video: (YouTube - http://youtu.be/Ak6lHdljnVA)

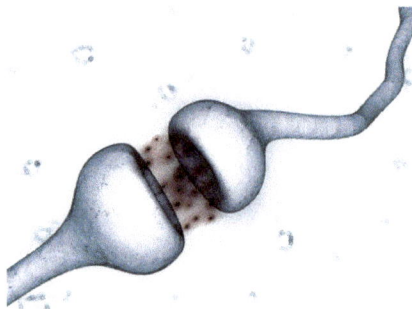

The *tibial nerve* is a branch of the *sciatic nerve*, that goes down the back of the calf muscles. This is a very important nerve that aids in pushing forward during your gait cycle. The *tibial nerve* passes through the *popliteal fossa*, and eventually through the arch of the *soleus* to the bottom of the foot.

The *tibial nerve* has both motor and sensory branches; the motor branches supply the back of the calf. When there is nerve entrapment in this area, the calf muscles are often reduced or atrophied. When there is compression of the sensory branches of the *tibial nerve*, you may experience numbness, tingling, and altered sensation along the back of the *calf*. Restrictions of this nerve will affect your ability to plantar flex the foot, or your ability to flex your toes downwards.

Nerve flossing exercises (combined with other protocols) can help you to resolve even chronic problems that have not responded to conventional therapy. Tibial nerve entrapment is often involved in cases of Plantar Fasciitis, wherein smaller branches of this nerve (medial and lateral Plantar nerves) can become irritated or inflamed due to soft tissue restrictions of the foot leading to plantar foot pain. The following exercises will help you to release a *tibial nerve* entrapment, which is commonly associated with foot and ankle weakness or pain.

- Tensioning the Tibial Nerve - Supine: ------ page 209.
- Mobilizing the Tibial Nerve - Seated ------ page 210.

Tensioning the Tibial Nerve - Supine: This exercise is similar to the Hamstring Stretch, but by everting and dorsiflexing the foot, you will be tensioning and adding tractional force to help pull and release the *tibial nerve* as it passes through the calf muscles.
Watch this video: (YouTube - http://youtu.be/Ak6lHdljnVA @1.16 min)

1

2

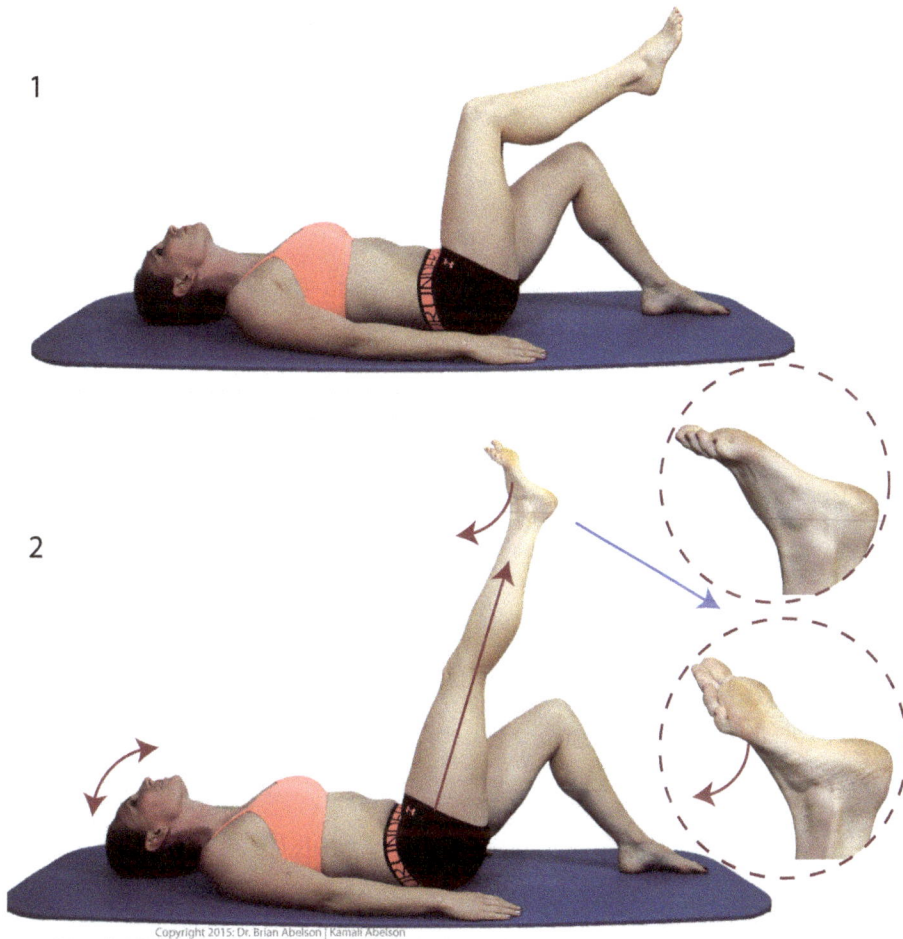

Copyright 2015: Dr. Brian Abelson | Kamali Abelson

1. Starting Position: Lie flat on your back, legs outstretched.
   - Bend one hip, and raise that leg up so that your hip and knees are bent at 90 degrees as shown in image 1.
2. Now straighten your leg at the knee and flex (dorsi-flex) your foot towards your shins, while tilting the foot outwards (eversion) at the same time.
   - Hold this position for two to five seconds to apply tension and traction on the *tibial nerve*, and to release the restrictions around it.
3. Bend your leg at the knee and relax your foot.
   - Keep your movements slow and controlled.
   - This a dynamic exercise, not a stretch.
4. Repeat this exercise five (5) to ten (10) times for each foot.

Mobilizing the Tibial Nerve - Seated: Tibial nerve entrapment is often involved in cases of Plantar Fasciitis, wherein smaller branches of this nerve (medial and lateral Plantar nerves) can become irritated or inflamed due to soft tissue restrictions of the foot leading to plantar foot pain.

Watch this video: (YouTube - http://youtu.be/Ak6lHdljnVA, 2.14 min)

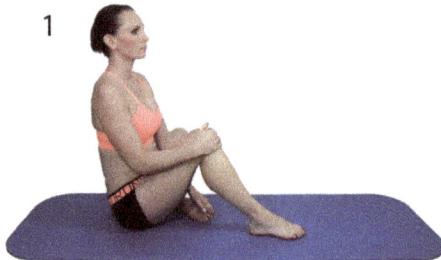

1

Copyright 2015: Dr. Brian Abelson | Kamali Abelson

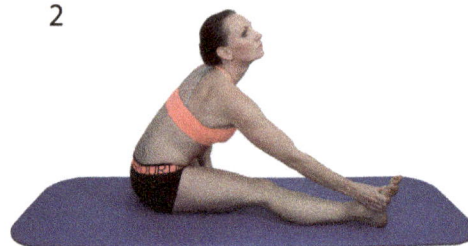

2

Evert the foot to floss the nerve.

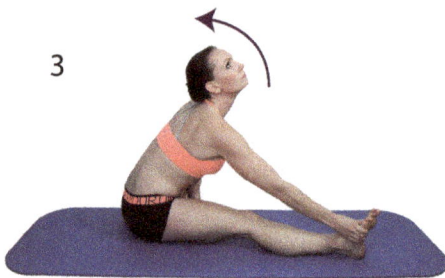

3

Mobilize the nerve through the tissues.

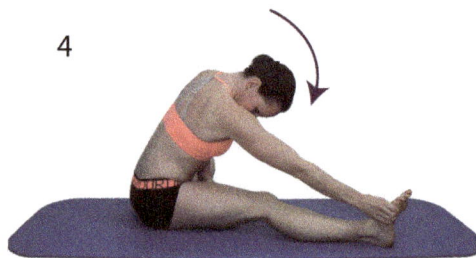

4

Increase tension on the nerve.

1. **Starting Position:**
   - Sit up straight, one leg folded in, and other outstretched as shown in image 1.
   - Bend the knee of outstretched leg so that the foot rests flat on the floor.
2. Straighten your leg at the knee and tilt your foot outwards (eversion), hold for one to two seconds (image 2).
   - To increase mobilization of the nerve so it glides through the tissues, tilt your head backward (extension) as shown in image 3.
   - To increase tension on the nerve, tip your head forward (flexing) as in image 4.
3. Bring the outstretched leg back to your body, and repeat step 2.
4. Repeat this action five to ten times for each foot.

Peroneal Nerve Flossing Exercises

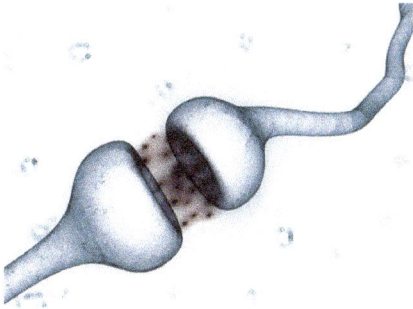

The following two exercises will help to release and mobilize an entrapped *peroneal nerve* by "flossing" it back and forth through the surrounding soft-tissues. The *peroneal nerve* can become trapped by, or can even adhere to, soft-tissue restrictions within the muscles and connective tissue of the lower leg. This entrapment can often lead to pain, burning or tingling sensations, muscle imbalances, and muscle weakness.

These are both great exercises to perform if you are suffering from a *peroneal nerve* entrapment.

- *Flossing the Peroneal Nerve - Supine Mobilization on page 212*.
- *Mobilizing the Peroneal Nerve - Seated Position on page 213*.

Watch this video: (YouTube - http://youtu.be/vk9YElLm57Y)

Flossing the Peroneal Nerve - Supine Mobilization: **The** *peroneal nerve* (also known as the *fibular nerve*) is a branch of the *sciatic nerve* (starting at the *fibular head*). There are superficial and deep branches to this nerve. Nerve compression of the *superficial peroneal nerve* often manifests as numbness and tingling along the outside of the lower leg. **Watch this video:** (YouTube - http://youtu.be/vk9YElLm57Y @ 2.12 min)

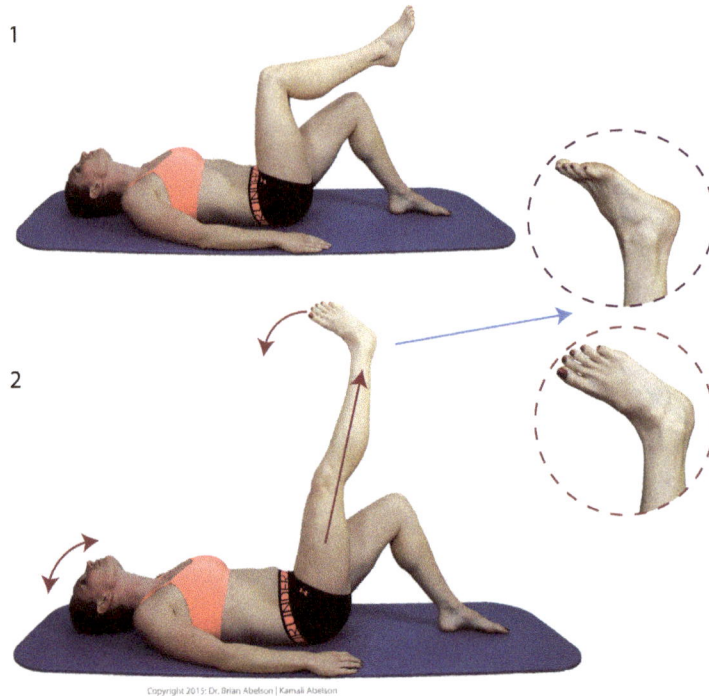

1. Starting Position: Lie flat on your back with your legs parallel to each other.
   - Raise your leg (bending at both the hip and knee) to 90 degrees as shown in Image 1.
   - Keep the leg in this raised position throughout the exercise.

2. To floss the *peroneal nerve*:
   - Straighten your knee and then turn your foot inwards (*inversion*) at the end of the motion.
   - As you straighten the knee, tuck your head in towards your chest to further tension the nerve through the tissues.

3. Slowly return to the starting position.
   - Drop your head back to the ground as you lower your leg.
   - Increase the mobilization of the *peroneal nerve* by tilting your head backwards (*extension*) to glide the nerve through the tissues.

4. Repeat this flossing action 6 to 8 times.
   - Keep your movements slow and controlled.
   - Maintain good form throughout all the repetitions.
   - Perform this exercise in a rhythmic manner - it is a dynamic exercise.

5. Repeat for the other leg.

Mobilizing the Peroneal Nerve - Seated Position: If you have experienced the phenomena known as '*foot drop*', then the most likely cause is entrapment or compression of the *deep peroneal nerve*. **Watch this video:** YouTube - http://youtu.be/vk9YElLm57Y, @ 2.59 min)

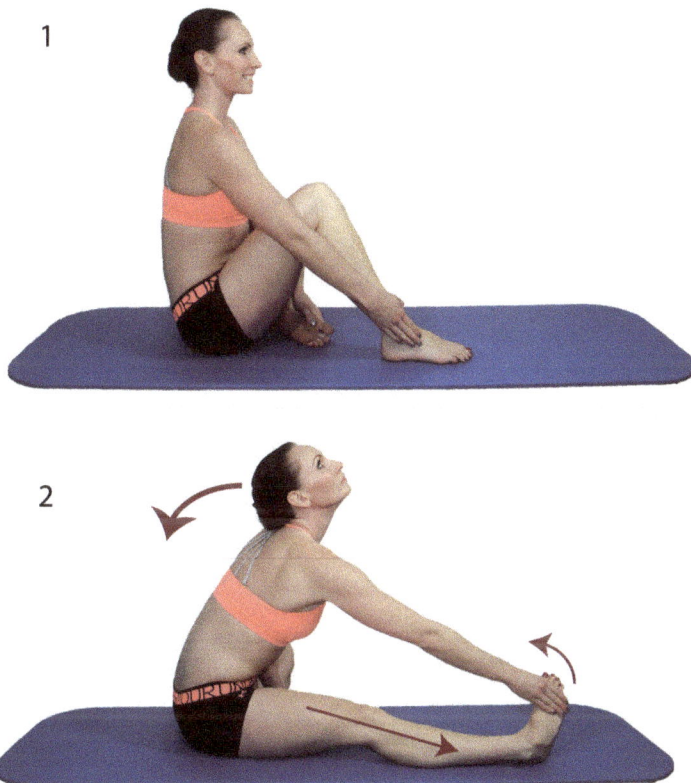

Copyright 2015: Dr. Brian Abelson | Kamali Abelson

1. Starting Position:
   - Sit on a mat, with one leg bent so that it's foot is flat on the ground.
   - Flex (dorsiflex) that foot towards your shin.
2. To floss the nerve:
   - Slowly extend the bent leg while turning the foot inwards (inversion).
   - To further tension the peroneal nerve through the tissues, tuck your head into your chest (as you straighten the knee).
3. Slowly return both your leg and head to the starting position.
   - Return your head to neutral position as you bring the knee to your chest.
   - Increase the mobilization of the *peroneal nerve* by tilting your head backwards at the end of the movement to help the nerve through the tissues.
4. Repeat this flossing action 5 to 6 times.
   - Keep your movements slow and controlled.
   - Maintain good form throughout all the repetitions.
   - Perform this exercise in a rhythmic manner - it is a dynamic exercise.
5. Repeat for the other leg.

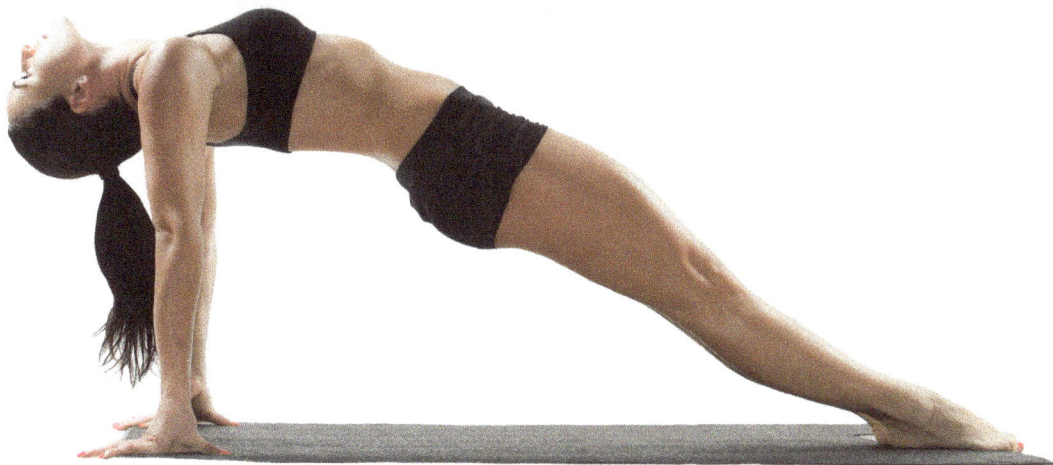

Strengthening Exercises for Plantar Fasciitis

In this chapter

This chapter describes the strengthening exercises that we recommend when treating Plantar Fasciitis. See the following topics (*Phase 1: Foundational Protocol for Plantar Fasciitis on page 107* and *Phase 2: Addressing Problems in the PF Kinetic Chain on page 149*) for more information about how to combine these individual exercises into effective routines for your particular condition.

Remember, the goal is to strengthen weaker muscles, while stretching over-active muscle groups.

For your convenience, we have divided the exercises into the following sections:

Foundational Strengthening Routine for PF:

Condensed Foundational Strengthening Routine for PF:

Lower Extremity Exercises for PF:

Basic Core Stabilization Routine for PF:

Intermediate Core Stabilization Routine for PF:

Advanced Core Stabilization Routine for PF:

Foundational Strengthening Routine for Plantar Fasciitis

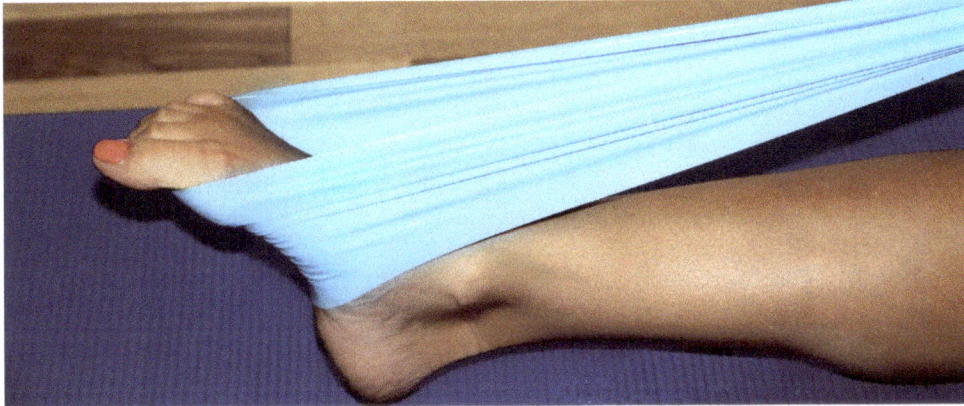

The Foundational Strengthening Routine must be performed by anyone suffering from Plantar Fasciitis, no matter what their test results indicate. This routine provides general strengthening of your foot and ankle, and should be performed on **Days 2, 4**, and **6 Strengthening Protocol**.

You will need a **Theraband**, a secure anchor, and an exercise mat (or towel) for many of these exercises. **Therabands** are easy-to-transport rubber sheets that you can use almost anywhere. They are an excellent tool for toning and strengthening the muscles of your body. Select a theraband that provides sufficient resistance, but which lets you complete at least eight repetitions of any of these exercises.

Note: If you have the time, we recommend that you perform these exercises for both feet, even if only one foot is involved in your Plantar Fasciitis. This will help to remove strength imbalances that commonly occur with Plantar Fasciitis.

The **Foundational Foot Strengthening Routine** (to be performed by everyone) includes the following five exercises:

- Theraband Strengthening of the Foot Routine ------ page 218.
- Salsa Towel Crunch ------ page 220.
- Pen and Loonie Exercise ------ page 221.
- Shin Strengthening Advancing to Dynamic Pulses ------ page 222.
- Eccentric Calf Raises ------ page 223.

Don't worry, although the book provides details about each exercise, and the list may seem long, the entire **Foundational Foot Strengthening Routine** only takes 10 to 15 minutes to perform.

Theraband Strengthening of the Foot Routine - **This exercise combines three different exercises into one routine. You will need a yoga/exercise mat and a 5-foot length of Theraband or rubber tubing. Watch this video:** (YouTube - http://youtu.be/YQKEHnKBr00o)

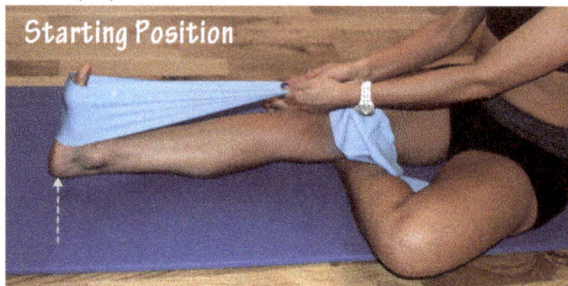

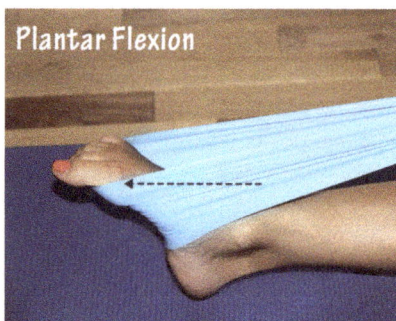

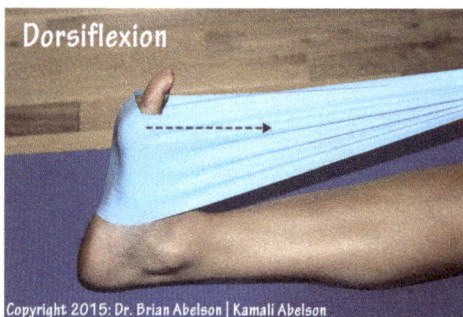

- First Exercise: Plantar Flexion/Dorsiflexion of the Foot ------ page 218.
- Second Exercise: Internal Rotation of the Foot ------ page 219.
- Third Exercise: External Rotation of the Foot ------ page 219.

First Exercise: Plantar Flexion/Dorsiflexion of the Foot:

Watch this video: (YouTube - http://youtu.be/YQKEHnKBr00o)

Copyright 2015: Dr. Brian Abelson | Kamali Abelson

1. Watch this video before performing the exercise.
2. Starting Position: Sit on the mat with your legs stretched out in front of you.
   - Cross one leg under, placing your foot underneath the thigh of the opposite outstretched leg (see Starting Position).
   - Wrap the Theraband or tubing around the arch of your foot and apply tension by holding and pulling on the two ends of the band or tubing.
   - Lift your heel up from the mat and maintain this "heel-up" position throughout the course of the exercise.
3. While maintaining tension, point your foot and toes away (*plantar flexion*) from you and then bring your foot back (*dorsiflexion*) towards your shin.
4. Perform 10-to-15 repetitions on each foot.

Second Exercise: Internal Rotation of the Foot:

Watch this video: (YouTube - http://youtu.be/YQKEHnKBr00o, @1.27 minutes)

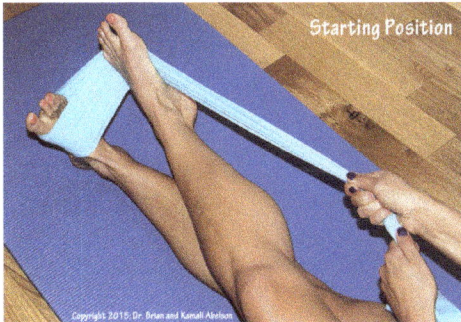

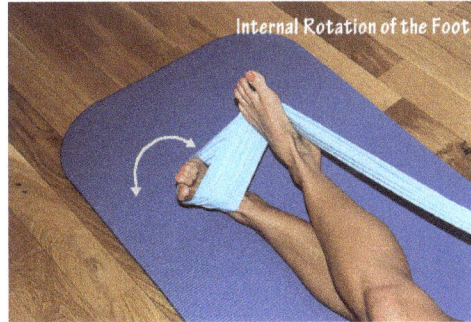

1. Starting Position: Sit on the mat with your legs stretched out in front of you.
   - Wrap the Theraband or tubing around the middle of your foot and apply tension by holding and pulling on the two ends of the band or tubing.
   - Cross the opposite foot over the shin of the outstretched leg making contact with the Theraband with the bottom of this opposite foot.
   - Bring the Theraband into tension.
   - Lift your heel up from the mat, and maintain this "heel-up" position throughout the exercise.
2. Turn your bottom foot inwards (internal rotation) as far as you can, and then return it to the starting position.
3. Perform 10-to-15 repetitions for each foot.

Third Exercise: External Rotation of the Foot:

Watch this video: (YouTube - http://youtu.be/YQKEHnKBr00o, @ 2.24 minutes)

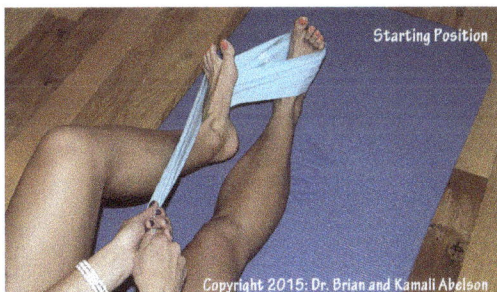

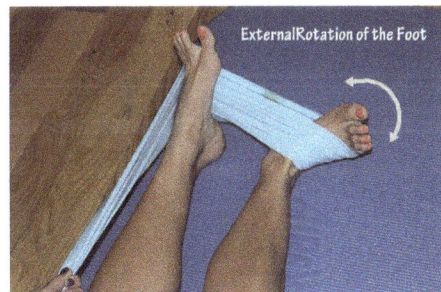

1. Starting Position: Sit on the mat with your legs stretched out in front of you.
   - Wrap the Theraband or tubing around the middle of your foot and apply light tension by holding and pulling on the two ends of the Theraband or tubing.
   - Slide the opposite foot under and over the Theraband or tubing.
   - Make contact with the Theraband using the outside part of your foot and stretch it so that your legs end up parallel to each other. See the illustration.
   - Lift your heel up from the mat and maintain this "heel-up" position throughout the course of the exercise.
2. Turn your foot outwards (*external rotation*) as far as you can and then return it to the starting position.
3. Perform 10-to-15 repetitions for each foot.

Salsa Towel Crunch - This fun little exercise is remarkably effective for increasing metatarsal stability. It also increases strength and neuromuscular control of the intrinsic muscles of the foot (*flexor digitorum brevis, abductor hallucis, abductor minimi, lumbricals, flexor hallucis brevis, adductor hallucis,* and the *flexor digiti minimi brevis* muscles). **Watch this video:** (YouTube - http://youtu.be/FQKLUi6rFqU)

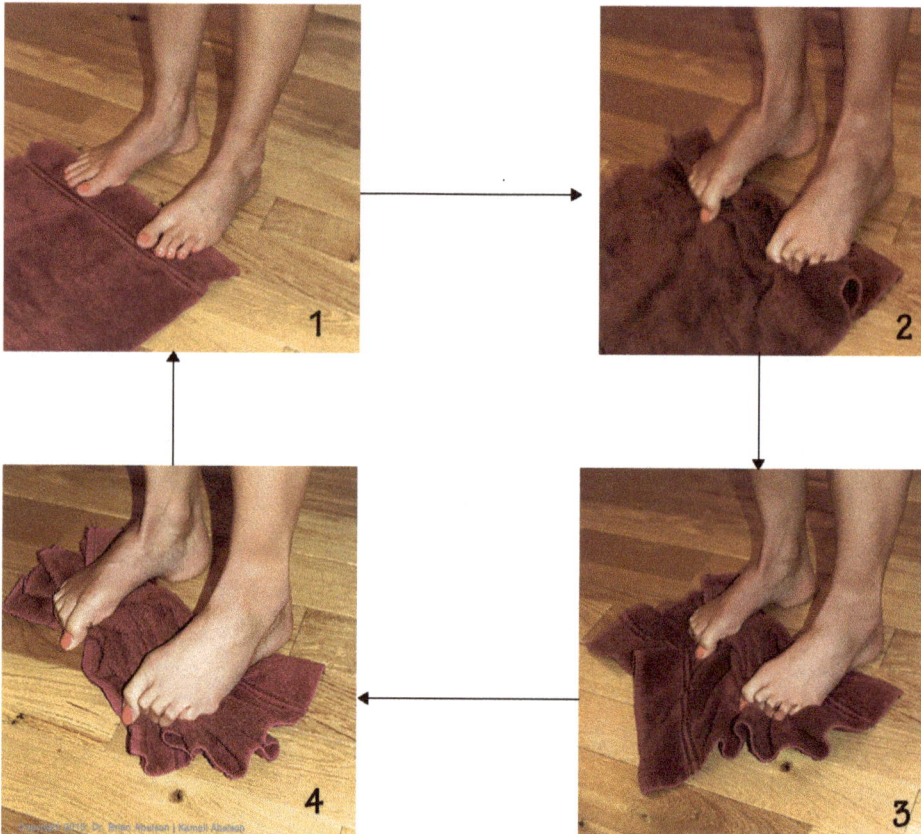

1. Place a light towel or paper towel on the floor under your toes.
2. Scrunch your toes to grab the towel and pull it under your feet.
3. At the same time, move your hips back-and-forth.
   Play some Salsa music to make it more fun!
4. Repeat this until all of the towel is under your feet.
5. Repeat 5-to-8 times.

Pen and Loonie Exercise - The intrinsic muscles of your foot, especially those under the arch, can become lazy from the shoes that we use. This exercise strengthens these intrinsic muscles, especially those that support the arch of the foot. You will need a large coin (quarter, loonie, dollar, etc) and a pen to perform this exercise.

Watch this video: (YouTube - http://youtu.be/dTOQG8Uf3oM)

Strengthening the Intrinsic Muscles of the Foot

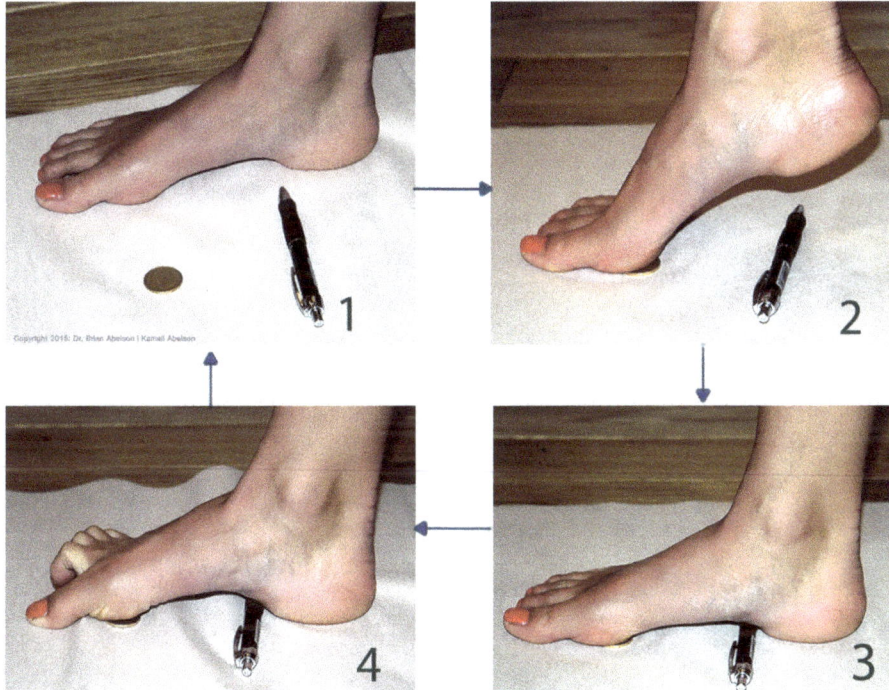

1. Starting Position.
   - From a standing position, place a coin under the joint of your foot just behind your big toe (*metatarsal phalangeal joint*).
   - Slide a pen under the arch of the foot.
2. Keep your heel on the ground and, while maintaining pressure on the coin, lift the arch of the foot. This will take a considerable amount of focus, but the end result and benefits are well worth the effort.
3. Perform 6-to-8 repetitions, for 2-to-3 sets, on each foot.

Lower Extremity Strengthening Exercises for PF

The exercises on the following pages address issues identified in the kinetic chain of your lower extremities. Add the appropriate exercises to your strengthening routine if you have failed the kinetic chain test for that area. See *Shin Strengthening Advancing to Dynamic Pulses - page 222* and *Eccentric Calf Raises - page 223* for more information.

Shin Strengthening Advancing to Dynamic Pulses - Even experienced marathon runners need this exercise. To truly resolve Plantar Fasciitis, it is essential to develop strong shins (your dorsi-flexors). Remember, it is through eccentric contractions that your shins control how your feet hit the ground when running or walking. This exercise will help to develop this ability. If you have identified problems in your shins, then add this exercise to your Day 2, 4, and 6 Strengthening Protocol.

Watch this video: (YouTube - http://youtu.be/7yAUZjV4t28, @ 1.48 minutes)

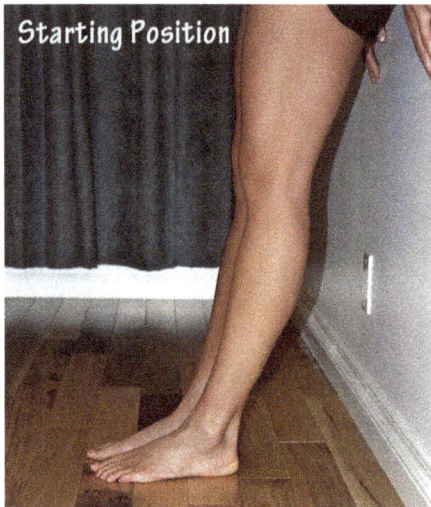

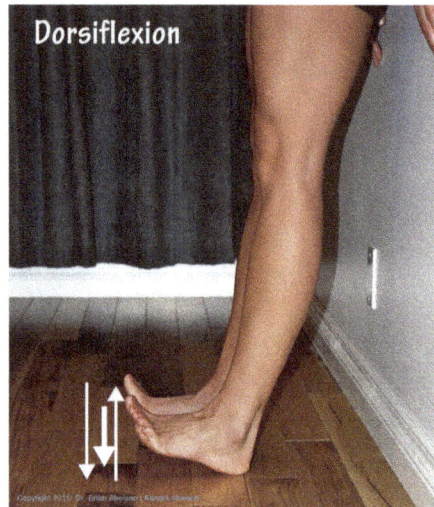

1. Starting Position:
   - Stand with your back against the wall.
   - Place your feet approximately 10 inches away from the base of the wall.

Slow Repetitions: Dorsiflexion Pulses: (YouTube - http://youtu.be/7yAUZjV4t28)

2. Pull your feet up towards your shins (**dorsiflexion**) so that you are standing on your heels.

3. **Hold** this position for a count of four (4) and then **lower** your feet back down again.

4. Perform 10 slow repetitions - holding each for a count of four (4) in the dorsiflexed position.

Fast Repetitions: Dorsiflexion Pulses: (YouTube - http://youtu.be/7yAUZjV4t28, @1.48 minutes)

After a period of two or three weeks of doing the slow repetitions, you can introduce the dynamic pulses described here. Do NOT do these pulses if you are in acute pain.

5. Now perform 10 fast repetitions by pulsing your feet dynamically.

6. The combination of 10 slow and 10 fast repetitions equals ONE set.
   - It is extremely important that you do not bend your knees when performing this exercise.
   - Your knees should not be in a hyper-extended position, but should be kept straight in a locked position.
   - Observe the video to see just how fast you should be able to perform this exercise.

7. Build up to 3 sets over a 3-week period.

Eccentric Calf Raises - This is a great exercise for increasing calf strength, without causing further injury. Weak calf muscles are one of the factors that lead to excessive pronation. Excessive pronation can cause increased stress in numerous soft-tissue structures of the lower extremity (*plantar fascia, Achilles tendon, IT band,* and *patellar tendon*).[40] **Watch this video:** (YouTube - http://youtu.be/yQ0F7Z8neAo)

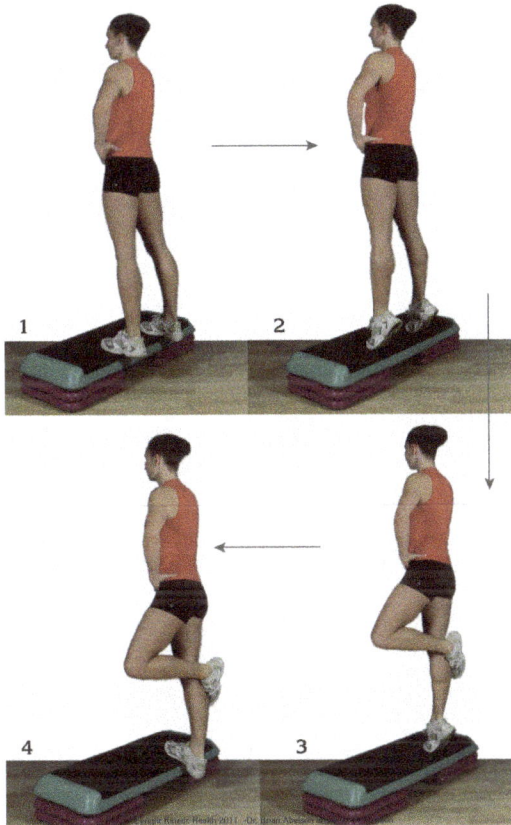

TIP: Make this exercise more challenging by using dumbbell weights (starting with 5-to-10 lb weights). Hold the dumbbell on the side for which you are performing the eccentric calf raises. Be sure that you have performed the **basic** version of this exercise for at least two weeks before adding weights to this exercise.

1. Starting Position:
    - Stand on the front of your feet, with your heels hanging over the edge of a stair.
    - If necessary, brace yourself by placing your hands on the adjacent wall or banister.

2. Rise up on both legs for one (1) count.

3. Cross one leg behind the other, and *slowly* drop down on the other leg for 3 counts. This is the most important part of this exercise, and must be performed in a *slow, controlled* manner. You are strengthening your calf muscles during the downward motion.

4. Perform 10 repetitions on each leg, then repeat on the other leg for one set.

5. Build up to 3 sets of this exercise.

40. Powers, C.M. (2003). *The influence of altered lower-extremity kinematics on patellofemoral joint dysfunction: a theoretical perspective.* Journal of Orthopedic & Sports Physical Therapy, 33:639-46.

Hip Strengthening Exercises

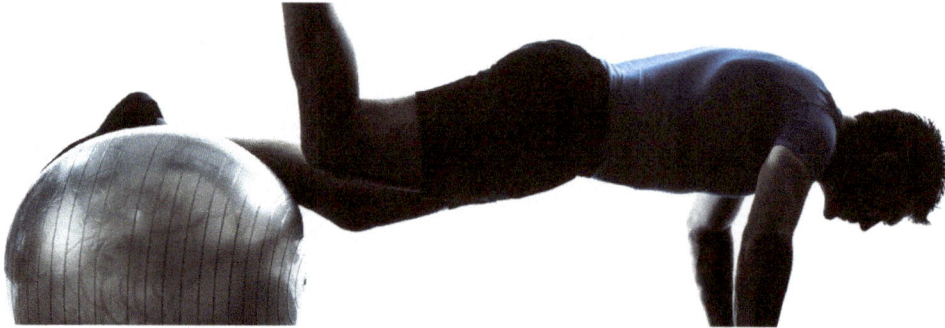

Hip stability has major effects on ALL the structures of the lower body. Research has shown that a lack of hip stability is a major factor in the cause and perpetuation of Plantar Fasciitis. Weak gluteal muscles cause:[41]

- Increased internal rotation of the leg (*femur*).
- The knee to veer inwards (*knee valgus*).
- The foot to excessively pronate.

All of these changes can cause abnormal motion patterns to develop, and result in increased stress being placed on the *plantar fascia*.

Add **one** of the following Hip Strengthening Exercises to your Day 2, 4, and 6 Strengthening Protocol,

- One Leg Split Squat - (Bulgarian Split Squat) ------ page 225.
- Strengthening Hip Abductors with the Suspended Clam Exercise ------ page 226.
- Pelvic Raise: Beginner to Intermediate ------ page 227.

---

41. Lephart SM, Ferris CM, Riemann BL, Myers JB, Fu FH. *Gender differences in strength and lower extremity kinematics during landing.*
Clin Orthop. 2002; 162-169.

One Leg Split Squat - (Bulgarian Split Squat) - The single leg split-squat or Bulgarian Split Squat is an excellent exercise for targeting the gluteal muscles. Standard double-leg squats often do not elicit effective activation of the gluteal muscles. This is often due to spending long hours sitting (or previous injuries) both of which create improper muscle-firing compensations in your hips.[42] The single leg split-squat helps to re-establish the correct movement patterns by turning your gluteal muscles back on. [43] A great side effect of this exercise is obtaining nicely rounded buttocks! The rear leg is only used for balance while your front leg performs the majority of the work. **Watch this video:** (YouTube - http://youtu.be/T--Sg-g0vnw)

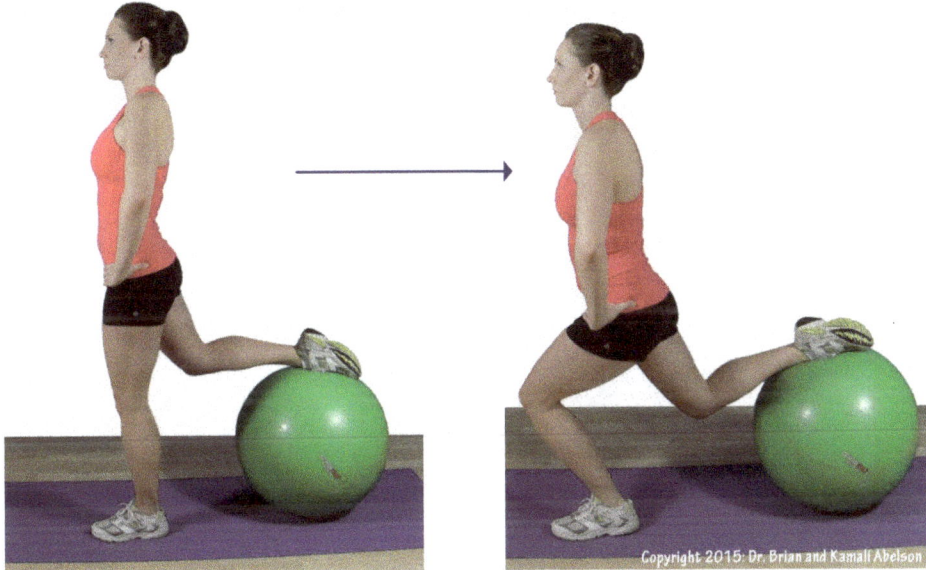

Copyright 2015: Dr. Brian and Kamali Abelson

1. Starting position: Place your shin and foot on top of a chair. You can also use a bench or Swiss Ball. Using a Swiss Ball will make this into a much more challenging exercise.

    ■ Face forward with the other foot firmly planted on the ground.
    ■ Brace your core and maintain an erect torso.

2. Drop down through your hips for a count of two as illustrated, and hold for a count of 2-to-4 seconds. Be sure to squeeze your gluteal muscles when you are in the down position in order to activate and strengthen these structures.

    ■ Reduce the depth of your squat if you experience knee pain while performing this exercise.
    ■ Use the back leg for balance and stabilization. Your front leg does the majority of the work.

3. Rise up to return to the starting position, and perform 10 repetitions for each leg.

TIP: We have shown this exercise with a Swiss Ball, but you may want to start with a stable bench or chair instead. You can also make this exercise more difficult by holding hand-weights in your hands.

42. Distefano LJ, Blackburn JT, Marshall SW, Padua DA, *Gluteal muscle activation during common therapeutic exercises.* J Orthop Sports Phys Ther. Jul;39(7):532-40, 2009.
43. Ayotte N, Stetts D, Keenan G, Greensway E. *Electromyographical analysis of selected lower extremity muscles during 5 unilateral weight-bearing exercises.* J Orthop Sports Phys Ther. 2007;37(2):48–55.

Strengthening Hip Abductors with the Suspended Clam Exercise - The clam exercise derives its name from the basic opening and closing hip motions that are involved in performing the exercise. This simple exercise strengthens your hip abductors (gluteus medius, gluteus maximus) and improves stability throughout your pelvis and legs. By incorporating some resistance by using a looped Theraband and lifting your feet, you can make this exercise more challenging and effective.
Watch this video: (YouTube: http://youtu.be/3B2IoSmixsE, @1.04 min)

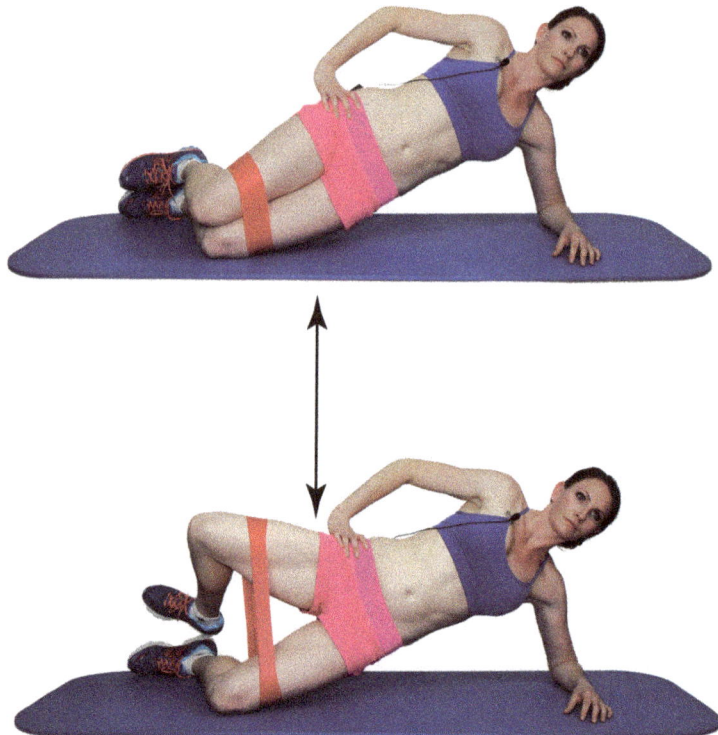

Copyright 2014: Kinetic Health | Dr. Brian Abelson

1. **Starting Position:**
    - Place a looped Theraband around your legs, just above your knees.
    - Lie on your side on the floor.
    - Ensure your hips and knees are bent at a 45 degree angle.
    - Keeping the knees and ankles together, lift both feet up off the ground into a modified side-bridge position as shown in image 1.

2. Open and close your knees (like a clam opening and closing its shell) by lifting the top knee up until it is in line with your hip and then bring it back to the starting position.
    - Keep your heels together throughout this exercise.
    - All movements should be controlled and smooth.
    - You should feel your gluteal muscles tighten as you perform this exercise.

3. Perform 10 to 16 repetitions. Work your way up to 3 sets.

4. Repeat this exercise for the opposite side.

Note: This exercise can be performed without a Theraband. But the Theraband makes it more challenging and effective.

Pelvic Raise: Beginner to Intermediate - The Pelvic Raise is a simple exercise that can strengthen and activate your hip and pelvic floor muscles. This exercise also strengthens the muscles of your lower back, abdominals, glutes, and hamstring.

This book provides two versions - Beginner and Intermediate. As you strengthen these structures, you can move forward into the intermediate version to continue to build a stronger core. Do NOT attempt the advanced version until you can successfully perform the beginner and intermediate versions with good form for several weeks.

Beginner Pelvic Raise: Start with this beginner version. Once you can easily do this version, you can then progress to the intermediate version. Be sure to maintain good form throughout all levels.
Watch this video: (YouTube - http://youtu.be/jd-6cgBsQt0)

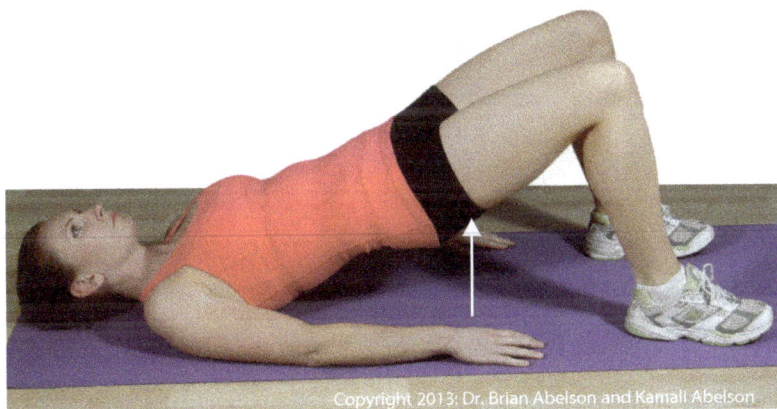

Copyright 2013: Dr. Brian Abelson and Kamali Abelson

1. Starting Position:
   ■ Lie flat on your back with your arms relaxed and slightly out to your sides, knees bent, and feet flat on the floor.
   ■ To make this more challenging, raise up onto your heels (to activate more of your hamstrings and glutes while you perform this exercise).

2. Exhale, and using the muscles of your hips, abdomen, and lower back, raise your pelvis up until you have created a flat surface with your abdomen and thighs.
   ■ Basically you are making a bridge out of your pelvis.
   ■ Ensure that your pelvis does not drop, tilt, or rotate to either side throughout the exercise.

3. Focus on keeping your gluteals squeezed together, and hold this raised position for a count of 4. Slowly drop back down to the floor.

4. Perform this exercise for 8-to-10 repetitions (one set).

5. Perform two to three sets of this exercise.

TIP: Once you can perform this beginner's exercise comfortably for 3 sets, move on to the Intermediate version.

Intermediate Pelvic Raise - Pillar March: Only perform this exercise *after* you can comfortably complete the *Beginner Pelvic Raise on page 227.*
Watch this video: (YouTube - http://youtu.be/jd-6cgBsQt0, @ 1.32 minutes)

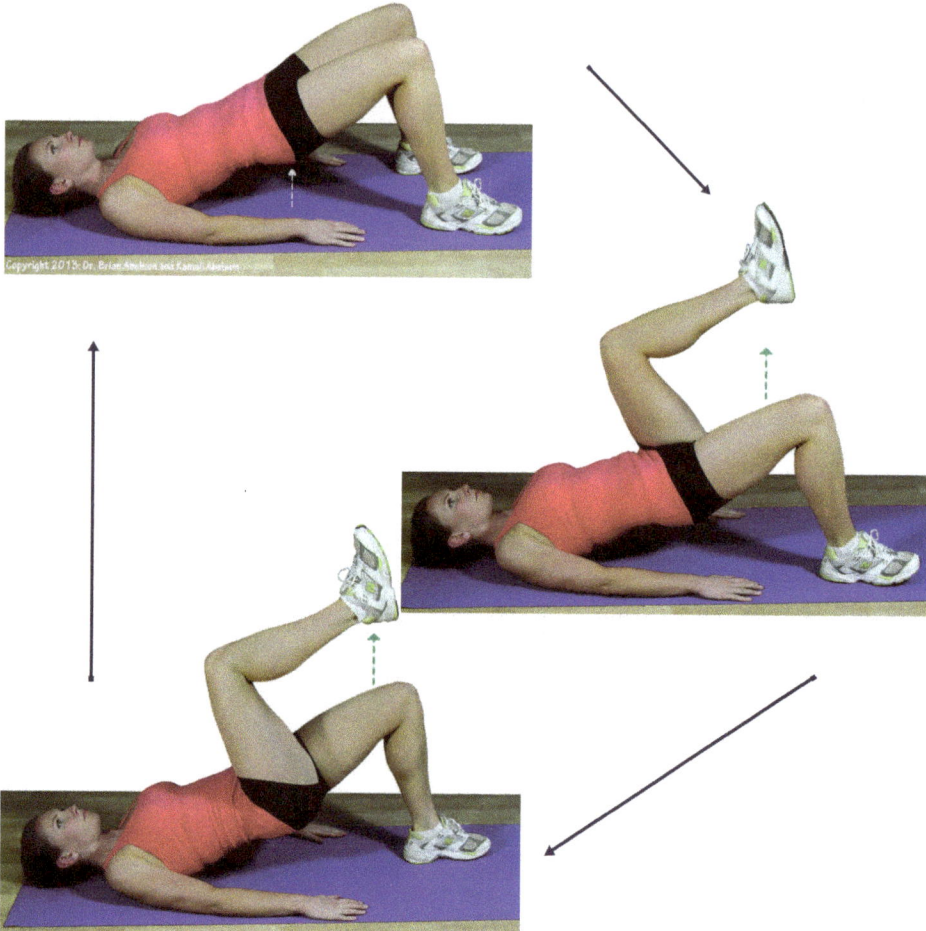

1. Watch the video before attempting this exercise.
2. Starting Position:
    - Lie flat on your back with your arms slightly out to your sides, knees bent, and feet flat on the floor.
    - To make this more challenging, raise up onto your heels (to activate more of your hamstrings and glutes while you perform this exercise).
3. Exhale, and using the muscles of your hips, abdomen, and lower back, raise your pelvis up until you have created a flat surface with your abdomen and thighs.
    - Basically you are making a bridge out of your pelvis.
    - Ensure that your pelvis does not drop, tilt, or rotate to either side throughout the exercise.
4. While maintaining this raised position, bring one knee up at a time, and start "marching" continuously in place for **20 seconds**.
5. Repeat this exercise 2 to 3 times.

Core Stabilization Exercises

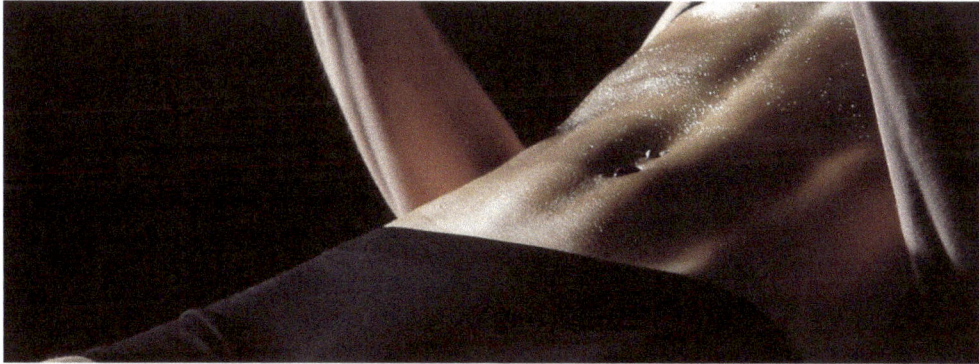

If you are unable to effectively perform the basic core tests, then you must perform exercises to strengthen your core. These exercises will activate the neuro-muscular connections that are required to develop a strong functional core. We recommend starting with the Beginner version of front and side planks, and then advancing progressively to the Intermediate and Advanced versions.

Basic Core Stabilization Exercise: For the *Basic Core Stabilization Routine*, do only the Beginner version of the video. As your core strengthens, you can progressively move into the more advanced versions in order to develop a stronger core.

- Front Plank - Beginner Core ------ page 230.
- Side Plank - Beginner Core ------ page 231.

Intermediate Core Stabilization Exercises: If you were able to perform the Core Tests, but failed some aspect (posture, timing, number of repetitions), then you should do the following intermediate exercises, but only if you can successfully and easily perform the exercises in the *Basic Core Stabilization Routine for PF - page 216*.

- Front Plank – Intermediate Core ------ page 232.
- Side Plank - Intermediate Core ------ page 233.

Advanced Core Stabilization Routine: The following are optional exercises you can add to your Core routine if you want something more challenging and difficult.

- High Plank Spider Crawl ------ page 234.
- Spider Crawl Pushup ------ page 235.

Caution: Do NOT do the advanced exercises unless you can successfully perform all the Core exercises in the *Basic Core Stabilization Routine for PF on page 216* and the exercises in the *Intermediate Core Stabilization Routine for PF on page 216*.

Front Plank - Beginner Core - The front plank is a wonderful exercise for strengthening the core of your body. It is a much more effective and safer exercise than sit-ups. Stuart McGill, a professor of spine biomechanics at the University of Waterloo, has done considerable research on how sit-ups can actually cause spinal injury. (This is why we do not include sit-ups in our core strengthening programs – the research does not support using them.) When performing the front plank, it very important to maintain a stiff rigid core, with perfect form to achieve optimal results.

Watch this video: (YouTube - http://youtu.be/gfj5MWBNxxU)

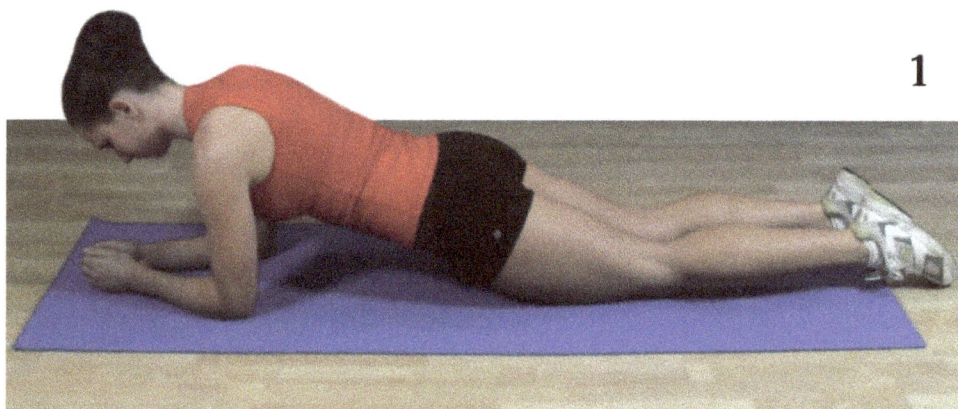

1. Lay flat on your stomach with your legs fully extended.
   - Place your elbows shoulder-width apart, with your forearms on the ground as illustrated.
   - Brace your core. See *How to Brace your Core on page 169* for more information.
2. Lift your body up off the ground so that only your **forearms** and **knees** are supporting the weight of your body.
   - Your body should form a straight line, from your head to your hips.
   - Do not allow your spine to curve down or up.
   - Do not sag, and always continue to brace your core.
   - Keep your shoulders relaxed and do not hunch.
   - Keep your neck in a neutral position.
3. Hold the plank position for 10 seconds, then lower yourself back to the ground.
   - Holding this for 10 seconds helps you to avoid oxygen debt in your tissues, and helps to increases the development of slow-twitch muscle fibers, which helps in developing stabilization of your core.
4. Repeat this exercise 6-to-10 times.

Side Plank - Beginner Core - This incredibly effective exercise activates all the muscles of your core. This is the beginner version. To make this exercise more difficult, you can try the straight-leg version (intermediate version). If you have any back pain, do the bent leg version.
Watch this video: (YouTube- http://youtu.be/P8-ppF2x9SU)

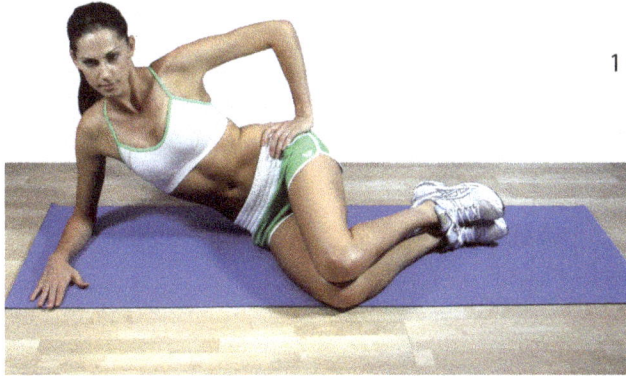

1

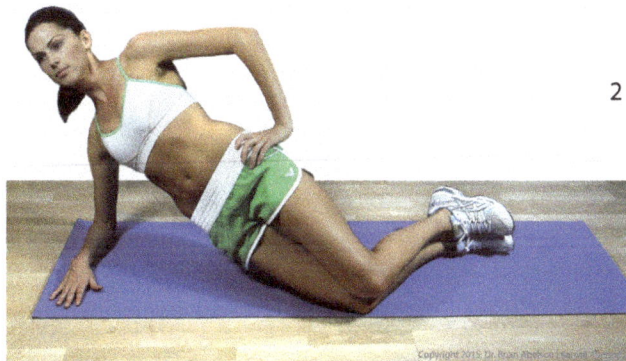

2

1. Lie on your side with your legs bent, and one arm bracing your body's weight, as shown in Image 1.

   ■ Bend your knees to a 90-degree angle.
   ■ Brace your core and inhale.

2. Exhale as you lift your body up off the ground so that only your arm and knees are supporting the weight of your body. See Image 2.

   ■ Your body should form a straight line, from your head to your knees.
   ■ Do not allow your spine to curve forward or back.
   ■ Do not sag, and always continue to brace your core.
   ■ Distribute your body weight between your bent elbow and bent knees.

3. Hold the bridge/plank position for 10 seconds, then slowly lower yourself back to the ground.

4. Repeat the exercise 6-to-10 times, on both sides.

TIP: Try the following variation if you find this exercise is too hard on your shoulders. Cross your free hand across your chest, and place it on top of your shoulder. Press in and down to provide additional support for the shoulder.

Front Plank - Intermediate Core - The front plank is a great exercise for strengthening multiple areas in your entire core. To achieve maximum benefits (maximum muscle activation) from this exercise, it is essential to maintain perfect form. This activates the abdominals and obliques, and is much more effective than sit-ups and other exercises for strengthening the core.

Watch this video: (YouTube- http://youtu.be/gfj5MWBNxxU, @1.43 min)

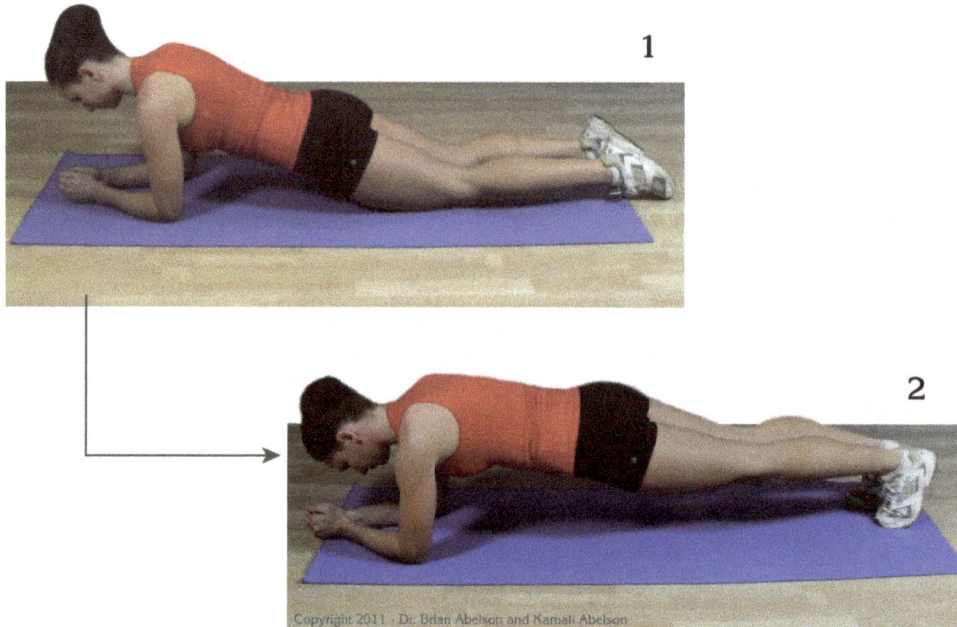

Copyright 2011 - Dr. Brian Abelson and Kamali Abelson

1. Lay flat on your stomach with your legs fully extended.
    - Place your elbows shoulder-width apart.
    - Brace your core. See *How to Brace your Core on page 169* for more information.
2. Lift your body up off the ground so that only your forearms and toes are supporting the weight of your body.
    - Your body should form a straight line, from your head to your toes.
    - Do not allow your spine to curve down or up.
    - Do not sag, and always continue to brace your core.
    - Keep your shoulders relaxed and do not hunch.
    - Keep your neck in a neutral position.
3. Start by holding the bridge/plank for 10 seconds, and build up to 30 seconds.
4. Repeat this exercise 4-to-10 times. The number of repetitions will vary based on your strength and the length of time that you are holding the plank position.

TIP: Initially (for at least the first 2 weeks), we ask you to hold the plank position for only a short duration of time (10 seconds), but with multiple repetitions. After this period of time you can increase your holding duration until you are able to hold the front plank position for at least 30 seconds, while still performing 3-to-5 repetitions. As you progress increase your rest times between repetitions to about 30 seconds.

Side Plank - Intermediate Core - The straight-leg side plank activates numerous deep muscles in your core. It will activate all your abdominals including the deep muscles in your lower back (*quadratus lumborum*) while strengthening your shoulders.
Watch this video: (YouTube- http://youtu.be/P8-ppF2x9SU, @ 1.10 min).

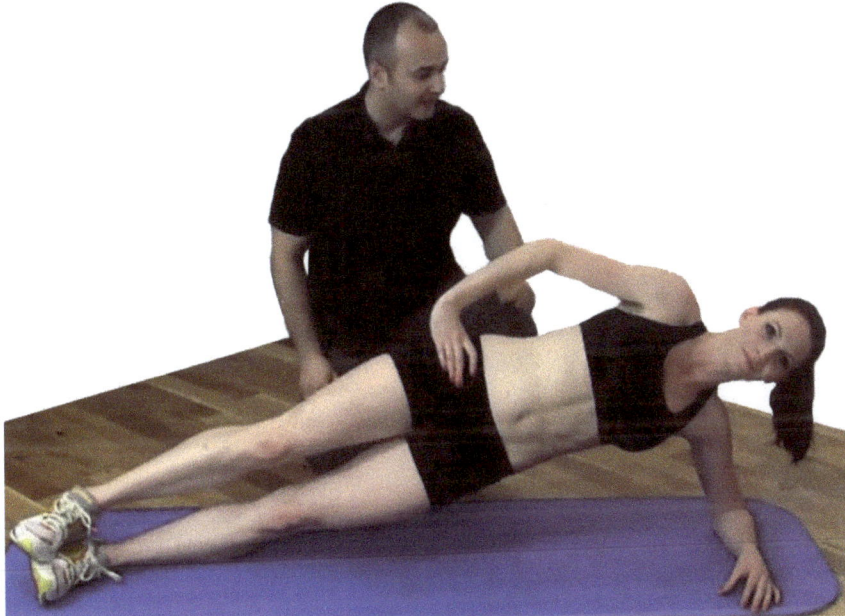

1. Starting Position:
   - Lie on your side with your legs stretched out, and stacked upon each other.
   - Keep one arm bent parallel to the floor. Keep the other hand braced on your hips.
   - Ensure your elbow is under the shoulder.
   - Brace your core. See *How to Brace your Core on page 169* for more information.

2. Exhale as you lift your body up off the ground so that only your arm and feet are supporting the weight of your body. *Maintain good form throughout this exercise.*
   - Your body should form a straight line, from your head to your knees. This straight line should be consistent when viewed from either the front (coronal view) or side view (sagittal view.)
   - Do not allow your spine to curve forward or back.
   - Do not sag, and always continue to brace your core.

3. Hold the bridge/plank for 10 seconds, and build up to 30 seconds.

4. Repeat the exercise 4-to-12 times, **on both sides**. The number of repetitions will vary based on your strength and the length of time that you are holding the plank position.

TIP: Initially (for at least the first 2 weeks), we ask you to hold the side-plank position for only a short duration of time (10 seconds), but with multiple repetitions. After this period of time you can increase your holding duration until you are able to hold the side-plank position for at least 30 seconds, while still performing 3-to-5 repetitions. As you progress increase your rest times between each repetitions to about 30 seconds.

High Plank Spider Crawl - This **optional** exercise is a great, advanced core exercise that works your abdominals, chest, shoulders, and triceps. You can do either this exercise, or the more advanced *Spider Crawl Pushup on page 235*. (You don't have to do either of these, but they have been included for those of you who want more of a challenge in your routines.) It is important to maintain good form throughout this exercise, and ensure that you keep your core and thigh adductors engaged throughout this action. Take a minute to watch the video before trying this exercise.

Watch this video: (YouTube -http://youtu.be/Gk-LOimCQ-o).

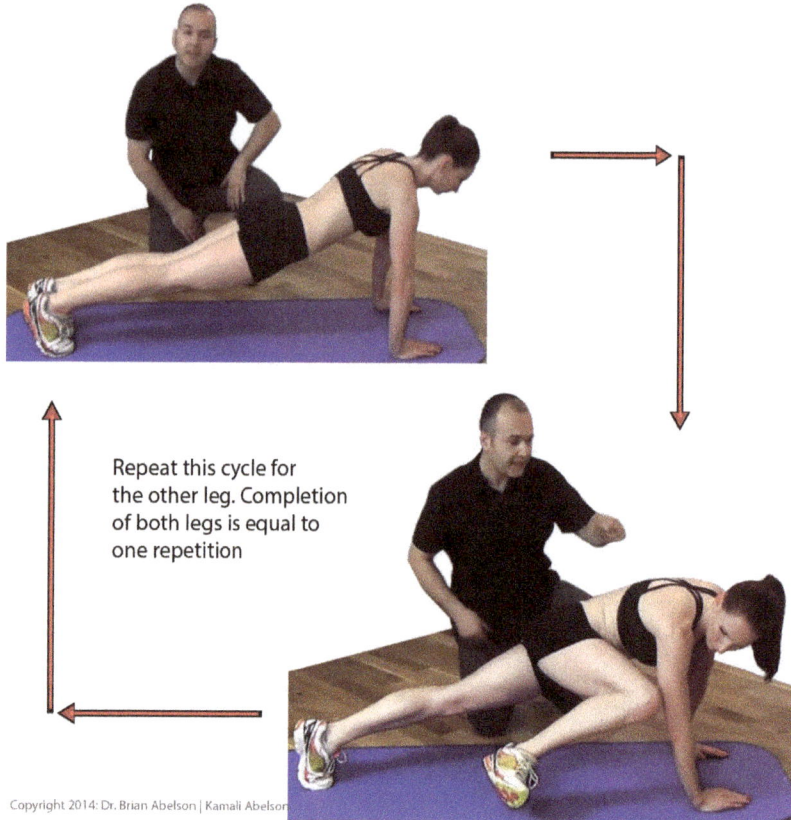

Repeat this cycle for the other leg. Completion of both legs is equal to one repetition

Copyright 2014: Dr. Brian Abelson | Kamali Abelson

1. Starting Position: Start in full, extended, high plank position, supporting your weight on your hands and toes. Feet should be together, and your body straight.

    - Wrists, elbows, and shoulders should be lined up.
    - Keep your pelvis flat and parallel to the floor
    - Engage your core muscles and the muscles on the inside part of your thighs throughout this exercise.

2. Bring your knee up to touch one arm as shown in this image Make sure you *look at the knee* as you bring the knee up. This will help you to engage your core more effectively.

3. Bring your leg back to the starting position.

4. Repeat step 2 for the other leg.

5. Do this continuously, 8-10 times, starting with one set, and building up to 2-to-3 sets. This is a challenging exercise, so it make take a few weeks before you can do three sets.

Spider Crawl Pushup - This exercise increases the intensity of work that your abdominals, chest, shoulders, and triceps must perform. It combines the spider crawl motion with pushups. You can do either this exercise, or the intermediate-level *High Plank Spider Crawl - page 234.* It is important to maintain good form throughout this exercise, and keep your core and thigh adductors engaged throughout this action.

Watch this video: (YouTube -http://youtu.be/Gk-LOimCQ-o, @ 1.19 minutes)

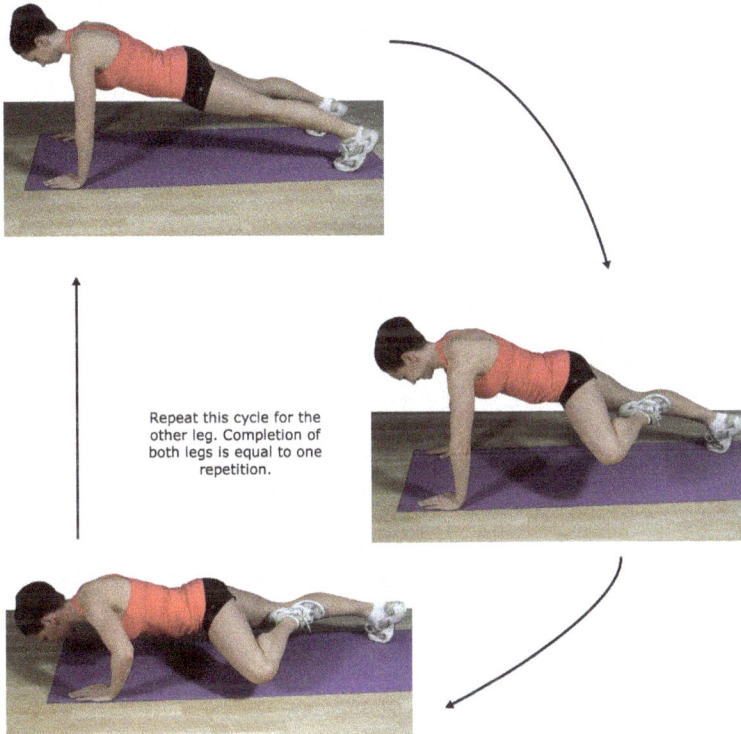

Repeat this cycle for the other leg. Completion of both legs is equal to one repetition.

1. Starting Position: Start in full, extended, high plank position, supporting your weight on your hands and toes. Feet should be parallel, and your body straight.
    - Wrists, elbows, and shoulders should be lined up.
    - Keep your pelvis flat and parallel to the floor
    - Engage your core muscles and the muscles on the inside part of your thighs throughout the exercise.

2. Bring your knee up to touch your elbow, while dropping down. You will not be able to look at the elbow when you are doing this action. The key is to maintain form. It is not necessary to drop your chest all the way to the floor.

3. Push up to the starting position as you return your leg to its starting position.

4. Repeat steps 2 and 3 for the **other leg.**

5. Do this continuously, 8-to-10 times, alternating legs, and start by completing one set. Build up to 2-to-3 sets. This is a challenging exercise, so it may take a few weeks before you can do three sets.

Plantar Fasciitis

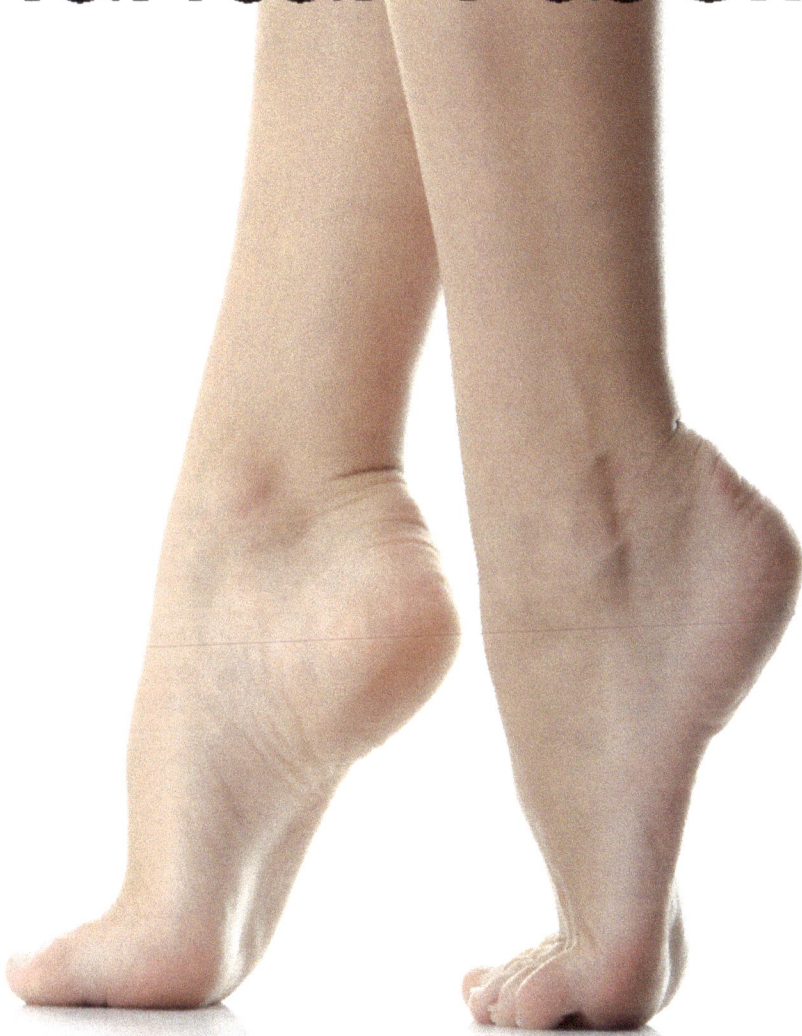

Self Care for

Plantar Fasciitis

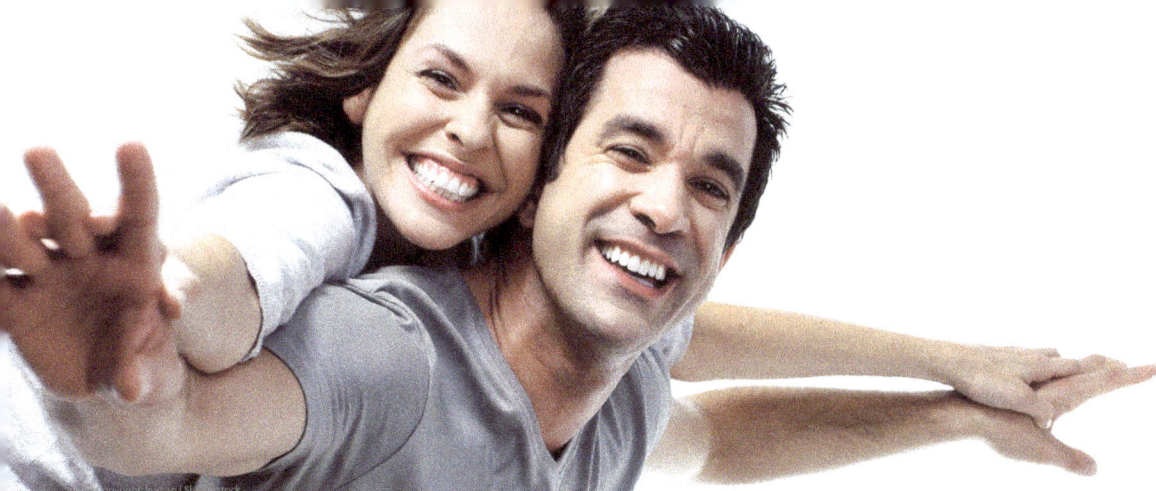

Self-Care Tips and Hints

Since soft-tissue and joint injuries are very common, it is good to know what you can do to take care of yourself when it happens. Rapid treatment is essential for ensuring quick recovery from these injuries.

The tips and hints we are providing in this chapter relate to the care of Plantar Fasciitis caused by repetitive actions, trauma, poor body mechanics, inflammation, excessive stress to the muscles and tissues of the body, and muscle imbalances within the kinetic chain. They do *not* apply to serious trauma or emergency situations.

Note: In this book, we are **not** talking about dealing with traumatic injuries involving open wounds, bleeding, impaled objects, extreme force injuries, etc. For such cases, seek immediate care from your medical practitioner.

For most non-traumatic soft-tissue injuries, start self-care with the following:

■ *Understanding the Inflammatory Process on page 240*.
■ *Heat Therapy - page 245*.
■ *Epsom Salt Baths - page 247*.
■ *Using a Night Splint for Plantar Fasciitis - page 248*.
■ *Why Exercise is Essential - page 159*.

Understanding the Inflammatory Process

Research has shown that when muscle fibers are damaged (as in an acute or strain/sprain injury), inflammatory cells *(macrophages)* stream into the injured area to remove damaged tissue and to stimulate the muscle fibers to regenerate.

These *macrophages* are present in your blood stream at all times. When you injure your body, your body releases histamines that increase blood flow into the injured area, this increased blood flow releases additional macrophages into this area to digest the damaged tissue (a process known as *phagocytosis*). Fluid then rushes into the area from which the damaged tissue was removed (this is the swelling that occurs in the inflammatory process). Then about 24 hours later *non-phagocytosing macrophages* come in and fill the area with *Insulin like Growth Factor (IGF-1)*. The IGF-1 spurs the damaged area to begin the formation of new tissue (precursor cells).[44] These precursor cells then join together to form the new tissue, replacing the old damaged tissue.

Without this important inflammatory process, healing and regeneration of the injured area does not occur.

As you can see, this process requires the body to be able to move fluids in and out of the injured or damaged tissue. Anything that blocks this movement can reduce the rate of healing

Differentiating Between Acute and Chronic Inflammation

It is important to differentiate between normal (*Acute Inflammation*) and run-away or abnormal inflammation (*Chronic Inflammation*).

Acute Inflammation refers to the type of inflammation that happens right after you injure yourself. It could be caused by trauma, strain, sprain, infection, or even by hard physical exercise. This type of inflammation is usually short in duration, and acts to speed up the healing process. Inflammation immediately after an injury is a GOOD thing; it is an indication that your body has moved into an accelerated healing mode.

In comparison, *Chronic Inflammation* is an over-reaction, it is the body attacking its own tissues. This includes a number of autoimmune conditions such as rheumatoid arthritis, hay fever, asthma, celiac disease, and many others. The

---

44.   H. Lu, D. Huang, N. Saederup, I. F. Charo, R. M. Ransohoff, L. Zhou. Macrophages recruited via CCR2 produce insulin-like growth factor-1 to repair acute skeletal muscle injury. The FASEB Journal, 2010; DOI: 10.1096/fj.10-171579

problem is that chronic inflammation is an out-of-control process. Unlike *Acute Inflammation* (which is short in duration), *Chronic Inflammation* just keeps going on and on. Even heart disease has been linked to chronic inflammation. The Chronic inflammatory process increases the production and availability of a substance called *myostatin* which *hinders* the regeneration of new tissue.

Cold Therapy

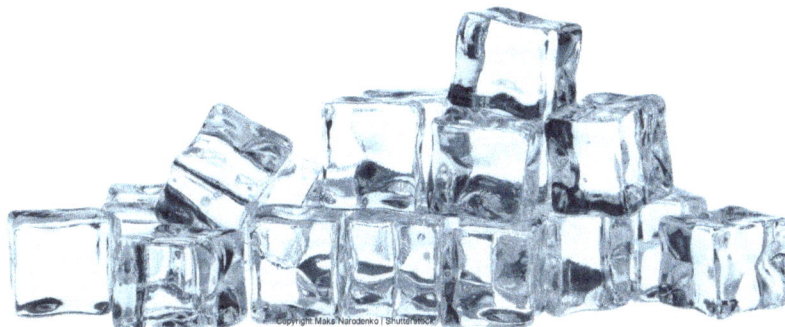

The standard advice that is given when you have a soft-tissue injury is to ICE immediately afterwards. Unfortunately, new research has shown that this may not be the best option for optimal healing. WHY? Read on!

What is the Impact of Icing on Inflammation and Healing?

Anytime you injure yourself with a soft-tissue injury, whether you strain a muscle, have muscle spasms, get a bruise, or cut yourself, your body uses the inflammatory process to heal itself. This inflammatory process also occurs when you break down, or stress muscle tissue after exercising.

Unfortunately, it has been shown that anti-inflammatory drugs or icing (cold therapy) will both suppress this healing process. As soon as you suppress this inflammatory process, you STOP the healing process.

Which brings into question, should you, or shouldn't you be using ice for post-workout muscle pain? My opinion, *don't use ice unless you absolutely have to!* Yes, ice does reduce pain, so after an extremely painful acute injury, it does help to reduce the pain experienced. On the other hand, icing also can *stop the healing process* and slow the regeneration of new muscle tissue. Using the same logic, you should NOT use non-steroidal anti-inflammatories (NSAIDS) either before or after your work out as they could inhibit the growth of new muscle tissue.

The Not So Good Standard Advice

The standard advice given after an acute injury is to both ice and start taking anti-inflammatory medications. I certainly gave my patients this same advice for years, based on my prior medical training and all the educational material available at that time. After all, swelling causes pain (nociceptive pain) by increasing the pressure on nerve endings, and you want to do your best to get your patients out of pain as soon as possible.

So the patient ices and the pain is diminished, this is a good thing right? Well yes and no. YES it's good because we have a reduction in pain and the patient can function, but NO because the healing process has now stopped.

So, When Should I Use Ice and Medication?

As the new research about inflammation and icing has come forward, it has caused me to change my opinion and perspectives on this subject. As my knowledge has grown, and my questions and doubts answered, I have come to the conclusion that you should only ice an injury for two purposes – *to reduce pain and control excessive swelling*, and even this, only when absolutely necessary

In fact, if we are talking about the normal soreness that results from working out, I would *avoid ice and cold therapy altogether*. It is simply not necessary for the majority of the time, As I mentioned earlier, this also includes avoiding all NSAIDS, since most of these medications sabotage tissue regeneration. Whether we are talking about tissue repair due to injury or trying to develop new muscle after exercise, both ice and anti-inflammatory medications can be counter-productive to injury recovery.

On the other hand if you are dealing with an extremely acute and painful situation, then ice is a great way to reduce that pain. Yes, you *will be inhibiting the healing process*, but only for a short period of time. If you need to take medication because of the pain, try acetaminophen (Tylenol), it will reduce pain but will not reduce the inflammation. Just be aware that all medications do come with side-effects, if you don't need the medications, don't take them.

You can find some great suggestions on how to naturally reduce chronic inflammation in our book about diet and nutrition – Choose Health!

Icing For Pain Relief!

If you are in severe pain, icing is a great way to *reduce that pain* (after an acute injury). I would recommend icing for no longer than the first 72 hours after the injury. If you feel that you don't need the ice, then don't use it.

This does not mean we are recommending that you heat the injured area right after an injury. Heat therapy does increase blood flow to an area, but this heat can cause an increase in inflammation, which in turn will cause an increase in pain. We need a certain amount of inflammation to heal, but too much inflammation will definitely be counter-productive.

Red Flags - When Not to Ice!

Do not use Cold Therapy if the person:

- Is unconscious, unable to communicate, or has no sensation in the injured area.
- Tends to develop a rash or blisters when exposed to cold.
- Has a circulatory problem.
- Has Raynaud's Disease, rheumatoid or gouty arthritis, or kidney malfunctions,

Tips and Hints for Icing

So, now that you know when to ice, and when to avoid icing, here are some tips on the best way to use cold therapy (icing) to reduce pain, and keep the healing pattern going!

- While icing, elevate the injured area – preferably to above the heart – to reduce swelling and move blood away from the affected area (using gravity as an aid).
- Ice every two to three hours, but always make sure that the area being iced has warmed up, and is no longer numb.
- Prevent frostbite by not allowing the ice pack to sit directly on your skin. Use a thin towel in-between.
- Our Kinetic Health Hot/Cold Paks have a cloth covering, and can go directly on your skin.

Icing with an Ice-Pack - First place a thin cloth over the injured area so that the ice-pack is not in direct contact with the skin.

1. Apply the ice-pack to the injured area.

2. Keep the ice-pack against the affected area until it feels numb.

3. You should first feel cold, then a burning sensation, followed by aching, then numbness. If you don't feel numb, then you haven't iced for long enough.
   - Allow the icing process to take a maximum of 15 to 20 minutes. Never longer!
   - Do NOT allow the skin to freeze...you are not trying to get frost-bite.

4. Leave a minimum of one hour between each icing session to give your tissues sufficient time to warm-up.

Using Ice Massage - Ice massage can be more effective than regular icing.

1. Fill small paper cups with water and keep them in your freezer till frozen.

2. Peel the top of the cup back to expose the ice.

3. Use the bottom of the cup, the paper covered part, as a handle.

4. Massage the ice over the injured area in small circular motions, allowing the ice to melt away.
   - Use a towel to catch the melting water.
   - To prevent tissue damage, only perform ice massage for a maximum of 7 to 9 minutes at a time.

Heat Therapy

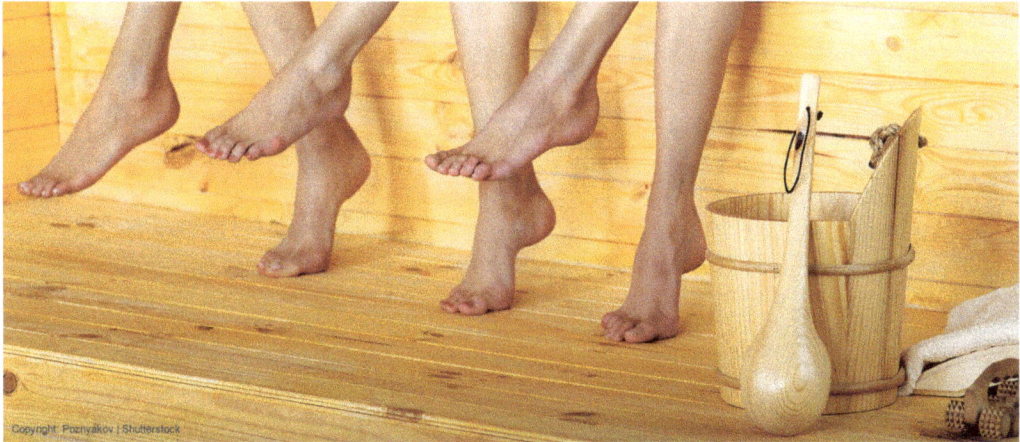
Copyright: Poznyakov | Shutterstock

Without a doubt, Heat Therapy feels much nicer and more comforting than Cold Therapy. But problems can arise when heat therapy is used too soon after an injury or trauma. In fact, the early use of heat therapy by our patients is often one reason for the increased time required to resolve their soft-tissue injuries.

Heat Therapy should only be used *after inflammation has subsided*. Never use heat therapy within the first 72 hours of an acute injury. Applying heat to soft tissues (muscles, ligaments, and tendons) while the area is still inflamed and swollen will only aggravate the injured tissues. During the first 72 hours, cold therapy provides much more effective and appropriate relief.

Benefits of Heat Therapy

Once the inflammation has subsided, you can apply heat to the affected area to help restore flexibility, relieve muscle cramping, reduce arthritic symptoms, and most of all, to increase the rate of healing by increasing blood-flow to the area.

The power of heat therapy comes from its depth of penetration and its ability to increase circulatory and neurological function. Increasing circulation results in increased delivery of oxygen and nutrients to the affected area while at the same time displacing waste by-products. Heat affects the nervous system by stimulating the sensory receptors in the skin. This has the effect of decreasing the transmission of pain signals to the brain, thereby reducing muscle spasms and episodes of acute pain.

Types of Heat Therapy

The effectiveness of heat therapy varies from individual to individual. Each person needs to experiment to determine which therapy is best suited to their condition. There are two primary types of heat therapy:

- **Moist Heat**: Moist heat therapy includes hot baths, heated whirlpools, hot packs, or hot moist towels. Many people feel they get better depth of penetration with moist heat.
- **Dry Heat**: Dry heat therapy includes dry saunas, electric heating pads, and heat lamps. These can be very effective forms of heat therapy but they also tend to dehydrate the individual, so remember to drink lots of fluids when you use dry heat therapy.

For how long should you apply heat therapy? For a minor, superficial injury you may only want to use heat therapy for 10 to 20 minutes. For chronic injuries, you may need to apply heat therapy for 20 to 35 minutes.

Heat Treatment with a Hot Towel

- Dampen an old, clean towel (towels may discolour with this process).
- Heat the moist towel in a microwave for one to two minutes. Check the temperature of the towel, and heat for another minute if necessary.
- Carefully remove the moist hot towel (don't give yourself a steam burn) and wrap the hot towel with a dry towel (to prevent burns, and to retain the heat).
- Apply the hot towel to the affected area until the muscles relax and warm up, and your skin turns slightly rosy.
- Stop after 15 to 20 minutes. Do not re-apply for at least 1 to 2 hours.

Attention: Always use caution with Heat Therapy. Use only moderate heat to avoid burning the soft tissue. Do not use heat treatment if you suffer from one or more of the following conditions: cancer, diabetes mellitus, tendency to hemorrhage, decreased sensations, peripheral vascular disease, acute inflammation, cognitive impairment, deep vein thrombosis, dermatitis, heart disease, hypertension (high blood pressure), skin lesions, or open wounds. If in doubt, consult your physician! Try to avoid using Heat Therapy at night, or when you are in bed. You are more likely to fall asleep with the heating pad, and that could be dangerous since it can cause burns and overheating.

Epsom Salt Baths

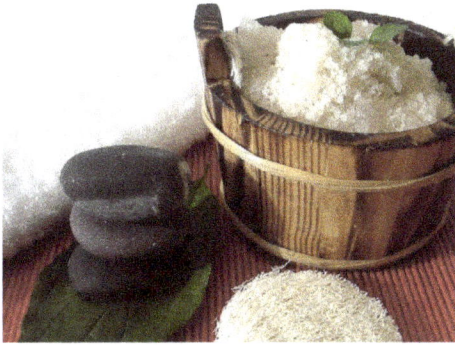

Grandmother's magic home remedy for aches and pains...**epsom salts**. Soaking in an epsom salt bath is one of the best things you can (and should) do for the body.

Epsom salts (magnesium sulfate) have a high concentration of magnesium, which helps to reduce muscle cramps, ease joint pain, and increase circulatory function.

But, remember that epsom salt baths is another form of Heat Therapy, and therefore all the rules that apply to Heat Therapy also apply to epsom salt baths.

Using Epsom Salts Locally

- Fill a bucket of hot water, add one cup of epsom salts, and soak your sore feet.
- Dip a wash cloth in epsom-salt-drenched water, and wrap it around your sore foot.
- Soak a cloth in epsom salt water, wring it out, and place it over a sore or painful area. Now wrap a tensor bandage or towel around everything to keep the heat in, and to hold the epsom-salt-soaked towel in place! It works wonders!

Make an Epsom Salt Bath:

Mix two (2) cups of epsom salts in lots of hot water.

Soak in the bath and let the Epsom Salts do their magic!

Using a Night Splint for Plantar Fasciitis

Some of you may find that no matter what you do, your feet are simply too painful, and do not allow you to perform the recommended exercises in this book. This is because those first few, painful steps in the morning often results in re-injury to the contracted and tight *plantar fascia* on the bottom of your feet. That is correct, your normal sleeping positions can actually injure your foot.

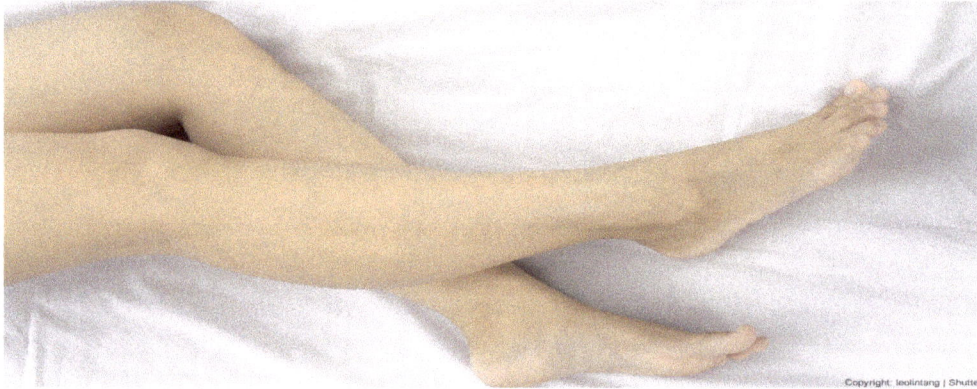
Copyright: leolintang | Shutter

Normally, most people sleep with their feet in a pointed position (plantar-flexed). Unfortunately, this means that over the course of the night, this position can cause the *plantar fascia* and other structures to become even tighter and more constricted. Your first steps in the morning can actually tear the tissue on the bottom of your feet with each step. This continual re-injury could be the reason you are unable to perform even the simple exercises in this book.

Under such circumstances, you may want to think about using a **Night Splint** for a few weeks.

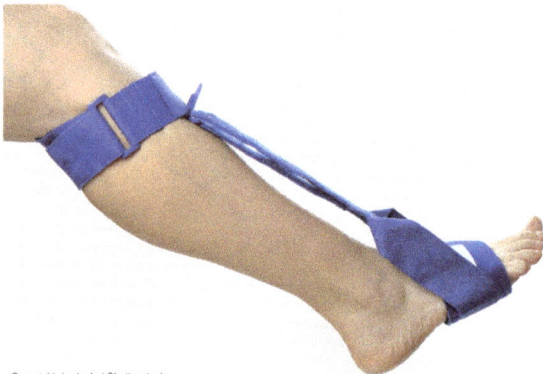
Copyright: jordache| Shutterstock

A Night Splint is used to keep the *plantar fascia* and *Achilles tendon* in a stretched, taut position while you sleep. A Night Splint can speed the healing process by keeping the plantar fascia relaxed while you sleep.

This would allow you to perform the exercises in this book, without being in constant acute pain.

Just don't get the idea that the Night Splint is a permanent solution, or a substitute for the exercises and therapies we have recommended. I have had patients come to me, who have had four or five reoccurrences of Plantar Fasciitis, simply because the ONLY therapy they used was the Night Splint.

Although a Night Splint is not a permanent solution, it can be used to break the cycle of constant re-injury. This tool could reduce the pain enough to allow you to perform the exercises (which are essential for a fully recovery).

Caution: It is important to remember that the Night Splint will NOT resolve the numerous biomechanical problems that are the actual cause of your Plantar Fasciitis. It is a *temporary* tool that can help to stabilize and rest the structures of your feet

---

Rest is Essential

Rest, in our busy world, is becoming an increasingly rare commodity. But it is an essential component for healing the body.

Your body needs rest and sleep in order to function properly and to repair itself. While you sleep, your body performs much of its maintenance and renewal functions.

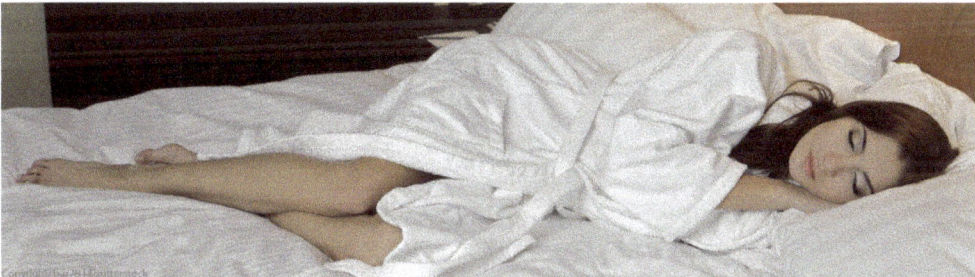

If you have any type of soft-tissue injury (caused by sports, career, home care, or just daily activities), you must *rest* that area to give it a chance to recover properly.

Lack of sleep results in decreased immune function, increased potential for disease (heart disease, stroke, cancer), decreased hormone production (human growth hormone), decreased tissue repair, decreased cognitive function, decreased fat metabolism, depression, increased inflammation, and even decreased life span.

Some very interesting research has come out of the National Academy of Science about the effects of sleep deprivation. Sleep deprivation causes an elevated level of the stress hormone, corticosterone. Increased levels of this hormone causes a reduction in the function of brain cells. This, in turn, has been directly related to problems in concentration and other possible cognitive issues. A little sad, but lack of sleep may even reduce cognitive function so much that you don't even realize the degree of your problem.

We have found that our patients' lack of rest and sleep is one of the primary reasons for a slow or delayed recovery from an injury. Avoid over-using an injured area before it is recovered as that can cause further injury, more inflammation, and increased healing time.

How much sleep you require will vary based on several factors, including your diet (good diet, bad diet), environmental factors (smoking, drinking), quality of sleep, genetics, and current injuries. Even the quality of light that you are exposed to will affect the amount of sleep you need (spending a long time in front of the computer disrupts your circadian rhythm). In general terms we recommend at least 7 to 8 hours of sleep per night. Bottom line: without proper sleep, your body will not repair itself, you decrease the overall quality of your life, and you may even decrease your life span.

By doing these simple steps, you provide your body with a critical element needed for self-healing...REST!

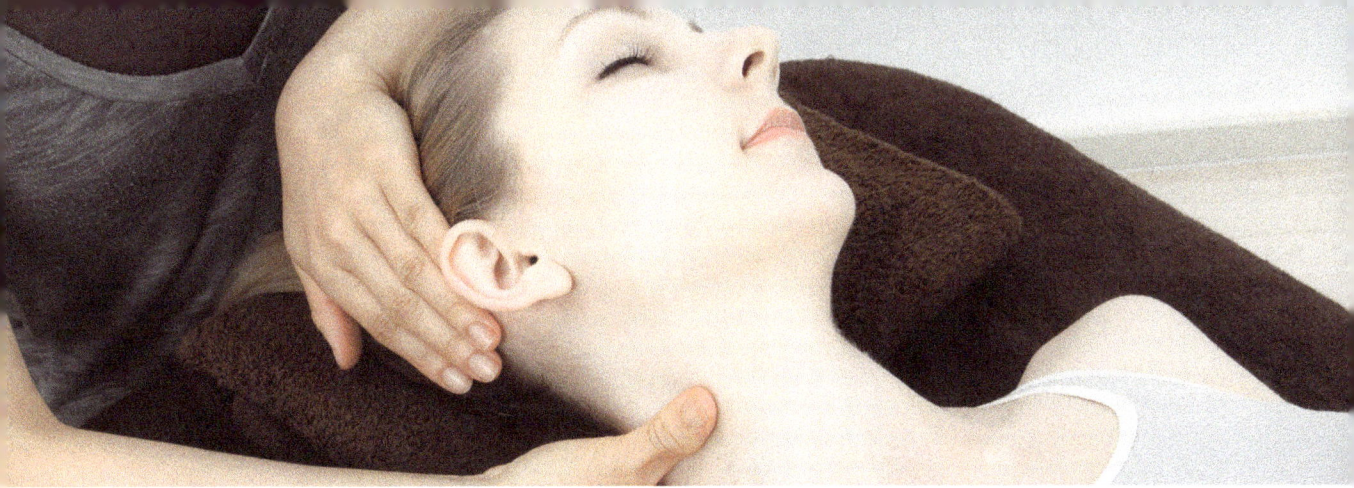

Phase 3: When Exercise is Not Enough

12

Active Release Techniques® (ART) ------ page 253
Instrument-Assisted Techniques ------ page 256
Joint Manipulation ------ page 257
Massage Therapy ------ page 259
Physiotherapy and Occupational Therapy ------ page 260
Acupuncture ------ page 262
Fascial Manipulation ------ page 264

In some cases, the combination of exercise and self-care are enough to completely resolve your case of Plantar Fasciitis, but in other cases more help is sometimes needed. This chapter is about the various therapies and procedures you can use (in conjunction with your exercise program) to help resolve your Plantar Fasciitis.

My disclaimer, this chapter is laced with my own personal opinions, which are based on over 20 years of clinical practice, as well as my experiences as an instructor in a variety of soft-tissue techniques. I believe that sharing this experience can help you make good choices about the best types of therapy to investigate, and which therapies to avoid.

Understanding Clinical Logic

Before making specific recommendations, I need to quickly go over what I consider to be a key factor in finding a good practitioner. This factor has nothing to do with the actual techniques performed, but instead focuses upon the logic that practitioners should apply to each of their cases.

Kinetic Health ®   251

The logic I am referring to is the same scientific principle that we all learned back in grade school. It is called the *Scientific Method.* In the Scientific Method you are first presented with a problem, then you do your research, come up with a hypothesis, perform an experiment, analyze the data, then draw logical conclusions from your data. If the results were good, your hypothesis was proven correct. If not, it is time to formulate another hypothesis that takes into account the new data collected.

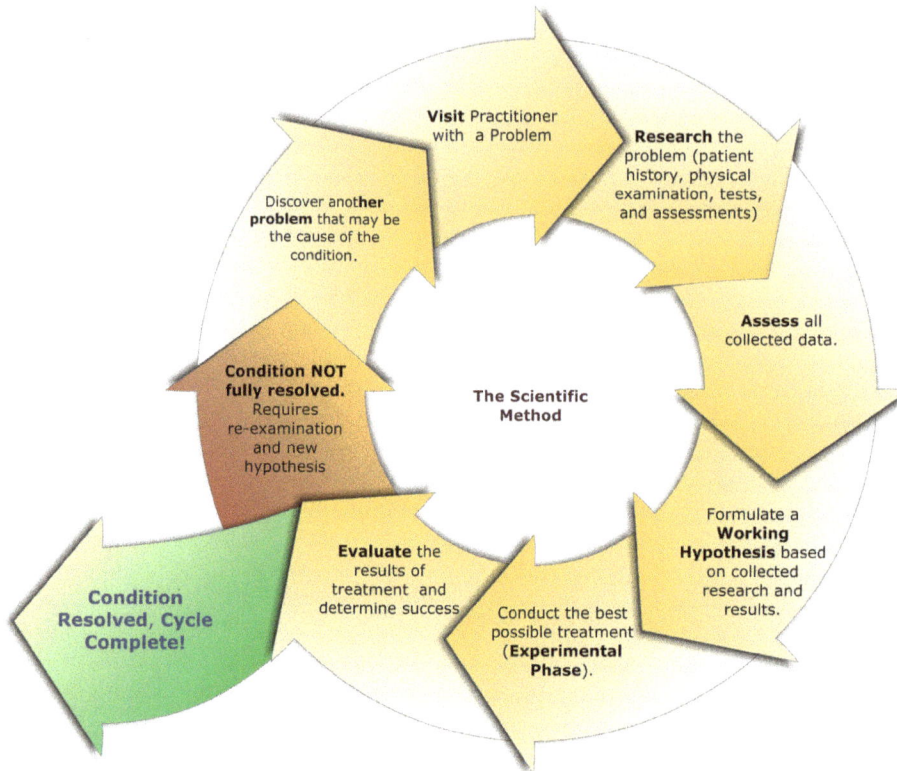

The Scientific Method

Visit Practitioner with a Problem

Research the problem (patient history, physical examination, tests, and assessments)

Discover ano**ther** **problem** that may be the cause of the condition.

Assess all collected data.

Condition NOT fully resolved. Requires re-examination and new hypothesis

Formulate a **Working Hypothesis** based on collected research and results.

Evaluate the results of treatment and determine success

Condition Resolved, Cycle Complete!

Conduct the best possible treatment (**Experimental Phase**).

Applying the Scientific Method from a clinical perspective means that you first go to a practitioner with a *problem* that needs to be solved. The practitioner then performs the appropriate *research* by obtaining a complete patient history, performing a physical examination (one that includes orthopedic, neurological, and biomechanical assessments) as well as a variety of other diagnostic procedures. Once he/she has collected this information, the practitioner can formulate a working diagnosis (or *hypothesis*) based on the collected results and information.

The *experimental stage* consists of treatment and exercise over a defined period of time. It has a specified start-date, and an expected end-date. Upon conclusion of the treatment, all results are reviewed and evaluated. This gives the practitioner the ability to draw a series of logical conclusions. The condition has either improved, resolved, not changed, or gotten worse. If the problem has not resolved, then it is time to explore some of the more unusual or rare causes of your condition.

This way, you have a game plan, and you understand the clinical process. Essentially it's a partnership between you and the practitioner working towards a mutual goal. Both of you have responsibilities, the practitioner to provide the best care they can, and you (the patient) must show up for all your appointments and perform all the prescribed exercises and treatment recommendations.

Bottom line, look for a practitioner who follows this process. Look for logic in the treatments they prescribe. There are lots of great, dedicated practitioners out there who can help you through this process. On the other hand, if you discover that a complete physical examination has not been performed, that treatments are rushed, or there is no set treatment and review times, then it may be time to consider other alternatives.

So let's take a look at some of the various therapies and techniques that I tend to recommend. Each of these therapies and techniques have their own strengths and weaknesses. In my own practice I have found that the best results often come by combining these various procedures.

Active Release Techniques® (ART)

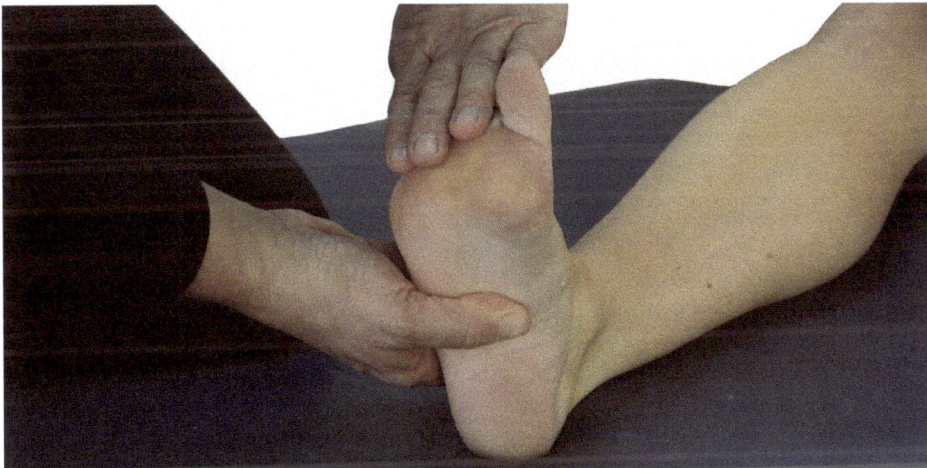

I helped to teach courses in Active Release Techniques (ART) for over ten years. In my opinion, ART is one of the **most** effective and reliable methods for releasing adhesions or restrictions between soft tissue layers. Just about any soft-tissue injury can be treated effectively with ART. This multidisciplinary technique was developed by Dr. P. Michael Leahy of Colorado Springs, Colorado.

Essentially, ART is a hands-on soft-tissue technique that can simultaneously locate and break up scar-tissue. The power of ART lies in how it combines patient motion with practitioner techniques to release the adhesions between tissue layers. This process restores mobility and relative motion to the soft tissue layers, increases circulatory function, and increases neurological function by breaking restrictive adhesions.

Effectiveness of Active Release Techniques

ART is one of the modalities at the top of my list for soft-tissue techniques, especially when it is performed correctly by a skilled practitioner. The key word is *skilled*! ART practitioners claim to have a 90% success rate, and this is quite true when the practitioner is both skilled, experienced, and combines their treatments with functional exercise protocols. The key is to find someone with both the training and experience you require.

It is extremely important to ensure that your ART practitioner focuses on treating more than just the feet. ART is designed to treat a larger kinetic chain. I have seen a lot of patients suffering from Plantar Fasciitis (PF) who have told me that they have tried ART, and obtained only minimal results. Upon questioning these patients, I usually discover that their practitioner had only treated a very limited area of the body (or they only received one or two treatments). This is a common mistake; the practitioner must often address all the key structures in the kinetic chain in order to obtain a full resolution of the problem.

Length of ART Appointments

Another key point is that soft-tissue adhesions require a certain amount of time before they release. If an ART practitioner has spent only two minutes with you during an appointment, then the results will be minimal at best. Adhesions need time to release, especially when multiple structures are involved.

Ask your practitioner about the length of each appointment. In our clinic, appointment times are broken up into 10, 20, and 30 minute slots. It is well worth getting a longer appointment, especially if multiple structures are involved.

It is very important to check out the certification levels of your selected ART practitioner. ART practitioners can take courses in *Upper Extremity, Lower Extremity, Spine, Complex Protocols, Long Nerve Entrapment, Biomechanics*, and *Palpation*. Make sure your practitioner is certified in at least the lower extremity (for Plantar

Fasciitis). In addition (as one of the writers of the *ART Online Biomechanics Course*), I can tell you that it is well worth your time to find someone who is also certified in biomechanics.

Finding an ART Practitioner

Chiropractors, physiotherapists, registered massage therapists, sports medicine practitioners, and some related health-care practitioners can practice this technique. Unfortunately, some people practice ART without ever taking a single course in the topic. ART takes training, time and experience, so make sure your practitioner is certified to perform this technique. To verify your ART practitioner's qualifications, visit the Active Release web site at www.activerelease.com.

No matter how effective ART treatments can be, they still need to be combined with a series of exercises. Tissue re-modeling takes time, and requires a combination of stretching, and strengthening exercises to obtain the best results. Read more about tissue remodeling in *Remodelling Tissues with Strengthening Exercises on page 162*.

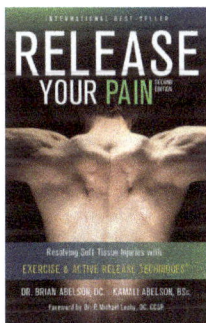

If you want to learn more about how ART can help resolve numerous soft-tissue injuries, you may want to read our best-selling book, **Release Your Pain** – *Resolving Soft Tissue Injuries with Active Release Techniques*. You can get your copy at www.releaseyourbody.com.

For more information about **Active Release Techniques**, you can also visit our websites at:

- www.activerelease.ca
- www.kinetichealth.ca
- www.releaseyourbody.com

Instrument-Assisted Techniques

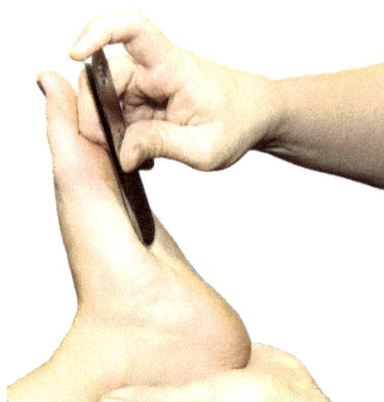

There are several forms of instrument-assisted soft-tissue techniques that can be very useful for treating Plantar Fasciitis. Some of the major techniques are *Graston, FAKTR*, and various *IASTM* instruments.

In each of these techniques, the instruments are used to separate and break down scar-tissue (collagen cross-links). This process increases circulatory function and helps the practitioner to mobilize, reduce, and re-organize fibrotic restrictions in the neuromuscular-skeletal system.

Researching across time, I have discovered that many of these techniques are very similar to an ancient form of Chinese Medicine known as Gua Sha. Gua Sha uses an instrument to scrape the surface of the skin, and release tightness and restrictions in the underlying soft-tissues. There has been well over a hundred studies done to evaluate the effectiveness of Gua Sha in the treatment of musculoskeletal problems; all demonstrating very good results.

Effectiveness of Instrument Assisted Techniques

With regard to Plantar Fasciitis, these instrument-based techniques can help to access severely restricted areas in your body, areas that the Practitioner's hands cannot always easily reach. For example, the Graston tools can be very effective for breaking up restrictions near the heel bone (calcaneus), an area which can otherwise be difficult to treat.

It is my opinion that instrument assisted techniques are most effective when used in conjunction with other hand-on techniques such as *Active Release Techniques, Chiropractic Manipulation, Fascial Release,* and *Massage Therapy.* Of course, it is still important to integrate *functional exercise programs* with the therapy in order to obtain the maximum benefits.

Note: With most instrument-assisted techniques, it is common to experience some discomfort during the procedure, and find some minor bruising afterwards. This is usually nothing to worry about as it is just part of the normal healing process.

Joint Manipulation

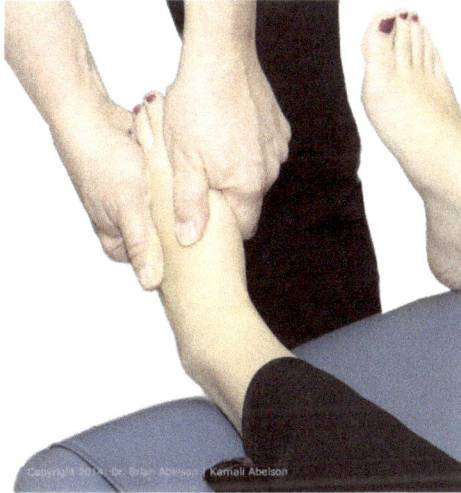

Joint restrictions are a component of Plantar Fasciitis that is often overlooked. Any type of joint restriction in the low back, hips, knees, ankles, or feet will create abnormal motion patterns.

Historical records show that manipulative therapies have existed for thousands of years. Manipulation has been documented in Chinese and Indian literature as far back as 2000 years ago. In China, manipulation has always been considered an effective form of therapy.

This statement holds more weight when you consider that these Chinese physicians were only paid when their patients remained healthy. Now that is what I call a proactive health care system.

Today the most common types of western manipulation are *Chiropractic* and *Osteopathic Manipulation*. Both professions have a colourful history with no lack of controversy. The key point here is that all that controversy is primarily historical! Today these medical professions are regulated by government bodies, and comply with strict medical criteria. Practitioners of both professions have no less than seven (7) years of post-secondary education. In fact, the first three years of their training is almost identical to that of any other medical professional.

There are some opponents to manipulation who would still have the public believe that these therapies are unsupported. This is complete nonsense since there are literally hundreds of peer-reviewed scientific articles proving and supporting the benefits of manipulation.

How Joint Manipulation Works

Essentially, practitioners of manipulation move joints in a manner that frees up or breaks the restrictions that are causing neurological or biomechanical problems. These releases occur across much more than just the joints; manipulation also has a significant effect upon the body's soft tissues. Essentially, once joint restrictions are released, it is much more effective and easy to work on their surrounding soft tissues.

Manipulation affects muscles by causing the stress receptors (*Golgi tendons*) in the muscles to temporarily inhibit all activity in the areas being adjusted. This reaction causes the muscle groups of the surrounding joints to go into an *instantaneous state of relaxation*. This intervention has a very important and positive effect when your practitioner is trying to break the pain-cycle. This approach to manipulation is strongly supported by scientific studies.

How Joint Restrictions Affect Plantar Fasciitis

Your body has 206 bones, with 52 of them in your feet. If just one of those bones becomes restricted in its ability to move, it can result in the development of abnormal motion patterns, which in turn could prevent a full resolution of your Plantar Fasciitis.

Let us look at just one example. In many cases of Plantar Fasciitis, the ankle is one of the most common areas where you will find restrictions. The ankle needs to be both mobile and stable, while at the same time allowing for both plantar and dorsiflexion of the foot. Poor ankle dorsiflexion can have a huge effect upon the entire kinetic chain. For example, restricted dorsiflexion of the ankle can cause the *subtalar joint* to evert, which then tightens the calf muscles (*gastrocnemius* and *soleus*), resulting in internal rotation of the knee (thus destabilizing the knee), and subsequently causing a variety of hip dysfunctions. The hip dysfunctions, in turn, destabilizes the entire lower extremity even more. As you can see, this single restriction can affect the entire kinetic chain of the body.

Joint manipulation is a great way to free up those restrictions and restore normal mobility.

Effectiveness of Joint Manipulation

Manipulation is generally very safe and effective when performed by a trained health-care professional. Look for practitioners that are trained and have experience in Lower Extremity Manipulation.

I have seen numerous cases of Plantar Fasciitis which would never have been resolved without joint manipulation. On the other hand, for manipulation to remain effective, treatments must be combined with appropriate exercise. When manipulation is combined with soft-tissue techniques (such as Active Release Techniques, Graston Techniques, or Massage Therapy) it becomes even more effective since both joint and soft-tissue restrictions are removed or released.

Note: Many practitioners are trained in both joint manipulation and soft-tissue techniques such as Active Release Techniques, Instrumented Assisted Techniques, Fascial Manipulation, and numerous others methodologies. This is a great combination of procedures; much more powerful than using just one approach. In my own practice, 99% of all our patients who receive joint manipulation also receive some type of soft-tissue therapy. However, as with all therapists. it is always advisable to first check out their current certification in these procedures.

Massage Therapy

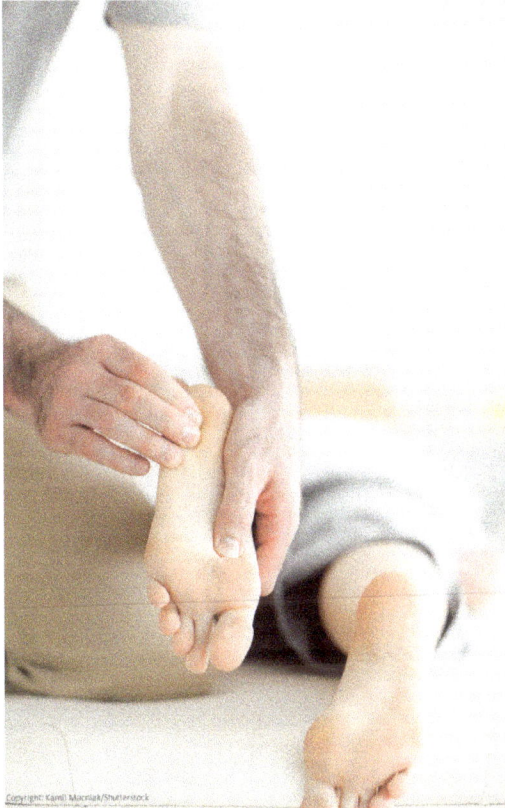

Massage is not just an effective approach to pain management and rehabilitation, it also has tremendous physical, biochemical, and psychological benefits. Massage increases circulatory function, increases blood oxygen levels, moves nutrients to needed areas, and displaces waste by-products. In fact, in terms of pain relief, some studies have shown that massage surpasses the effectiveness of numerous medications, without any of the negative side-effects.

Massage therapy has consistently been shown to help patients in dealing with their pain. This includes common muscle and joint pain as well as stress and pain arising from pregnancy, osteoarthritis, rheumatoid arthritis, and even cancer.

Massage therapy also provides huge psychological benefits in its ability to decrease stress and anxiety. Even stressed premature babies notice the difference; on average, premature babies who receive regular massages gain *47% more weight* than those who do not receive massage.

Effectiveness of Massage

Massage Therapy is very safe and highly recommended. Trained *Registered Massage Therapists* are very effective at treating and providing relief for a wide range of conditions such as Plantar Fasciitis, migraine headaches, tendonitis, arthritis, osteoporosis, sports injuries, and a broad range of other common soft-tissue conditions.

Finding a Massage Therapist

Since there are literally hundreds of different modalities that could be labeled as massage, there is no single governing body for the regulation of massage therapy. When you look for a Registered Massage Therapist, check for the following:

- Does the therapist have any experience in dealing with your particular type of soft-tissue injury?
- Does the Registered Massage Therapist have at least 2200 hours of training (or equivalent in practice)?
- How long has the Massage Therapist been practising?
- Is the Massage Therapist licensed?
- Where did the Massage Therapist receive training?
- Does the Massage Therapist have any training in advanced or specific massage techniques?
- What experience does the Massage Therapist have in treating your condition.

Physiotherapy and Occupational Therapy

Physiotherapists and Occupational therapists are professionals who aim to rehabilitate and improve the condition of people who suffer from movement disorders.

To achieve their results, both professions can use a combination of several different modalities such as:

- Therapeutic exercises.
- Electrotherapeutic and mechanical agents such as ultrasound, laser, shock-wave, TENS, short wave diathermy, and interferential.
- Functional training and some manipulation of joints and soft tissues.

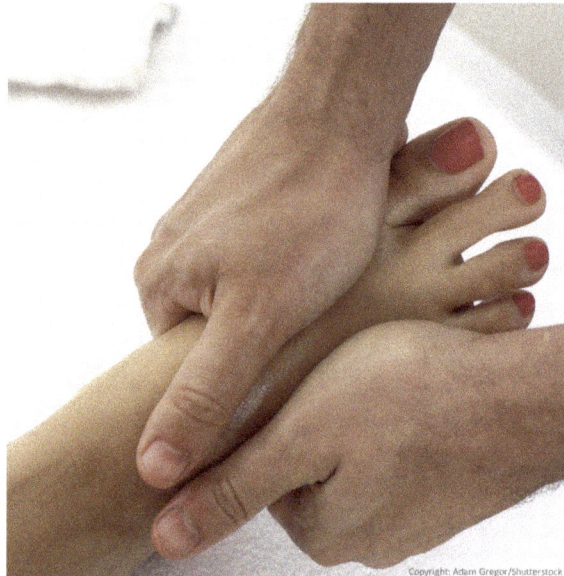

Copyright: Adam Gregor/Shutterstock

Many of these therapists also take additional training in other techniques such as *Acupuncture*, IMS (*Intermuscular Stimulation*), *Active Release Techniques*, *Instrument Assisted Techniques*, and a wide array of other procedures.

Over the years, it has been my pleasure to work closely with, and train some great Physical and Occupational Therapists. These individuals are usually very hands-on in their treatment approaches and provide their patients with individualized treatment programs. They can truly be great resources of information, and as a patient, you could greatly benefit from treatments with this type of practitioner.

Effectiveness of Physiotherapy & Occupational Therapy

Depending on the treatment protocol practiced by your therapist, you may find that the treatment is either *extremely effective* or that it borders on what I would call *completely ineffective*.

The best therapists I have met in both these fields tend to be *very hands-on*. They are deeply involved in every aspect of their patient's treatments, the exercise programs, and tend to closely monitor the progress. These therapists tend to achieve great results.

On the other hand, I have found that the majority of patients (who come to our clinic) that have experienced only *minimal to no positive changes*, tend to come from therapists whose primary treatment method consisted of only *electrical modalities*. In most of these cases, the patient experienced next to no hands-on therapy. Therapists whose treatment protocols focus primarily on electrical and heat modalities *rarely succeed in resolving these conditions*.

The following is obviously my own personal opinion, but there is a very good reason for having ultrasound, interferential, and tens machines collecting dust in our clinic. I have not seen great results with these modalities. Twenty some years ago, when I got out of school, I used these machines every day, but have found that my results from that time were nothing compared to the successes we achieve daily today. In fact, during those early days, I found myself increasingly frustrated at the poor outcomes I was achieving for my patients, despite my best efforts.

In my opinion, the therapists MUST get into (hands-on) the involved tissue structures. Our hands are full of tactile receptors that no machine can duplicate. Our hands let us know where the restriction is, when one layer of tissue is not translating over another, and most importantly when the involved tissue begins to change and return to a normal functional state.

So bottom line, yes, I highly recommend these practitioners. Just make sure that they provide more than just electrical modalities in their treatment protocol!

Acupuncture

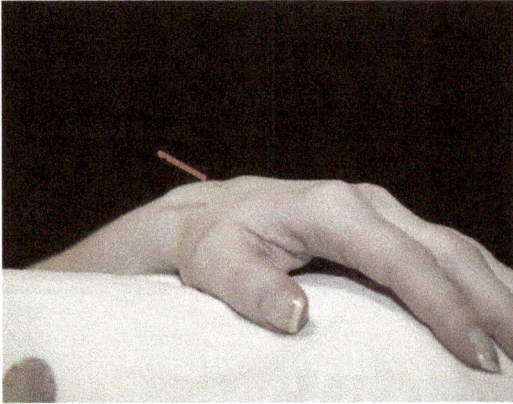

"Acupuncture regulates multiple physiological systems and achieves diverse therapeutic effects!"

Western medicine is only just beginning to understand how acupuncture actually works.

With our patients, I often obtain very effective results by combining acupuncture with Active Release Techniques, Fascial Manipulation, and Joint Manipulation. In many cases, by performing acupuncture during the initial phases of treatment, I am able to reduce the pain sufficiently so that I can then get into and perform myofascial release on previously over-sensitive areas.

Acupuncture and the Body's Fascial Planes

Chinese Medicine speaks about maintaining the balance of energy throughout the body. But, there is also another interesting explanation coming out of the world of fascial research, from researchers such as *Dr. Helene M. Langevin* of *Harvard Medical School.*

This new understanding has to do with **fascial planes**. About 80% of all acupuncture points are located along connective tissue planes. These fascial planes are full of nerves and circulatory structures that run between muscles and bones, and surround and support circulatory structures.

It is postulated that when an acupuncture needle is inserted into one of these fascial planes, the needle is transmitting a mechanical force that is affecting both neurological and circulatory function. This is easier to understand if we consider the normal technique used in needle insertion.

Once the acupuncture needles are inserted into specific points, they are *rotated* numerous times. The practitioner performs this action until he or she can feel the needle being grabbed onto by the underlying connective tissue. This '*grab*' can actually be measured by special machines– it is known as '*tug response*'. This 'tug' on the connective tissue also serves to stretch the surrounding connective tissue (this action has been confirmed by ultrasound imagery). Essentially, this means that as long as there is an acupuncture needle in the tissue, the tissue is experiencing a sustained stretch. Holding this sustained stretch for 30 to 45 minutes can have a considerable effect on both neurological and circulatory function.

Effectiveness of Acupuncture for Treating Plantar Fasciitis

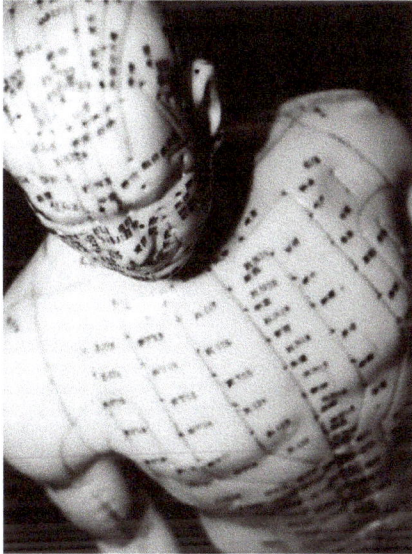

I have found Acupuncture to a be a very important *adjunctive therapy* when treating Plantar Fasciitis. It will not replace exercise, nor help with tissue remodeling, or even free up joint restrictions, but it can provide considerable pain relief, especially during very acute cases.

In cases of Plantar Fasciitis, the connective tissue becomes thicker, more fibrotic, and does not glide over other adjacent tissues very well, reducing overall mobility. The thickening of the fascia also affects sensory nerve function. This may be one of the reasons why acupuncture seems to reduce pain so dramatically. The sustained stretch of connective tissue could actually be affecting sensory nerve function.

At our clinic, for cases where the foot is so sensitive that it cannot be touched, we often use acupuncture on the **opposite side** of the body to ease the pain. An example would be using a point known as the *HE-8 (shaoyin point)*.

Depending on the patient's tolerance, local points on the foot may also be used. Needling is often focused directly into the *plantar fascia*, or in close proximity to the insertion of the *plantar fascia* into the heel (*calcaneus*). These points are referred to as *Shi mian* points.

In acupuncture, when extreme heel pain is present, practitioners often use points (*KID7, KID8*) to stimulate what is known as the '*kidney meridian*' to reduce this pain. Other acupuncture points would be applied to affect tendon and ligament function (*LIV3*). While yet other points will be used to work on the calf muscles (*BL56,BL57*).

As you can see, acupunture can be used to affect structures throughout the entire kinetic chain.

Fascial Manipulation

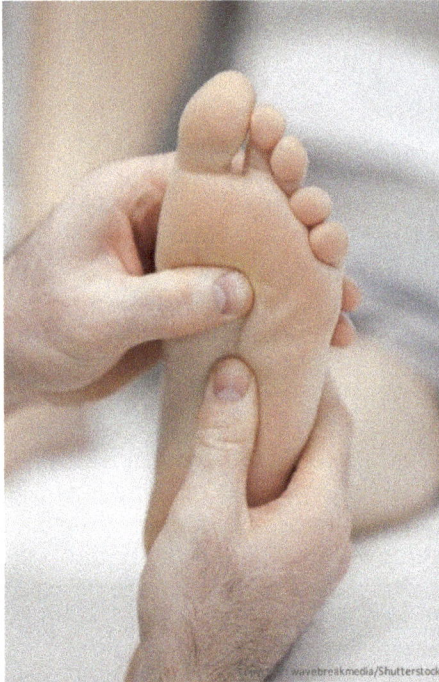

Fascia is everywhere, weaving through, and interconnecting every component of our body. Muscle fibers originate from, and insert into, fascial fibers. These fascial fibers, in turn, insert into multiple regions of the bone, and even into adjacent muscles. These additional points of contact and control provide the muscle with the ability to generate force in multiple directions.

One of the key components of treating Plantar Fasciitis, is to take into consideration all the fascial inter-connections to the structures that are involved in performing and coordinating the motions of your foot's kinetic chain.

Fascial manipulation does this by determining the plane of motion in which your body has developed restrictions, then uses hands-on procedures to break those restrictions.

This process involves taking a complete history of injuries throughout a person's life, biomechanical analysis to look for abnormal motion patterns, the balance of opposing fascial lines (Tensegrity), and extensive palpatory investigation.

I received my training in **Fascial Manipulation** in north-eastern Italy, from some of the pioneers in this technique– the Stecco family - *Luigi Stecco PT, Dr. Carla Stecco*, and *Dr. Antonio Stecco*. In addition to the Stecco Group, you can also find Fascial practitioners that have been trained either by *Thomas Myers* of *Anatomy Trains*, or *Rolfers* such as *Robert Schleip of Ulm University*.

There are several types of fascial manipulation that can help you. Again, the key is to find someone who is fully trained and has experience in treating Plantar Fasciitis.Also, if you can find a practitioner who integrates the kinetic chain concepts behind fascial manipulation into their methodology, then you will definitely increase the odds of completely resolving your condition.

I have found that I get the most powerful and effective results when I combine the methodologies of *Fascial Manipulation* with *Active Release Techniques*, *Instrument Assisted Techniques*, and *Manipulation*.

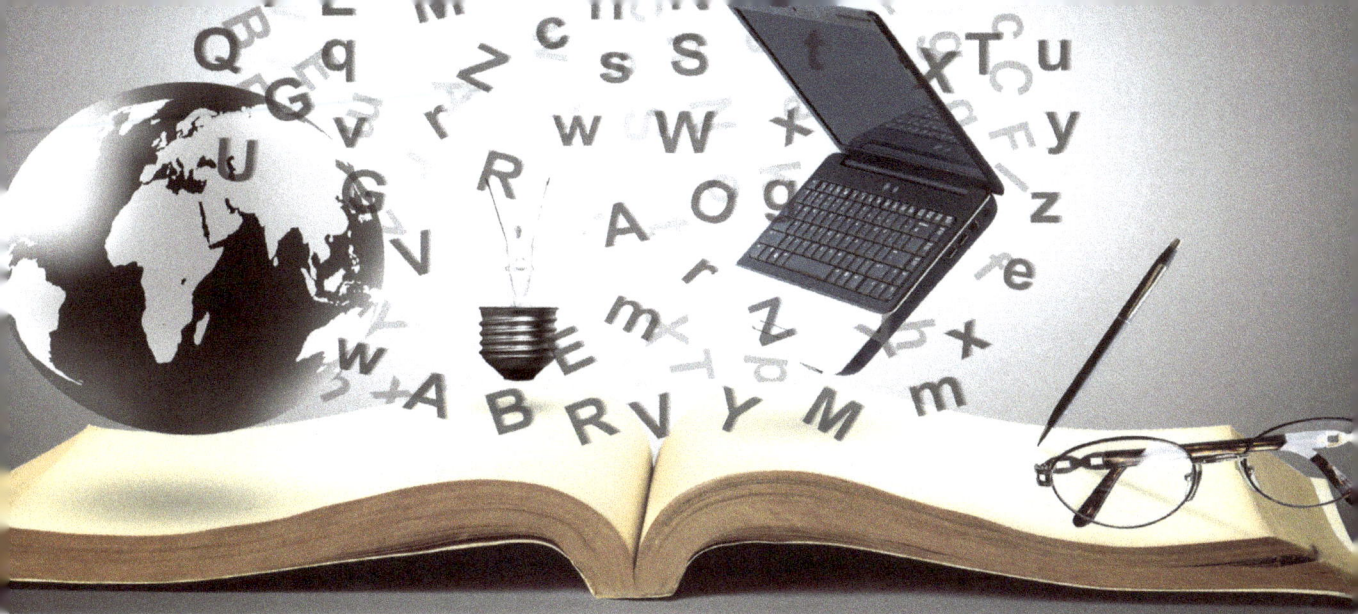

Index

B

C

heat therapy
  benefits of **245**
  epsom salts **247**
  types of **246**

heel bone (see calcaneous) **55**

heel spurs
  not a cause of Plantar Fasciitis **34**

hip
  extension of **74**
  flexion of **74, 80**
  flexors **79, 82, 83**
  internal rotation **80**
  muscles of **82**
  problems from tight flexors **83**
  role of gluteals **85**

hip flexors
  about hip **82**
  image of **82**
  myofascial routine **201**
  stretching **202, 203**
  stretching routine **201**

hip stability
  kinetic chain impact **31**

hips
  strengthening **226, 227**

hula-hoop **169**

human growth hormone **162**

hyaluronic acid **29**

hyperalgiesia **87**

I

icing
  ice massage **244**
  ice pack usage **244**
  impact on healing **241**
  pain relief **243**
  red flags **243**
  tips and hints **243**
  traditional advice **242**
  when not to ice **243**
  when to ice **242**

iliacus **26, 83, 84, 202**
  role of **84**
  stretching **202**

iliopsoas **83, 84, 201**
  antagonist of gluteals **83**

impingements
  effect of **38**

infection
  red flags **109**

inflammation
  impact of icing **241**
  relation to fats **99**
  traditional advice **242**
  when to ice **242**

injuries
  impact on kinetic chain **38**

injury phases
  regenerative **160**

interossei **64**

inversion
  foot **28**

ischial tuberosity **76**

IT band **223**

J

joint manipulation
  benefits of **28, 257**
  effect on Plantar Fasciitis **258**
  effectiveness of **258**
  how it works **257**

joints
  ankle joints **54**
  foot **51**
  increase mobility of the big toe **206**
  manipulation of **257**
  restrictions **28, 50**
  restrictions of **28**
  subtalar joint **55**

muscles
    biomechanics of contraction **42**
    fascial inter-relationships **42**
    standard perspectives for motion **42**

muscular compensations
    effect on kinetic chain **38**

myofascial release **8**
    calf muscles **198, 199, 200**
    peroneals **194**
    releasing nerves **27**
    shins **192**
    tibialis anterior **191**

N

navicular bone **54**

nerve compression syndromes **27**
    common sites for PF **87**
    compression vs common PF **89**
    hyperalgiesia **87**
    paresthesia **87, 88**
    peroneal nerve testing **147**
    red flags **109**
    tibial nerve **147**
    tibial nerve testing **146**

nerves
    flossing the peroneal nerve **212, 213**
    flossing the tibial nerve **209, 210**
    image of foot innervation **88**
    lateral plantar nerve **88**
    medial plantar nerve **88**
    pain patterns for PF **88**
    sciatic nerve **88**
    testing function **146, 147**
    tibial nerve **88**

neurological mechanisms
    fascial control **41**

neuromuscular compensations
    effect on kinetic chain **38**

neuromuscular grooving **168**

night splint
    using **248**

nutrition
    impact of **33**
    role in healing **98**

O

obesity
    effect on healing **99**
    fat equation **99**

occupational therapy **260–261**

osteopathic manipulation **257**

P

pain
    red flags **109**

paresthesia **87, 88**

patellar
    ligament **78**
    tendon **223**

patellofemoral syndrome **80**

pectineus **80, 81**

peroneal nerve
    entrapment **147**
    flossing **211, 212, 213**

peroneus
    brevis **71, 72, 193**
    longus **63, 71, 72, 193**
    stretching **193**
    tertius **67, 71**

phalangeal bones **52**

phalanges
    role in gait **52**

physiotherapy **260–261**

pin and stretch of the
    foot **188**

plantar aponeurosis **34**

plantar fascia **39, 44, 177, 223, 224**
    about **22, 39, 49, 56**
    description of **39**
    gait cycle **57**
    how it works **39**
    inflammation of **22**
    stress caused by **52**
    windlass mechanism **39**

Q

R

S

W

More Publications from Kinetic Health and Release Your Body

Written by the internationally best-selling authors of **Release Your Pain,** these books and exercise routines can help you release your pain, rehabilitate injuries, and help you achieve your best in both sports and daily life. Get your copy from Bookstores, Online Book Retailers, and at www.releaseyourbody.com.

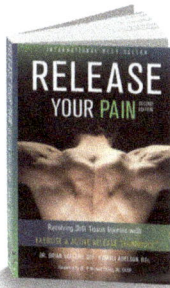

Release Your Pain - Resolving Repetitive Strain Injuries with Active Release Techniques
by Dr. Brian Abelson and Kamali T. Abelson

This international best seller has helped thousands of people resolve pain caused by repetitive strain and soft-tissue injuries, and is a great introduction to how the highly effective soft-tissue treatment method - Active Release Techniques - can help you recover from your soft-tissue injuries.
Available Now in Bookstores and at www.releaseyourbody.com!

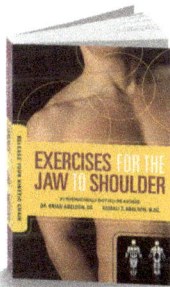

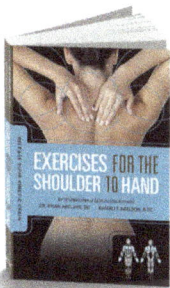

Exercises for the Jaw to Shoulder - Release Your Kinetic Chain by Dr. Brian Abelson and Kamali T. Abelson

If you suffer from headaches, jaw pain, TMJ, chronic neck pain, whiplash injuries, rotator cuff pain, shoulder pain, or other soft-tissue injuries of the jaw, neck, or shoulder, then this book may be exactly what you need.   Instead of working with just the area of injury, these routines work with the Kinetic Chain, and can help you to take a key step towards resolving long-standing soft- tissue injuries and neuromuscular problems.
Available Now in Bookstores and at www.releaseyourbody.com!

Exercises for the Shoulder to Hand - Release Your Kinetic Chain by Dr. Brian Abelson and Kamali T. Abelson

If you suffer from Shoulder Pain, Golfers Elbow, Tennis Elbow, Rotator Cuff Syndrome, carpal tunnel syndrome, wrist pain, or other hand injuries, this book reveals how everything you do – from working at your desk, to swinging a golf club - impacts the complex kinetic chain relationships within your soft tissue structures. The exercises are designed to help build and strengthen these neuromuscular relationships – a key step to resolving long-standing soft-tissue injuries, and improving strength, power, and sports performance.

Available Now in Bookstores and at www.releaseyourbody.com!

Author Biographies

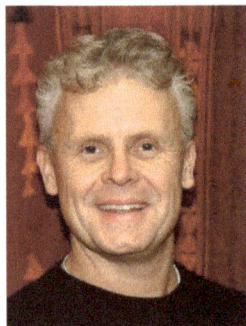

Dr. Brian Abelson DC - Brian's incredible, interdisciplinary knowledge of anatomy, physiology, human biomechanics, kinetic chain relationships, and exercise made these books possible. Just ask any of his patients, and they will fill your head with exclamations about how he can somehow *bring it all together* to solve their musculoskeletal problems!

He brings an integrated approach to health care (merging multiple soft tissue techniques, osseous manipulation, functional exercise programs and nutrition) in his daily practice.

Brian is a highly proficient Instructor and successful Practitioner (20+ years). He has a background in athletic performance and has participated in a wide variety of sports himself: Ironman Triathlons, Marathons, Competitive Cycling, Mountaineering, Latin Dance and Martial Arts. One of Brian's greatest passions is travel and experiencing new cultures. Brian is a devoted father, husband, and eternal optimist.

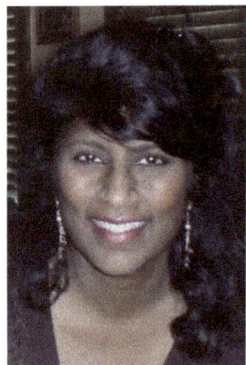

Kamali T. Abelson BSc - Kamali's long experience in the technical communication and publishing industry (25+ years) definitely came in handy as we wrote these books. Especially as they grew from the original vision of a 50-page booklet, into a multi-volume set of books, each over 250 pages, packed with new illustrations, photos, and exercises.

Kamali enjoys the company of her friends, being a mom and wife, running, hiking, travelling, dancing, and the arts. Given the opportunity, she would be spending most of her time travelling to distant corners of the world, taking dance and art lessons, meeting new people, and absorbing new cultures, thoughts, and ways!

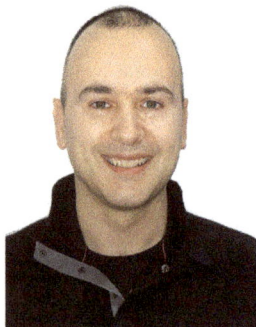

Dr. Evangelos Mylonas DC - Evangelos is articulate, engaging, and passionate about healthcare. In his practice, he daily merges his rich international experience and the ability to communicate in multiple languages with his extensive knowledge of anatomy, biomechanics, soft-tissue techniques, chiropractic and functional rehabilitative exercises.

He passionately pursues knowledge, travel, and continual learning. Over the past few years he has worked with Dr. Abelson in producing a number of books and videos on a wide variety of health and exercise related topics. His clinical experience and expertise have been invaluable through the editing and development processes of this book.

www.ingramcontent.com/pod-product-compliance
Lightning Source LLC
Chambersburg PA
CBHW041016280326
41926CB00094B/4657